ACE®
FITNESS NUTRITION MANUAL

AMERICAN COUNCIL ON EXERCISE®

NATALIE DIGATE MUTH, M.D., M.P.H., R.D.

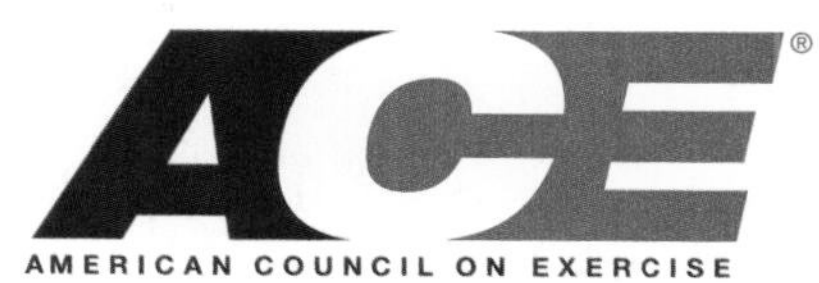

Library of Congress Control Number: 2013935353

ISBN 9781890720476

Printed in the United States of America

E F G H

Distributed by:
American Council on Exercise
4851 Paramount Drive
San Diego, CA 92123
(858) 576-6500
FAX: (858) 576-6464
ACEfitness.org

Project Editor: Daniel J. Green
Technical Editors: Cedric X. Bryant, Ph.D., FACSM, and Sabrena Jo, M.S.
Art Direction: Karen McGuire
Production: Nancy Garcia
Photography: hype-media.com
Stock photo images: iStock

Index: Kathi Unger
Chapter Models: Lisa Acevedo, Linda S. Chemaly, Michael Davis, Patricia A. Davis, Natalie Digate Muth, Jetta Starr Eveland, Nancy Garcia, Robert Garcia, Helen Koules, Valerie O'Neill, Michael Marsh, Brittany McCall, Anthony Padilla, Jesse Patton, Mary Saph Tanaka, Pam Wright

Acknowledgments:
Thanks to the entire American Council on Exercise staff for their support and guidance through the process of creating this manual.

NOTICE

The fitness industry is ever-changing. As new research and clinical experience broaden our knowledge, changes in programming and standards are required. The authors and the publisher of this work have checked with sources believed to be reliable in their efforts to provide information that is complete and generally in accord with the standards accepted at the time of publication. However, in view of the possibility of human error or changes in industry standards, neither the authors nor the publisher nor any other party who has been involved in the preparation or publication of this work warrants that the information contained herein is in every respect accurate or complete, and they are not responsible for any errors or omissions or the results obtained from the use of such information. Readers are encouraged to confirm the information contained herein with other sources.

P16-018

TABLE OF CONTENTS

REVIEWERS

LAURA J. KRUSKALL, PH.D., RD, CSSD, FACSM, is the director of nutrition sciences at University of Nevada, Las Vegas, and the director of the Dietetic Internship. Her areas of expertise are sports nutrition, weight management, and medical nutrition therapy, and her research interests include the effects of nutrition or exercise intervention on body composition and energy metabolism. Dr. Kruskall holds a certification in Adult Weight Management, Level 2, from the Academy of Nutrition and Dietetics. She is a member of the editorial board for *ACSM's Health & Fitness Journal,* is a Certified ACSM Health/Fitness Specialist, and is a nutrition consultant for Canyon Ranch Spaclub and Cirque du Soleil in Las Vegas.

MICHELLE MURPHY ZIVE, M.S., RD, is an executive director at University of California, San Diego, of large community health projects that encourage consumption of fruits and vegetables and physical activity. She also works with residents to improve access to healthy food and physical-activity opportunities in their communities and leads health initiatives that focus on changing the policies, systems, and environment to support healthy lifestyles. Her research interests include obesity prevention, community health, and food security. She is especially interested in finding ways to apply what is learned in controlled research studies and translating it into useful strategies in the community. Zive is a frequent contributor to ACE, serving as a subject matter expert on exam committees and contributing to ACE publications, including the *ACE Health Coach Manual.*

FOREWORD

One of the greatest stumbling blocks for many fitness professionals involves knowing exactly how to handle questions from clients concerning nutrition. The American Council on Exercise (ACE) has addressed this issue many times over the past 25+ years—first in the *ACE Lifestyle & Weight Management Consultant Manual* and then with the 2012 release of the *ACE Health Coach Manual.* This text synthesizes that information in a way that enables fitness professionals to easily understand the boundaries of their scope of practice, thereby allowing them to confidently provide safe and appropriate nutrition education and service to their clients.

All fitness professionals know that the achievement of optimal health and weight management entails not only the physical activity they are so passionate about, but also healthy and balanced nutritional intake—the "calories in" portion of the "calories in/calories out" equation. In addition to educating readers about the various resources available to them, including the *Dietary Guidelines for Americans* and MyPlate, this text provides practical tools that can be used with clients.

Imagine the impact on your business and the success of your clients if, after a client mentions not being able to eat healthy dinners due to a lack of time or cooking skill, you offer grocery shopping and meal planning templates, a guided tour of the local grocery store, meal preparation tips, and even some simple yet healthy recipes. You suddenly become the ultimate resource in your clients' quest for better health!

Fitness professionals play an integral role in helping to empower individuals to live their most fit lives, particularly those impacted by obesity. Use this text wisely and effectively and you will broaden the range of services you offer to your clientele and dramatically improve their chances of long-term success—the ultimate goal of any fitness or lifestyle-change program.

Scott Goudeseune
President & CEO
American Council on Exercise

INTRODUCTION

The *ACE Fitness Nutrition Manual* takes an application-based, interactive approach to presenting theoretical nutrition concepts in way that will enable fitness professionals to provide practical, actionable tips to their clients while staying within the boundaries of their scope of practice. For example, Chapter 2: Basic Nutrition and Digestion features an "Expand Your Knowledge" box entitled The Truth Behind High-fructose Corn Syrup that teaches readers the science behind this sweetener, why it is preferred by manufacturers, and the controversy regarding its impact on weight gain and metabolic disorders. This feature is immediately followed by a "Think It Through" box that asks readers how they would respond to specific questions from a client regarding replacing foods containing high-fructose corn syrup with foods with other sweeteners. This approach is taken throughout the text, forcing the reader to apply complex content to real-life scenarios.

Chapter 1: Scope of Practice tackles the all-important question that concerns all fitness professionals—what they can and cannot do in terms of offering safe and effective nutrition advice to clients without overstepping their scope of practice and putting themselves and their clients at risk. This chapter features the all-new "ACE Position Statement on Nutrition Scope of Practice for Fitness Professionals."

Chapter 2: Basic Nutrition and Digestion provides the foundational knowledge all fitness professionals need in order to truly understand how the body turns food into fuel. In addition to outlining the essentials of digestion and absorption, this chapter explains the various macronutrients and micronutrients, as well as engineered foods, alcohol, drugs, and stimulants.

Chapter 3: Governmental Nutrition Guidelines and Recommendations forms the core of what ACE Fitness Nutrition Specialists should use as resources when providing nutritional guidance to their clients. After explaining the Dietary Reference Intakes, this chapter presents the *Dietary Guidelines for Americans* and MyPlate, which together with the numerous online tools provided by the federal government, offer a wealth of knowledge that all fitness professionals can share with their clientele. This chapter also features instruction on how to teach clients to understand and compare food nutrition labels so they are able to make healthier choices when selecting their food.

Chapter 4: Nutrition for Special Populations is divided into three sections. The first covers nutrition and hydration for sports and fitness, including how consumption of each of the three macronutrients should be modified for athletes. The second section explains how nutritional needs change over the course of a person's life, from childhood to old age. A woman's nutritional needs during pregnancy and lactation are also covered. The final section of this chapter explains the nutritional requirements of individuals with special dietary needs, ranging from vegetarianism and obesity to osteoporosis and anemia.

Chapter 5: Nutrition Coaching begins with an overview of the initial interview with a new client and provides tools for collecting nutrition information and obtaining a diet history. This chapter also covers motivational interviewing and the art of effective goal-setting.

Chapter 6: Essentials of Meal Selection and Preparation presents some practical tips that can help clients who claim they do not have time to cook or simply do not know how to put together a healthy meal. Included in this discussion are grocery shopping fundamentals, tips for putting together simple, tasty, and healthy meals, and how to make wise choices when eating out. Incorporating these lessons into your fitness business will broaden your ability to make a meaningful impact on clients' lives.

Chapter 7: Essentials for Growing Your Business teaches readers to revise their existing business plan once they have incorporated more nutrition-based offerings into the business. To be successful and expand their businesses, fitness professionals must be able to identify their vision and update their brand as they acquire new skills and expand the scope of what their business can offer. Finally, this chapter ends by teaching readers how to "sell" nutrition services to existing and new clientele.

This text closes with a collection of simple, nutritious, and delicious recipes that fitness professionals can share with their clients, whether they are vegetarians, trying to eat gluten-free, or following the Mediterranean diet (among other options).

We are confident that the *ACE Fitness Nutrition Manual* will help fitness professionals turn what has long been a perceived obstacle—not fully understanding scope of practice and being fearful about overstepping its boundaries—into not only an opportunity for business growth, but also a means of providing clients with the very best chances for long-term health and wellness.

Cedric X. Bryant, Ph.D., FACSM
Chief Science Officer

Daniel J. Green
Project Editor

Sabrena Jo, M.S.
Exercise Scientist

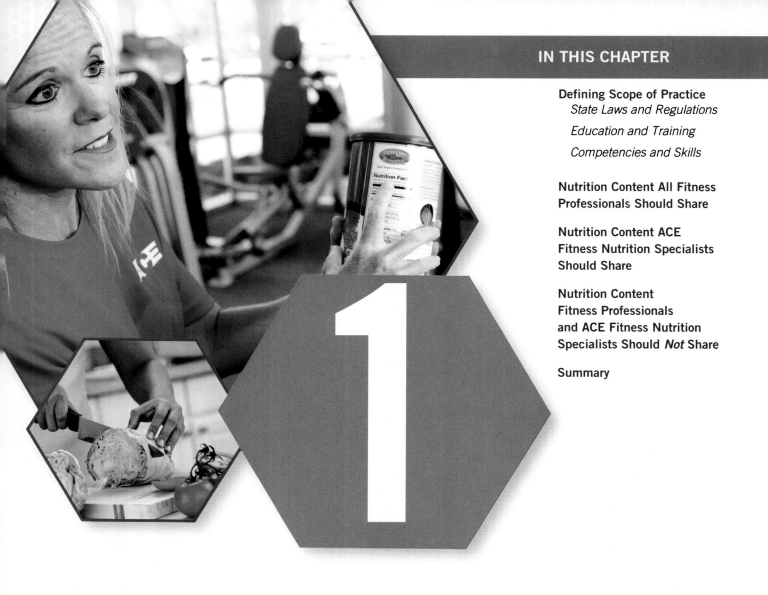

IN THIS CHAPTER

LEARNING OBJECTIVES

AFTER READING THIS CHAPTER, YOU WILL BE ABLE TO:

- OUTLINE THE SCOPE OF PRACTICE AS IT RELATES TO NUTRITION FOR AN APPROPRIATELY QUALIFIED FITNESS PROFESSIONAL WHO IS NOT A LICENSED NUTRITIONIST, LICENSED DIETITIAN, OR REGISTERED DIETITIAN
- DESCRIBE NUTRITION-RELATED ACTIVITIES THAT ARE CLEARLY WITHIN THE SCOPE OF PRACTICE OF A QUALIFIED FITNESS PROFESSIONAL
- DESCRIBE NUTRITION-RELATED ACTIVITIES THAT MAY OR MAY NOT BE WITHIN THE SCOPE OF PRACTICE OF A QUALIFIED FITNESS PROFESSIONAL BASED ON STATE STATUTES AND REGULATIONS
- DESCRIBE NUTRITION-RELATED ACTIVITIES THAT ARE CLEARLY OUTSIDE THE SCOPE OF PRACTICE OF FITNESS PROFESSIONALS

SCOPE OF PRACTICE

ACE POSITION STATEMENT ON NUTRITION SCOPE OF PRACTICE FOR FITNESS PROFESSIONALS

It is the position of the American Council on Exercise (ACE) that fitness professionals not only can but *should* share general nonmedical nutrition information with their clients.

In the current climate of an epidemic of obesity, poor nutrition, and physical inactivity paired with a multibillion dollar diet industry and a strong interest among the general public in improving eating habits and increasing physical activity, fitness professionals are on the front lines in helping the public to achieve healthier lifestyles. Fitness professionals provide an essential service to their clients, the industry, and the community at large when they are able to offer credible, practical, and relevant nutrition information to clients while staying within their professional scope of practice.

Ultimately, an individual fitness professional's scope of practice as it relates to nutrition is determined by state policies and regulations, education and experience, and competencies and skills. While this implies that the nutrition-related scope of practice may vary among fitness professionals, there are certain actions that are within the scope of practice of all fitness professionals.

For example, it is within the scope of practice of all fitness professionals to share dietary advice endorsed or developed by the federal government, especially the *Dietary Guidelines for Americans* (www.health.gov/dietaryguidelines) and the MyPlate recommendations (www.ChooseMyPlate.gov).

Fitness professionals who have passed National Commission for Certifying Agencies (NCCA)– or American National Standards Institute (ANSI)– accredited certification programs that provide basic nutrition information, such as those provided by ACE, and those who have undertaken nutrition continuing education, should also be prepared to discuss:

- Principles of healthy nutrition and food preparation
- Food to be included in the balanced daily diet
- Essential nutrients needed by the body
- Actions of nutrients on the body
- Effects of deficiencies or excesses of nutrients
- How nutrient requirements vary through the lifecycle
- Information about nutrients contained in foods or supplements

Fitness professionals may share this information through a variety of venues, including cooking demonstrations, recipe exchanges, development of handouts and informational packets, individual or group classes and seminars, or one-on-one encounters.

Fitness professionals who do not feel comfortable sharing this information are strongly encouraged to undergo continuing education to further develop nutrition competency and skills and to develop relationships with registered dietitians or other qualified health professionals who can provide this information. It is within the fitness professional's scope of practice to distribute and disseminate information or programs that have been developed by a registered dietitian or medical doctor.

The actions that are outside the scope of practice of fitness professionals include, but may not be limited to, the following:

- Individualized nutrition recommendations or meal planning other than that which is available through government guidelines and recommendations, or has been developed and endorsed by a registered dietitian or physician

- Nutritional assessment to determine nutritional needs and nutritional status, and to recommend nutritional intake
- Specific recommendations or programming for nutrient or nutritional intake, caloric intake, or specialty diets
- Nutritional counseling, education, or advice aimed to prevent, treat, or cure a disease or condition, or other acts that may be perceived as medical nutrition therapy
- Development, administration, evaluation, and consultation regarding nutritional care standards or the nutrition care process
- Recommending, prescribing, selling, or supplying nutritional supplements to clients
- Promotion or identification of oneself as a "nutritionist" or "dietitian"

Engaging in these activities can place a client's health and safety at risk and possibly expose the fitness professional to disciplinary action and litigation. To ensure maximal client safety and compliance with state policies and laws, it is essential that the fitness professional recognize when it is appropriate to refer to a registered dietitian or physician. ACE recognizes that some fitness and health clubs encourage or require their employees to sell nutritional supplements. If this is a condition of employment, ACE suggests that fitness professionals:

- Obtain complete scientific understanding regarding the safety and efficacy of the supplement from qualified healthcare professionals and/or credible resources. *Note:* Generally, the Office of Dietary Supplements (ods.od.nih.gov), the National Center for Complementary and Alternative Medicine (nccam.nih.gov), and the Food and Drug Administration (FDA.gov) are reliable places to go to examine the validity of the claims as well as risks and benefits associated with taking a particular supplement. Since the sites are from trusted resources and in the public domain, fitness professionals can freely distribute and share the information contained on these sites.
- Stay up-to-date on the legal and/or regulatory issues related to the use of the supplement and its individual ingredients
- Obtain adequate insurance coverage should a problem arise

Fitness professionals are increasingly faced with a bombardment of nutrition questions from clients, friends, and acquaintances. From the merits of specific **vitamins** and performance-enhancing supplements to popular diets, nutrition methods to improve athletic performance, and how to eat to lose those "last 5 pounds," the public wants nutrition information. Who better to give it than a trusted fitness expert, whom, the consumer supposes, is equally well-versed in nutrition?

The question often arises: When is it appropriate for fitness professionals to respond to these questions and when should they refer the client to a **registered dietitian (RD)**? The questions surrounding the nutrition-related **scope of practice** for the fitness professional have been the source of numerous industry discussions, debates, and expert panels.

This manual is designed to help prepare fitness professionals to take full advantage of their experience and education while staying within their scope of practice. Fitness professionals will learn how to provide clients and the general public with credible and practical nutrition information so that clients can make their own informed decisions. Fitness professionals will also learn to clearly identify when a client is best served by referral to a registered dietitian and how to develop strong relationships with these nutrition experts, who are allies in the pursuit to optimize a client's nutritional status.

Without a clear understanding of what is and is not within their scope of practice, fitness professionals may miss an important opportunity to provide education and guidance to their clients. When trainers defer all nutrition questions, many clients may get their nutrition information from unreliable sources like consumer publications and salespersons at supplement stores. On the other hand, when fitness professionals say too much, they may put the client and themselves at risk.

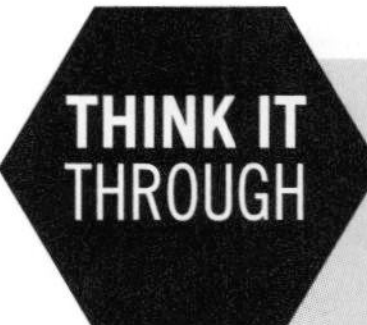

Continuing your education by becoming an ACE Fitness Nutrition Specialist is an excellent step toward providing sound, nutrition-related coaching services to your clients. What steps will you take to ensure that you do not overstep the boundaries of scope of practice as a fitness professional when teaching your clients about nutrition?

DEFINING SCOPE OF PRACTICE

Scope of practice refers to the range and limit of responsibilities normally associated with a position, job, or profession, as determined by rules and regulations defined by state laws and statutes, the roles and responsibilities as outlined by a certifying or accrediting body, and an individual's education and training.

State Laws and Regulations

Most states have laws regulating the practice of dietetics (Commission on Dietetic Registration, 2012). Forty-seven states regulate nutritionists and/or registered dietitians in one of the following three manners (Figure 1-1):

- *Licensure:* This involves a state statute that articulates a clearly defined scope of practice. Providing nutrition education or counseling without the requisite training and possession of a license is illegal. In these states, individuals who practice the profession without a license and who are not specifically exempt are subject to legal action. At the time of this publication, 35 states require licensure, in addition to Washington, D.C., and Puerto Rico. Fitness professionals practicing in these states who plan to integrate nutrition coaching into their practice may consider consultation with an attorney to fully understand that state's specific regulations.

Figure 1-1
State regulations regarding scope of practice

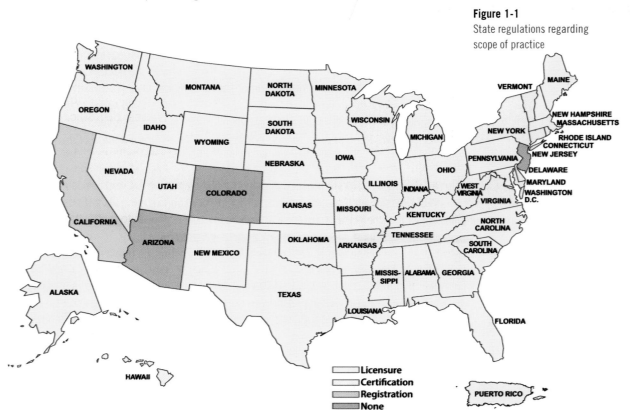

Note: Kentucky requires licensure of dietitians and certification of nutritionists.

- *Statutory certification:* In these states, individuals must meet specific requirements to be eligible for certification. However, non-certified individuals can still practice the profession. Eleven states require certification. Though the rules are much less stringent in these states compared to those states that require licensure, laws are constantly changing. It would be prudent for a fitness professional practicing in these states to carefully review the legislation with the assistance of an attorney to ensure full compliance with the rules.
- *Registration:* In this case, the state statute limits who is allowed to refer to him- or herself as a "registered dietitian" or "dietitian," but does not limit who can practice the profession. Only one state—California—requires registration.

Only three states—Arizona, Colorado, and New Jersey—do not have any laws regulating the field of nutrition.

Note that state laws are constantly evolving and changing. A fitness professional who plans to incorporate nutrition coaching into a practice is well-advised to review the standing legislation in his or her state, ideally with the assistance of an attorney in that state. Classification may have changed from the time of this publication. Up-to-date information is available on the Commission for Dietetic Registration website (www.cdrnet.org).

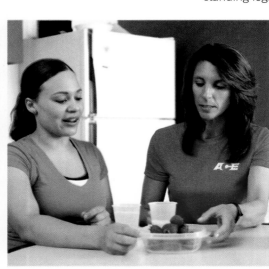

In states without licensure, anyone can legally provide nutrition services, though it may be considered unprofessional or unethical for individuals without the appropriate education and training or competencies and skills to do so. Ultimately, state requirements take precedent in determining minimal scope of practice requirements. For example, while a fitness professional in Colorado may legally be allowed to call himself a "nutritionist" and provide nutrition counseling, a fitness professional with the same education, experience, and fitness certification in Illinois could face a $5,000 penalty each for calling him- or herself a "nutritionist" and for providing nutrition counseling.

To ensure optimal client safety and to maintain the highest ethical standards, this text defines the scope of practice based on the regulations of the most restrictive states in combination with the successful mastery of the fundamental nutrition information contained herein. However, laws are subject to change and all fitness professionals should review their own state requirements, rules, and regulations before promoting their nutrition-related services. *In no way does this text intend to provide legal advice or substitute for the advice of an attorney.*

Education and Training

The limitations of scope of practice dictated by state laws trump the other determinants of scope of practice such as education and training or expertise and skill level. However, regardless of the presence or absence of legal restrictions, any services offered should be consistent with a fitness professional's education and training.

Most fitness certifying bodies and professional organizations include a statement outlining the professional's scope of practice. For example, the ACE position statement pertaining to nutrition that opened this chapter specifically notes that recommending supplements is outside the scope of practice of a fitness professional and states that ACE strongly encourages continuing education on diet and nutrition for all fitness professionals.

Beyond their fitness-related certification, many fitness professionals recognize the value in receiving additional training or certification in nutrition. In these cases, they have spent many hours learning about nutrition and likely have expanded their ability to effectively and accurately answer clients' questions. While education may broaden one's expertise, fitness professionals should be careful to follow the scope of practice guidelines set forth by the certifying or professional organization that offered the advanced training and recognize the limitations to their education and training. In some cases, a fitness professional may choose to pursue even further training to become an RD or attain an advanced degree in nutrition, which further expands scope of practice.

EXPAND YOUR KNOWLEDGE

How to Become a Registered Dietitian

Fitness professionals with a strong interest in nutrition may consider going back to school to become an RD. According to the Academy of Nutrition and Dietetics (A.N.D., 2013), "Registered dietitians (RDs) are food and nutrition experts who have met the following criteria to earn the RD credential:

- Completed a minimum of a bachelor's degree at a U.S. regionally accredited university or college and course work accredited or approved by the Accreditation Council for Education in Nutrition and Dietetics (ACEND) of the Academy of Nutrition and Dietetics.
- Completed an ACEND-accredited supervised practice program at a healthcare facility, community agency, or a foodservice corporation or combined with undergraduate or graduate studies. Typically, a practice program will run six to 12 months in length.
- Passed a national examination administered by the Commission on Dietetic Registration (CDR). For more information regarding the examination, refer to the CDR's website at www.cdrnet.org.
- Completed continuing professional educational requirements to maintain registration."

Competencies and Skills

Fitness professionals should work within their own set of competencies and skills. For example, while one fitness professional may have a special interest and expertise in **obesity** prevention, another may work primarily with athletes and be interested in nutrition to improve sports performance. Prior to sharing a piece of information or initiating a nutrition discussion, fitness professionals should ask themselves whether or not the activity is within their scope of practice, training, and skill set. If the answer is "no" or if one is unsure, referral is probably warranted.

Figure 1-2 provides a scope of practice decision tree as a reference tool to further assist fitness professionals in evaluating this essential topic.

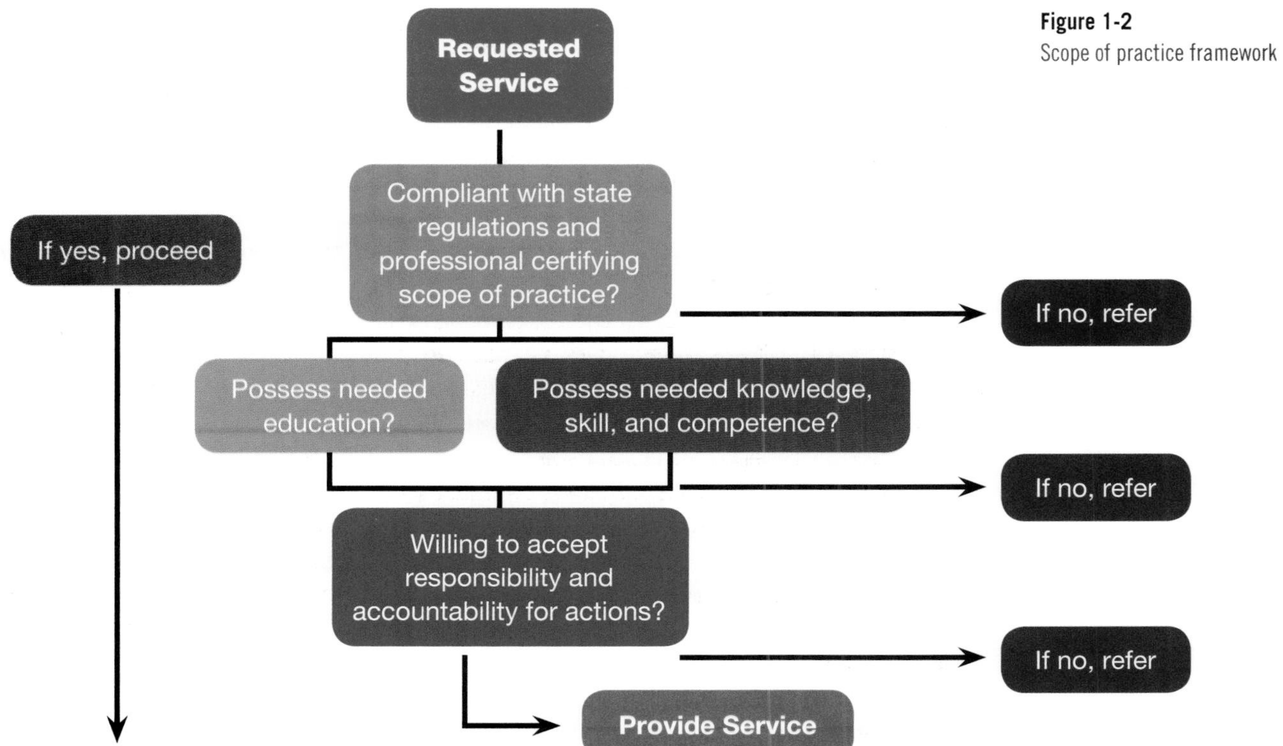

Figure 1-2
Scope of practice framework

NUTRITION CONTENT ALL FITNESS PROFESSIONALS SHOULD SHARE

As a fitness professional considers what nutrition information is or is not appropriate to incorporate into sessions with clients, it is important to highlight certain actions that are well within the scope of practice of nearly all qualified fitness professionals and not only *can* be shared with clients, but *should* be shared in order to provide the highest quality service.

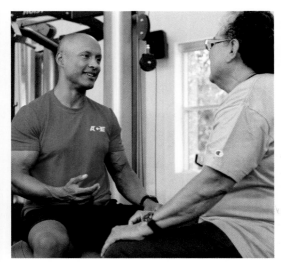

Given the alarming obesity epidemic [i.e., approximately 36% of American adults are obese and the rate is estimated to climb to 40% by 2015 (Flegal et al., 2012; Wang & Beydoun, 2007)]; the high motivation of the general population to learn more about nutrition; and the large amount of nutrition misinformation readily available and perpetuated online, in magazines, and through misinformed and unqualified individuals, fitness professionals should be prepared to discuss nutrition with their clients. All fitness professionals should share the dietary recommendations and guidelines endorsed by the federal government, especially the *Dietary Guidelines for Americans* and the MyPlate recommendations. The details of these food guidance systems are presented in Chapter 3. While historically many fitness professionals have considered these guidelines to be limited and basic, in reality, they contain a wealth of nutrition information and resources. In fact, if most people followed these recommendations—only 3% of Americans eat healthfully, engage in regular physical activity, maintain a healthy weight, and do not smoke (Sandmaier, 2007)—the nutritional status of Americans would be very good and far fewer people would be **overweight** or obese.

NUTRITION CONTENT ACE FITNESS NUTRITION SPECIALISTS SHOULD SHARE

While most of the states that require licensure of nutritionists emphasize what non-licensed persons *cannot* do, Ohio's statute serves as a useful example to help clarify scope of practice for "non-licensed individuals"—that is, individuals like ACE Fitness Nutrition Specialists, who have opportunities to discuss nutrition but do not hold the registered dietitian credential and state license. In Ohio, non-licensed individuals can provide "general nonmedical nutrition information," which includes, but is not necessarily limited to, the following:

- Principles of good nutrition and food preparation
- Food to be included in the normal daily diet
- Essential nutrients needed by the body
- Recommended amounts of essential nutrients
- Functions of **nutrients** in the body
- Effects of deficiencies and excesses of nutrients
- Food and supplements that are good sources of essential nutrients

Non-licensed individuals also may freely disseminate nutrition information, including information on **vegetarian** diets, alternative diet philosophies, and government or agency nutrition literature, books, and articles. Non-licensed individuals may also deliver a weight-management program that has been approved in writing by a physician or registered dietitian (Ohio Board of Dietetics, 2004).

While this statute legally applies directly only to the fitness professionals living in the state of Ohio, ACE believes these general guidelines serve as a useful and constructive outline from which to build knowledge and competency for ACE Fitness Nutrition Specialists. As such, the guidelines form the foundation for the ACE Fitness Nutrition Specialty Certification and the content contained within this manual and the ACE nutrition scope of practice position statement. ACE Fitness Nutrition Specialists are encouraged to share this information through a variety of venues, including cooking demonstrations, recipe exchanges, development of handouts and informational packets, and individual or group classes and seminars.

NUTRITION CONTENT FITNESS PROFESSIONALS AND ACE FITNESS NUTRITION SPECIALISTS SHOULD *NOT* SHARE

Certain nutrition information is best provided by a qualified nutrition professional who holds the necessary training and credentialing to ensure the client's safety and to best meet the client's needs. This information includes:

- *Medical nutrition therapy:* **Medical nutrition therapy** refers to the provision of individualized nutrition assessment and dietary recommendations to help manage a disease or medical condition, such as **diabetes.** Medical nutrition therapy is recognized by Medicare as the domain of the registered dietitian. Clients who have underlying medical diagnoses and illnesses should be encouraged to undergo a nutritional assessment from a registered dietitian. The ACE Fitness Nutrition Specialist may then help the client follow the dietitian's nutrition recommendations made to the client.
- *"Nutrition assessment," "nutrition counseling," or individualized nutrition recommendations:* The assessment of an individual's nutritional status and the provision of individualized nutrition recommendations or counseling are outside the fitness professional's scope of practice. A registered dietitian takes into consideration the client's full medical history, medications, background and family history, and many other factors when developing a dietary program. The fitness professional is often not privy to this information and not trained in how to interpret and manage abnormal findings. However, the fitness professional can use government resources such as the USDA's SuperTracker (www.supertracker.usda.gov) to help healthy, disease-free clients access a personalized eating plan based on the *Dietary Guidelines.*
- *Supplement guidance and recommendations:* Supplement use is widespread among health enthusiasts, athletes, and other individuals who seek the services of the fitness professional. In addition, many fitness facilities promote and sell supplements. As such, fitness professionals frequently field questions about supplements from clients. Due to the potential risks of supplement use, fitness professionals should *never* advise a client to take a supplement. However, fitness professionals *can* share information about supplement regulation, and the efficacy and safety of supplements. When doing so, it is important that the client understands that the fitness professional is not recommending or endorsing the supplement. Clients who are considering supplement use should be referred to a qualified medical professional or registered dietitian.
- *Promotion of credentials as a "nutritionist" or "dietitian":* Most states prohibit promotion of oneself as a "nutritionist" or "dietitian" without verification of specific credentials. Any fitness professional who does not hold these credentials and has not been verified by the state licensing or registration board should *not* refer to him- or herself or promote him- or herself as a nutritionist or dietitian. Upon successful completion of the ACE Specialty Certification in Fitness Nutrition, a fitness professional may state that he or she is an ACE Fitness Nutrition Specialist.

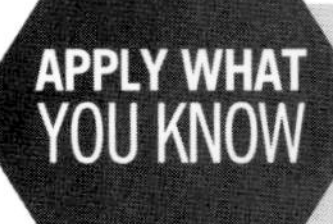

Referral to a Registered Dietitian

One of the most important ways that an ACE Fitness Nutrition Specialist can gain credibility among other allied health professionals and develop strong relationships with registered dietitians is to "speak the language" of the other professional and thereby establish an effective referral process. This four-step plan will help fitness professionals get started.

- *Identify a qualified professional:* The first step to initiating a referral is to identify a nutrition professional who you trust. You may identify this person through word of mouth and a recommendation from another allied health professional, through the database of registered dietitians maintained by the A.N.D. (available at www.eatright.org), through the facility where you work, or through other venues.
- *Establish a connection:* Before referring clients to an individual, it is helpful to establish a connection and relationship with that person. Not only does this communication help to increase the likelihood of success for the client, but it may also help to have a ready contact for future referral and generate return referrals in exchange. There are several ways to establish this connection: a brief introductory phone call or email, following up on a recommendation from another professional or client, or networking through professional meetings, joint acquaintances, or organized networking events, for example.
- *Make the referral:* Once you have determined to whom to refer a client, the next step is to make the referral. To be most effective, it is important to make the referral in writing. The referral letter should include (1) your name, credentials, and contact information; (2) a brief one- or two-line background about the client; and (3) the reason for referral.
- *Follow up:* Follow up with both the registered dietitian and your client after the client has visited with the registered dietitian. You can play an important role in helping to reinforce the messages and recommendations provided by the registered dietitian and also help to monitor the client's progress. To strengthen your relationship with the registered dietitian, write a brief follow-up letter acknowledging that you received the recommendations and will fulfill your intended role by helping the client achieve success with the recommendations. This follow-up letter helps to improve care for the client and demonstrates your professionalism.

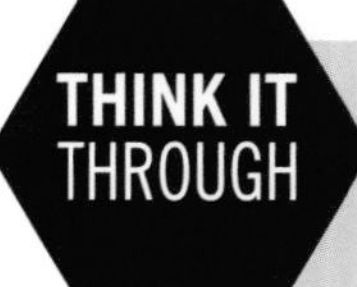

To better serve their clients, fitness professionals should develop a referral network that includes a variety of healthcare providers, including nutrition professionals. What steps will you take to develop and strengthen your relationship with a qualified nutrition professional in your community?

SUMMARY

As nutrition and exercise are both critical to achieve optimal health and wellness, fitness professionals are encouraged to share nutrition information with their clients. In those cases in which a client requests individualized nutrition information or when a client has a medical diagnosis that requires special nutrition recommendations, fitness professionals may serve their clients best by referring them to a physician and/or a registered dietitian for an individualized eating plan. The fitness professional still plays an important role in providing support and encouragement for the client to follow the recommended plan. Ultimately, when allied health professionals work together to help clients reach their goals, everyone benefits: the client receives the best care while both professionals strengthen their networks and increase their credibility.

REFERENCES

Academy of Nutrition and Dietetics (2013). *Registered Dietitian Educational and Professional Requirements.* Retrieved January 6, 2013: www.eatright.org/BecomeanRDorDTR/content.aspx?id=8143#.UOpcsoYySSo

Commission on Dietetic Registration (2012). *Laws That Regulate Dietitians/Nutritionists.* Retrieved October 26, 2012: www.cdrnet.org/certifications/licensure

Flegal, K.M. et al. (2012). Prevalence of obesity and trends in the distribution of body mass index among US adults, 1999–2010. *Journal of the American Medical Association*, 307, 5, 491–497.

Ohio Board of Dietetics (2004). *Bulletin # 8: General Non-medical Nutrition Information.* Retrieved October 26, 2012: www.dietetics.ohio.gov/bulletins/bulletin8.pdf

Sandmaier, M. (2007). *The Healthy Heart Handbook for Women.* Bethesda, Md.: U.S. Department of Health and Human Services: National Institutes of Health, National Heart, Lung, and Blood Institute. nhlbi.nih.gov/health/public/heart/other/hhw/hdbk_wmn.pdf

Wang, Y. & Beydoun, M.A. (2007). The obesity epidemic in the United States: Gender, age, socioeconomic, racial/ethnic, and geographic characteristics: A systematic review and meta-regression analysis. *Epidemiologic Reviews*, 29, 6–28.

SUGGESTED READING

Commission on Dietetic Registration (2012). *Laws That Regulate Dietitians/Nutritionists.* Retrieved October 26, 2012: www.cdrnet.org/certifications/licensure

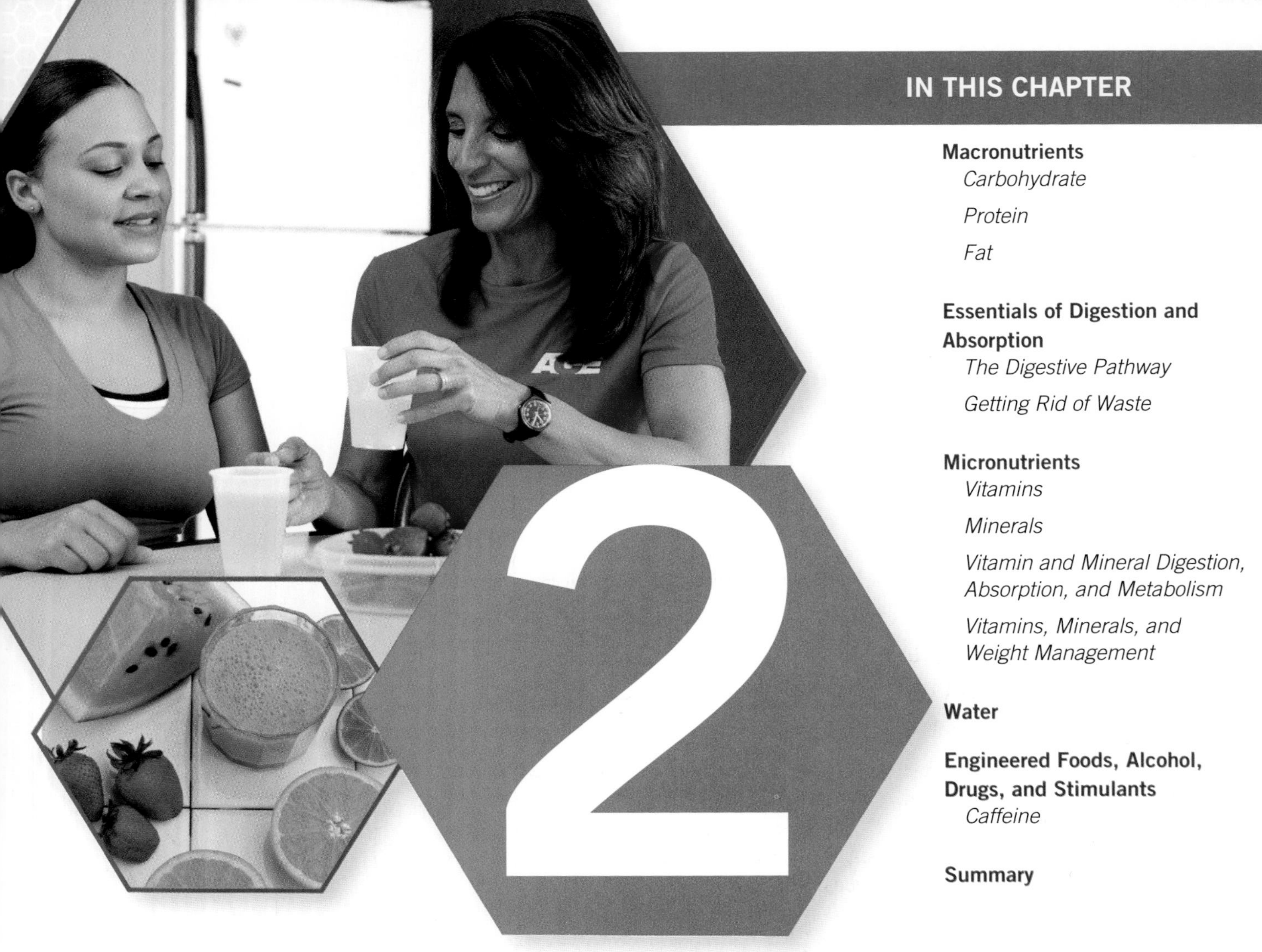

IN THIS CHAPTER

LEARNING OBJECTIVES

AFTER READING THIS CHAPTER, YOU WILL BE ABLE TO:

- DESCRIBE THE STRUCTURE AND FUNCTION OF THE MACRONUTRIENTS (CARBOHYDRATES, PROTEIN, AND FAT)
- DESCRIBE THE FUNCTION OF THE MICRONUTRIENTS (VITAMINS AND MINERALS)
- DESCRIBE THE IMPORTANCE OF WATER
- OUTLINE THE PROCESSES OF DIGESTION AND ABSORPTION

BASIC NUTRITION AND DIGESTION

Clients know that eating a healthful diet is good for their bodies. What they may not understand is why certain foods are considered healthier than others or how different food groups work differently in the body, such as how **protein** helps build muscle or why **carbohydrate** is the best energy source for endurance training.

An understanding of basic nutrition, **digestion,** and **absorption** will help an ACE Fitness Nutrition Specialist better explain nutrition recommendations and suggestions; provide clear answers to clients' questions; and have a broader knowledge base when they attend continuing-education classes, read about scientific findings in relevant articles, and communicate with their colleagues. From a discussion of the processes of **nutrient** digestion and absorption to **macronutrient** and **micronutrient** structure and function, this chapter provides a foundation of knowledge in nutritional sciences, an exciting scientific field that encompasses biology, chemistry, biochemistry, physiology, and psychology.

From a carbohydrate-rich and nutrient-packed citrus fruit to a protein-dense, fat-laden, and iron-loaded cut of steak, every food and beverage that a person eats or drinks gets broken down into its component parts—macronutrients (carbohydrate, protein, and **fat**), micronutrients (**vitamins** and **minerals**), and water. These nutrients enable the body to carry out numerous and complex functions, such as giving energy to fuel activity, providing structural components that comprise muscles and other tissues, and protecting vital organs. Every nutrient serves an essential role in the body, which is why it is so important to consume a nutrient-rich and varied diet.

MACRONUTRIENTS

The macronutrients, which by definition are needed by the body in large amounts, include carbohydrate, protein, and fat. Through the digestive process, the macronutrients are broken down into their basic building blocks of **monosaccharides, amino acids,** and **fatty acids.** They are then absorbed by the body and delivered to the cells to support the body's many vital functions.

Carbohydrate

Carbohydrates not only are the body's preferred source of immediate energy—and, in fact, the only energy source for the brain and red blood cells—carbohydrates also store energy, and in the case of **fiber,** may help improve digestive health and **cholesterol** levels.

Structure

Carbohydrates are built from subunits of monosaccharides, sugar compounds made up of carbon with water attached (as the name implies: "hydrated carbon," or carbohydrate). Three monosaccharides found in nature can be absorbed and utilized by humans—**glucose, fructose,** and **galactose.** Glucose is the predominant sugar in nature and the basic building block of most other carbohydrates (Figure 2-1). Fructose, or fruit sugar, is the sweetest of the monosaccharides and is found in varying levels in different types of fruits. Galactose is most often found joined with glucose to form **lactose,** which is a **disaccharide** and the principal sugar found in milk. Each of the carbohydrates contains 4 calories per gram.

Monosaccharides are rarely found free in nature. Instead, they are usually found joined together as disaccharides, **oligosaccharides,** or **polysaccharides.** Lactose, maltose (two glucose molecules bound together), and sucrose [table sugar (or granulated sugar)], which is formed by glucose and fructose. Most caloric sweeteners are disaccharides. Raw sugar, granulated sugar, brown sugar, powdered sugar, and turbinado sugar (Sugar in the Raw®) are all sucrose. Honey is a natural form of sucrose that is made from plant nectar and harvested by honeybees, which secrete an **enzyme** that hydrolyzes sucrose to glucose and fructose. Thus, honey is a mixture of fructose, glucose, and a bit of sucrose dissolved in water. Corn sweeteners, such as the corn syrup commonly found in sodas, baked goods, and some canned products, are a liquid combination of primarily glucose with much smaller amounts of maltose. Sorbitol, which is used in many diet products, is produced from glucose and found naturally in some berries and fruits. It is absorbed by the body at a slower rate than sugar.

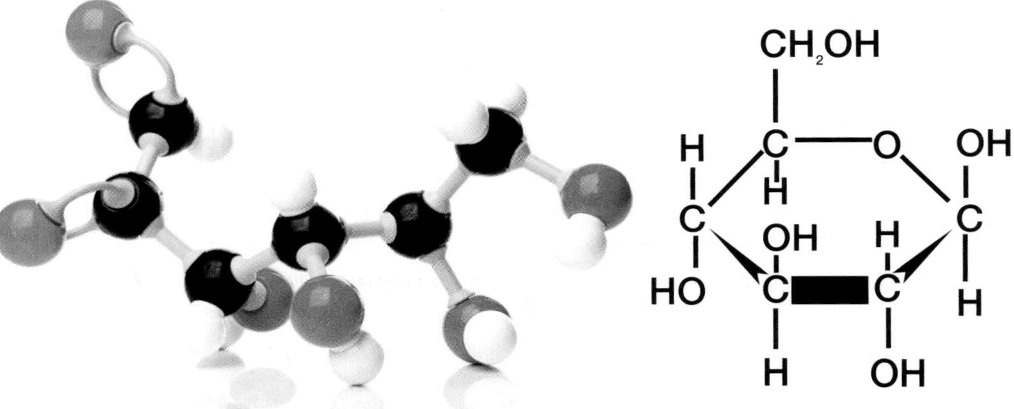

Figure 2-1
Glucose, which is also known as dextrose or grape sugar, has as its molecular formula $C_6H_{12}O_6$.

Note: Carbon is represented by the black balls, oxygen by the red balls, and hydrogen by the white balls.

EXPAND YOUR KNOWLEDGE

The Truth Behind High-fructose Corn Syrup

Corn syrup can be enzymatically converted to change some of its glucose to fructose, yielding high-fructose corn syrup (HFCS). HFCS first made its debut in the American food supply around 1970, when it accounted for about 0.5% of total sweetener use. It is produced when corn syrup undergoes processing to convert glucose to fructose. By the mid-2000s, almost half of all sweetened foods were sweetened with HFCS. HFCS makes up a large proportion of added sweeteners in beverages and processed and packaged foods, including many canned foods, cereals, baked goods, desserts, flavored and sweetened dairy products, candy, and fast food. Two forms of HFCS are used in the U.S. food supply: HFCS-55, which is found mostly in carbonated beverages and is 55% fructose, 41% glucose, and 4% glucose polymers, and HFCS-42, which is found mostly in processed foods and contains slightly less fructose (42% fructose, 53% glucose, and 5% glucose polymers) (Duffey & Popkin, 2008). Food manufacturers prefer HFCS to pure sugar (which is comprised of the sugar sucrose) due to its long shelf-life and cheap cost, which is in large part due to corn subsidies and other policies aimed to increase corn production that have led to corn prices that are actually less than the cost of production. In addition, high tariffs on imported sugar cane make sweetening with all-natural sugar costly.

After the publication of several animal and human studies suggested that HFCS may contribute to **obesity, insulin resistance** and **diabetes,** and decreased feelings of fullness after consumption, health advocates and the media became alarmed that HFCS may contribute to negative health outcomes, including the surge in obesity. Most human studies have found that HFCS is not associated with an increased risk of **overweight,** obesity, or metabolic disorders like diabetes when fructose is consumed in reasonable amounts [less than 50 g of fructose (or approximately 10% of total calories) per day] (Sievenpiper et al., 2012; Rizkalla, 2010). However, the number of long-term high-quality controlled studies is limited. This is an area of ongoing research and controversy. Of course, this is not to say that clients can eat all the HFCS they want without risk of ill consequence. Rather, HFCS probably does not increase health risk more than sugar or other sweeteners. That said, the typical American still consumes about 16% of daily calories from added sugars [U.S. Department of Agriculture (USDA), 2010], which is approximately 320 extra **empty calories** per day that provide minimal nutritional value. Add it up and the typical American eats about 20 pounds (9 kg) worth of added sugar over the course of a year.

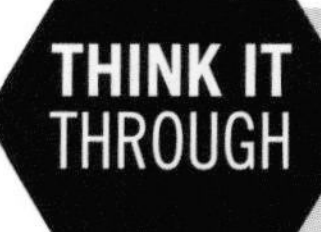

During your initial meeting, a new client, Jen, a 20-year-old college student, tells you that she is surprised that she has not lost weight in recent months because she stopped eating foods with high-fructose corn syrup and replaced them with snacks with other sweeteners. How would you respond to this statement, and what advice would you give Jen to facilitate better weight management in the future?

Artificial and Plant-based High-intensity Sweeteners

Noncaloric sweeteners—which are calorie-free because the body cannot metabolize them—also are used to add sweet taste to foods and beverages. Aspartame, also known as Equal® in packaged sweeteners and NutraSweet® in foods and beverages; Acesulfame K, which is called Sunett® in cooking products and Sweet One® as a tabletop sweetener; saccharin; sucralose (Splenda®); and neotame all are approved for use in the United States. While early studies found that certain sweeteners may cause bladder cancer in laboratory rats, subsequent studies have found no association in humans (Weihrauch & Diehl, 2004). Sugar extracted from the stevia plant is now a widely available natural alternative to artificial sweeteners.

Whether noncaloric sweeteners actually contribute to weight loss is a source of debate and controversy. While in theory the decreased caloric intake resulting from use of a noncaloric sweetener instead of a high-calorie sugar should result in fewer calories consumed and therefore weight loss, some studies have shown an opposite effect. Ultimately, research into the effects of noncaloric sweeteners on appetite, energy balance, and weight control is ongoing with mixed results (Mattes & Popkin, 2009).

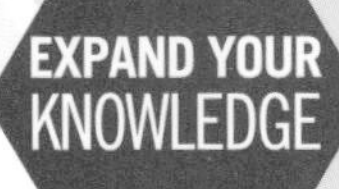

In Stores Now: Stevia—The All-natural Plant-based Sweetener

Once limited to the health-food market as an unapproved herb, the plant-derived sweetener known as stevia is now widely available and rapidly replacing artificial sweeteners in consumer products. Thirty times sweeter than sugar and with no effect on blood sugar and little aftertaste, stevia sales are predicted to reach about $700 million in the next few years according to the agribusiness finance giant Rabobank (Rabobank Group, 2009).

Stevia's history goes back to ancient times. Grown naturally in tropical climates, stevia is an herb in the Chrysanthemum family that grows wild as a small shrub in Paraguay and Brazil, though it can easily be cultivated elsewhere. Paraguayans have used stevia as a food sweetener for centuries, while other countries including Korea, Japan, China, and much of South America also have a shorter, though still long-standing, record of stevia use. There are more than 100 species of stevia plant, but one stands out for its excellent properties as a sweetener—Stevia rebaudiana, which contains the compound rebaudioside A, the sweetest-flavored component of the stevia leaf. Rebaudioside A chemically acts very similar to sugar in onset, intensity, and duration of sweetness and is free of aftertaste. Most stevia-containing products are made with extracted rebaudioside A with some proportion of stevioside, which is a white crystalline compound present in stevia that tastes 100 to 300 times sweeter than table sugar (Kobylewski & Eckhert, 2008).

Though widely available throughout the world, in 1991 stevia was banned in the U.S. due to early studies that suggested the sweetener may cause cancer. A follow-up study refuted the initial study, and in 1995 the U.S. Food and Drug Administration (FDA) allowed stevia to be imported and sold as a food supplement, but not as a sweetener (FDA, 1995). Several companies argued to the FDA that stevia should be categorized similarly to its artificial sweetener cousins as "Generally Recognized as Safe (GRAS)." Substances that are considered GRAS have been determined to be safe through expert consensus, scientific review, or widespread use without negative complications. They are exempt from the rigorous approval process required for food additives. In December 2008, the FDA declared stevia GRAS, and allowed its use in mainstream U.S. food production (Goyal, Samsher, & Goyal, 2010). It has taken food manufacturers a few years to work out the right stevia-containing recipes, but stevia is now present in a number of foods and beverages in the U.S., such as Gatorade's® G2, VitaminWater® Zero, SoBe® Lifewater Zero, Crystal Light®, and Sprite® Green. Around the world it has been used in soft drinks, chewing gums, wines, yogurts, candies, and many other products. Stevia powder can also be used for cooking and baking (in markedly decreased amounts compared to table sugar due to its high sweetness potency).

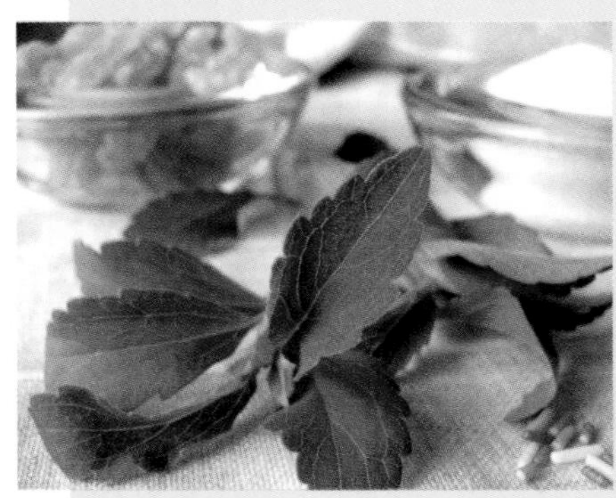

Stevia is marketed under the trade names of Truvia® (Coca-Cola® and agricultural giant Cargill®), PureVia® (Pepsi-Cola® and Whole Earth Sweetener Company®), and SweetLeaf® (Wisdom Natural Brands®). Though it is known by three different names, the sweetener is essentially the same product, though the different versions contain slightly different proportions of rebaudioside A and stevioside. Both Coke and Pepsi intend to use stevia as a soft-drink sweetener in the U.S., but have not yet unveiled their stevia-version Coca-Cola or Pepsi (although they have trialed it with a few of their less popular products such as Coke's Sprite Green).

Few long-term studies have been done to document stevia's health effects in humans. A review conducted by toxicologists at UCLA that was commissioned by nutrition advocate Center for Science in the Public Interest raised concerns that stevia could contribute to cancer (Kobylewski & Eckhert, 2008). The authors noted that in some test tube and animal studies, stevioside (but not rebaudioside A) caused genetic mutations, chromosome damage, and DNA breakage. These changes presumably could contribute to malignancy, though no one has actually studied if these compounds cause cancer in animal models. Notably, initial concerns that stevia may reduce fertility or worsen diabetes seem to have been put to rest after a few good studies showed no negative outcomes. In fact, one study of human subjects showed that treatment with stevia may improve glucose tolerance. Another found that stevia may induce the pancreas to release insulin, thus potentially serving as a treatment for **type 2 diabetes.** (These studies are reviewed in Goyal, Samsher, & Goyal, 2010.) After artificial sweeteners were banned in Japan more than 40 years ago, the Japanese began to sweeten their foods with stevia. Since then, they have conducted more than 40,000 clinical studies on stevia and concluded that it is safe for human use. Still, there is a general lack of long-term studies on stevia's use and effects.

All in all, stevia's sweet taste and all-natural origins make it a popular sugar substitute. With little long-term data available on the plant extract, it is possible that stevia in large quantities could have harmful effects. However, it seems safe to say that when consumed in reasonable amounts, stevia may be an exceptional natural plant-based sugar substitute.

Oligo- and Polysaccharides

An oligosaccharide is a chain of approximately three to 10 simple sugars. **Fructooligosaccharides,** which are found in fruits such as bananas and in vegetables like asparagus and soybeans, are oligosaccharides that are mostly indigestible, may help relieve constipation, improve **triglyceride** levels, and decrease the production of foul-smelling digestive by-products.

A long chain of sugar molecules is referred to as a polysaccharide. **Glycogen,** the storage form of carbohydrate found in meat products and seafood, and **starch,** a plant carbohydrate found in grains and vegetables, are the only polysaccharides that humans can fully digest. Both are long chains of glucose and are referred to as **complex carbohydrates** (vs. **simple carbohydrates,** which are short chains of sugar). Historically, much debate has centered on whether consumption of simple or complex carbohydrates is better for athletic performance. The role of a particular carbohydrate in athletic performance may be better determined by its **glycemic index (GI)** than its structure. GI ranks carbohydrates based on their blood glucose response: High-GI foods (e.g., white bread and graham crackers) break down rapidly, causing a large glucose spike, while low-GI foods (e.g., oatmeal and strawberries) are digested more slowly and cause a smaller glucose increase. The glycemic index is described and evaluated in more detail in Chapter 4.

Metabolism and Storage

Animals store excess carbohydrates as glycogen. Although glycogen can be found in animal products, most glycogen stores are depleted before meat enters the food supply. Plants store carbohydrates as starch granules. Edible plants make two types of starch: amylase (a small, linear molecule) and the more prevalent amylopectin (a larger, highly branched molecule). Because starches are longer than disaccharides and oligosaccharides, they take longer to digest. Still, humans are able to easily break down and digest starches with specific self-produced enzymes. However, the rest of the plant, which is formed largely of the carbohydrate cellulose and other fibers such as hemicellulose, lignin, gums, and pectin, is indigestible. This fiber passes through the human body undigested, as humans do not produce the necessary enzymes to break the sugar bonds, though some fiber does undergo fermentation in the **large intestine,** thereby providing a small amount of energy for normal gut bacterial growth. While other carbohydrates contain 4 calories per gram, fiber probably contributes about 1.5 to 2.5 calories per gram [Institute of Medicine (IOM), 2005].

Fiber is classified as **dietary fiber** and **functional fiber.** Dietary fiber is that fiber obtained naturally from plant foods, while functional fiber is obtained in the diet from isolated fibers added to food products. Together they comprise “total fiber.” **High-viscosity fibers** (typically those that used to be referred to as **soluble fiber**) include gums (found in foods like oats, legumes, barley, and guar, which is a type of bean), pectin (found in foods like apples, citrus fruits, strawberries, and carrots), and psyllium seeds. These fibers slow **gastric emptying,** or the passage of food from the stomach into the intestines. Consequently, they help to increase feelings of fullness. Also, the delayed gastric emptying slows the release of sugar into the bloodstream. The slow and steady release of sugar into the bloodstream, rather than a rapid surge, helps to avert a resulting insulin spike. High levels of insulin are associated with weight gain (and, for many, insulin resistance as a consequence of weight gain) and increased risk of **cardiovascular disease.** By binding bile acids in the **small intestine,** fiber also interferes with the absorption of fat and cholesterol and the recirculation of cholesterol in the liver. Once bound to fiber, the unabsorbed cholesterol can then be excreted in feces, which may decrease cholesterol levels.

Low-viscosity fibers (previously referred to as **insoluble fibers**) such as cellulose (found in whole-wheat flour, bran, and vegetables), hemicellulose (found in whole grains and bran), and lignin (found in mature vegetables, wheat, and fruit with edible seeds like strawberries and kiwi) play an important role in increasing fecal bulk and provide a laxative effect. Clearly, fiber serves many important and beneficial roles in the human body. Still, most people get nowhere near the recommended 14 grams/1,000 calories per day, or the approximately 25 to 35 grams per day for most adults (children over two years old should eat their age plus 5 grams per day) (IOM, 2005). With increased consumption of fruits, vegetables, legumes, and whole grains, most Americans could easily achieve this fiber goal.

Digested and absorbed carbohydrates that are not immediately used for energy are stored in the liver and muscle as glycogen. Approximately 90 grams of glycogen is stored in the liver. A minimum of 150 grams of glycogen is stored in muscle, though this amount can be increased up to fivefold with physical training (Mahan, Escott-Stump, & Raymond, 2011). **Carbohydrate loading** also increases glycogen stores (see Chapter 4). Because glycogen stores many water molecules with it, it is large and bulky and therefore unsuitable for long-term energy storage. Thus, if a person continues to consume more carbohydrates than the body can use or store, the body will convert the sugar into fat for long-term storage.

Protein

Proteins form the major structural component of muscle, as well as that of the brain, nervous system, blood, skin, and hair. This macronutrient serves as the transport mechanism for iron, vitamins, minerals, fats, and oxygen within the body, and is the key to acid–base and fluid balance. Proteins form enzymes that speed up chemical reactions and create **antibodies** that the body uses to fight infection. In situations of energy deprivation, the body can break down proteins for energy, yielding 4 calories per gram of protein.

Structure

Proteins are built from amino acids, which are carbohydrates with an attached nitrogen-containing amino group and, in some cases, sulfur. Proteins form when amino acids are joined together through **peptide bonds.** The completed protein is a linear chain of amino acids. These structures fold, creating a unique three-dimensional polypeptide. Individual polypeptides may remain free-standing or bind together to form a larger complex. Figure 2-2 illustrates the peptide bond and folding protein.

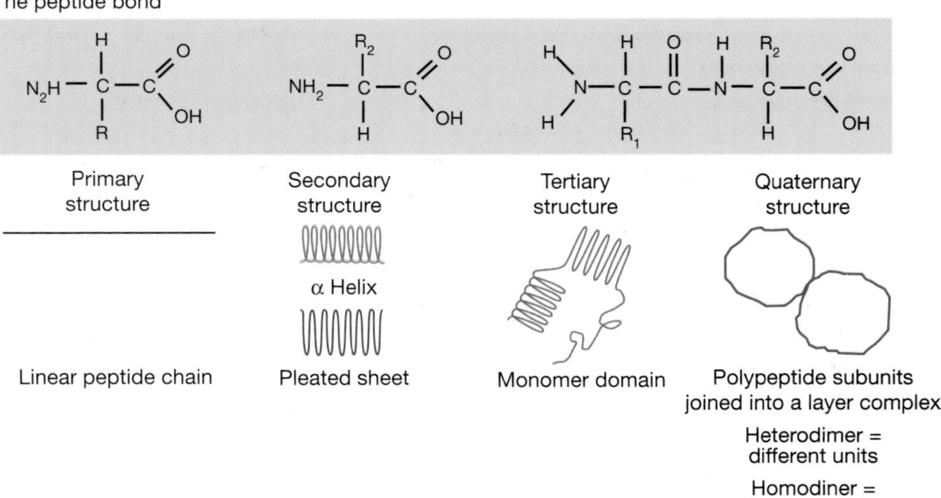

Figure 2-2
The peptide bond and folding protein

Reprinted with permission from Mahan, L.K., Escott-Stump, S., & Raymond, J.L. (2011). *Krause's Food and the Nutrition Care Process* (13th ed.). Philadelphia: W.B. Saunders Company.

The body can produce most of the amino acids that make up proteins, but there are eight to 10 **essential amino acids** that, by definition, are amino acids that cannot be made by the body and must be consumed in the diet. The others are called **nonessential amino acids** because they can be made by the body. A specific food's protein quality is determined by assessing its essential amino acid composition, digestibility, and **bioavailability,** which is the degree to which an amino acid can be used by the body. Generally, animal products contain all of the essential amino acids in amounts proportional to need (called **complete proteins**), whereas plant foods do not and are called **incomplete proteins** (low in one or more essential amino acids). Two notable exceptions are soy and chia seeds, which are both plant-based complete proteins. Vegetarian clients can boost protein quality and get all the essential amino acids they need by eating soy and chia seeds and/or by combining complementary incomplete plant proteins. Excellent combinations include grains-legumes (e.g., rice and beans) and legumes-seeds (e.g., falafel) (Figure 2-3).

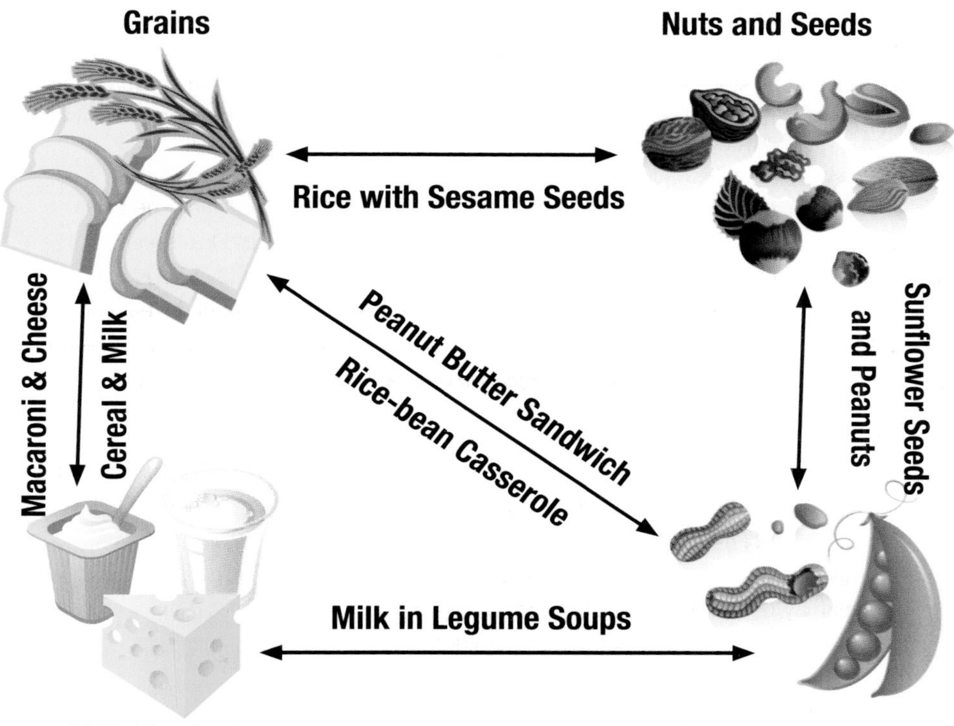

Figure 2-3
Protein complementarity chart

Adapted with permission from Lappé, F.M. (1992). *Diet for a Small Planet.* New York: Ballantine Books.

EXPAND YOUR KNOWLEDGE

How Many Essential Amino Acids Are There?

ACE texts, as well as many other reference texts and articles, often state that there are eight to 10 essential amino acids. But what exactly does that mean? It seems that it should be easy to determine whether an amino acid is essential (i.e., not produced by the body) or nonessential (i.e., produced by the body). So, why the confusion? Is the correct number eight, nine, or 10?

Eight amino acids are essential for everyone: valine, leucine, isoleucine, methionine, phenylalanine, threonine, tryptophan, and lysine. Historically, the amino acid histidine was thought to only be essential to infants and children; however, a culmination of studies seems to suggest that it is also essential for adults (Nutrition Reviews, 1975). The amino acid cysteine is nonessential for most people, but the body is unable to produce cysteine in the elderly, infants, and some individuals with certain chronic diseases, making cysteine an essential amino acid for these special populations.

What Are Chia Seeds?

Loaded with fiber, **polyunsaturated fatty acids,** protein (including all of the essential amino acids), calcium, and several other minerals, chia seeds are hitting the supermarkets and health food stores with promises of weight loss, improved athletic performance, decreased risk of cardiovascular disease, and a variety of other health benefits.

Chia seeds come from the plant *salvia hispanica,* a flowering plant from the mint family. The seeds are native to Mexico and Central America and were probably a staple in the Mayan and Aztecan diets. While commonly consumed in Mexico and the Southwestern United States, it was not until recently that the chia seed gained widespread attention as a potential "superfood." Few other foods provide as dense of a source of **omega-3 fatty acids** or as rich content of fiber (over 40% of the recommended daily amount in a 1 ounce serving).

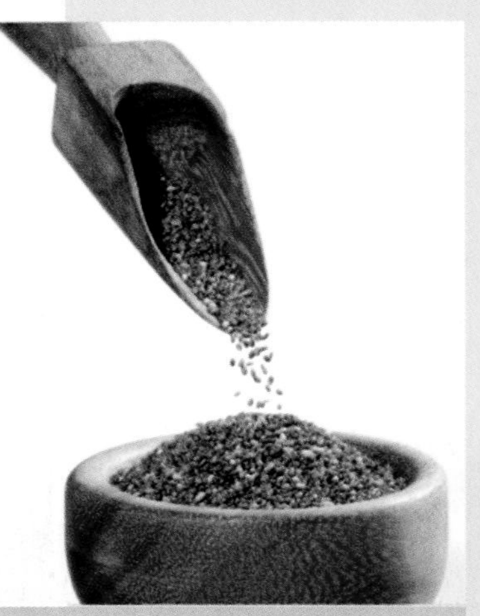

THE NUTRITIONAL CONTENT OF 1 OUNCE OF CHIA SEEDS

Calories: 137
Fat: 9 g
Polyunsaturated fat: 7 g
Protein: 5 g
Carbohydrate: 12 g
Fiber: 10 g
Calcium: 180 mg
Magnesium: 95 mg
Phosphorus: 244 mg
Potassium: 115 mg

Source: USDA Nutrient Database for Standard Reference (http://ndb.nal.usda.gov/)

The research evaluating whether the chia seed provides substantive, measurable health benefits lags behind the public interest in this latest purported miracle food. While study results continue to be released, so far the data is mixed. One study of 75 overweight adults randomized half of the participants to a chia seed group while the other half were given a placebo. The chia seed group consumed 25 g twice per day for 12 weeks; the control group took a placebo supplement. The researchers predicted that the chia seed group would have increased weight loss and improved cardiovascular risk profile due to the chia seed's high levels of satiety-inducing fiber and heart-healthy omega-3 fatty acids. While the chia seed group did have higher levels of alpha-linoleic acid, the omega-3 precursor to the heart-healthy EPA and DHA, levels of EPA and DHA as well as other markers of cardiovascular risk and **body composition** were no different between the two groups (see "Fat" on page 20 for information on the various forms of omega-3 fatty acid). The researchers concluded that the chia seeds provided no measurable benefit over the 12-week study (Nieman et al., 2009). However, it is possible that a longer-duration study, different amounts of chia seeds, or an evaluation of different variables could lead to different results.

Other researchers were interested in whether chia seeds could help improve performance of endurance exercise lasting longer than 90 minutes by serving as a source of carbohydrate loading. They compared carbohydrate loading with Gatorade to carbohydrate loading with 50% chia seeds and 50% Gatorade in six trained male athletes. Each study participant engaged in a one-hour run on a treadmill followed by a 10 K time trial on a track with both carbohydrate loading with Gatorade and carbohydrate loading with the Gatorade–chia seed mix with a two-week washout period in between. Performance measures were equal with both regimens, suggesting that chia seeds could provide a healthier source of carbohydrate for endurance athletes (Illian, Casey, & Bishop, 2011). However, the researchers did not measure degree of gastrointestinal distress, which could be higher with the chia seed group given the high fiber content of the seeds.

A systematic review conducted to evaluate the evidence to date to support the health claims for chia seeds concluded that there is little scientific evidence to support the effectiveness of chia seeds in providing any health benefits (Ulbricht et al., 2009). That is not to say that chia seeds do not provide benefit; it is simply that there is too little quality research available to make any definitive conclusions or recommendations. Importantly, the data to date suggest that consumption of chia seeds is generally safe and without major health risk, other than for those individuals who are allergic to chia seeds (Ulbricht et al., 2009).

Overall, the chia seed could be an exceptional addition to a healthy and balanced eating plan. Simply substitute chia seeds for eggs or oil by mixing a tablespoon of chia seeds with ¼ cup of water; use as a thickener for soups and puddings; or add chia seeds to an herb, seed, or granola mix.

Metabolism and Storage

The body's need for dietary proteins results from the constant breakdown and regeneration of the body's cells. The immediate supplier of amino acids for cell regeneration comes from the cell's free amino acid pool, which is made of dietary amino acids and the recycled amino acids from cell turnover. Because amino acid recycling is inherently inefficient, dietary amino acid intake is necessary to replace losses.

Unlike carbohydrate and fat, the body does not store protein. The continuous recycling of amino acids through the removal and addition of nitrogen allows the body to carefully regulate protein balance. Protein balance is measured in terms of **nitrogen balance,** which is a measure of nitrogen consumed (from dietary intake protein) and nitrogen excreted (from protein breakdown). In a healthy body, the amount of protein taken in is matched by the amount of protein lost in feces, urine, and skin. The muscle tissues undergo continual breakdown and resynthesis, with a fraction of muscle protein destroyed and an equal fraction rebuilt daily using amino acids from the amino acid pool. Negative nitrogen balance, in which the body breaks down more protein than it can create (**catabolism**), occurs during times of high stress such as with severe infections and trauma. Positive nitrogen balance, in which the body produces more protein than it breaks down (**anabolism**), occurs in times of growth such as childhood, pregnancy, recovery from illness, and in response to resistance training when overloading the muscle promotes protein synthesis. Importantly, just because an athlete consumes a high-protein diet does not necessarily mean that he or she will be in positive nitrogen balance and experience muscle growth. Case in point: an endurance athlete who consumes a high-protein, low-carbohydrate diet (and thus has minimal glycogen stores) will rely heavily on muscle protein for fuel, putting him in a negative nitrogen balance; as a result, he will experience decreased athletic performance and worsened muscular strength and endurance.

EXPAND YOUR KNOWLEDGE

Myth: You Cannot Eat Too Much Protein

Myth: As far as weight is concerned, you cannot eat too much protein. Anything beyond what your body needs will get excreted in urine.

Rationale: Because the body has little capacity to store proteins, it makes sense that anything consumed beyond what the body immediately needs will just get removed in the urine (similar to water-soluble vitamins).

The science: It is true that the body has a limited ability to store protein. It is also true that a portion of the protein does get excreted in the urine (the nitrogen group that shows up in urine as urea). However, the other portion of the protein (the carbon group) is readily converted to glucose or fat, depending on the body's current needs. Ultimately, protein consumed beyond what the body needs has the same fate as carbohydrate or fat consumed beyond what the body needs—conversion into stored fat.

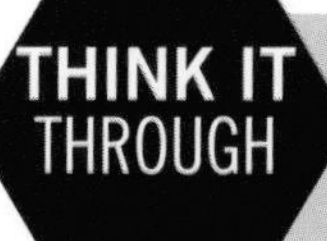

Your new client, Ashley, has just graduated from college and would like your help with staying physically active since she will no longer be playing on her collegiate volleyball team. She informs you that her next fitness-related goal is to run a marathon within the next six months. In your initial interview, you discover that Ashley eats a low-carbohydrate, high-protein diet because she believes it helps her burn more body fat and helps her better manage her weight versus eating a diet with more carbohydrates. What would you say to Ashley to help educate her about the role of carbohydrates in the diets of endurance athletes, such as marathon runners?

Fat

The most energy-dense of the macronutrients, fat provides 9 calories per gram, which is 2.25 times more calories than both carbohydrate and protein (4 calories per gram). Because of this high caloric value, foods that are high in fat should be consumed in moderation if weight control is the goal, but they should not be avoided altogether. **Monounsaturated fats** and **polyunsaturated fats** (such as those found in olive oil and salmon, respectively) are heart-healthy and excellent sources of essential nutrients (though still calorie-dense).

Fats serve many critical functions in the body, including insulation, cell structure, nerve transmission, vitamin absorption, and hormone production.

Structure

To understand how various fats function in the body, first consider their structure (Figure 2-4). All fats are made up of hydrogen, carbon, and oxygen, and all fats are insoluble in water. Beyond that, they are a very **heterogeneous** group of molecules.

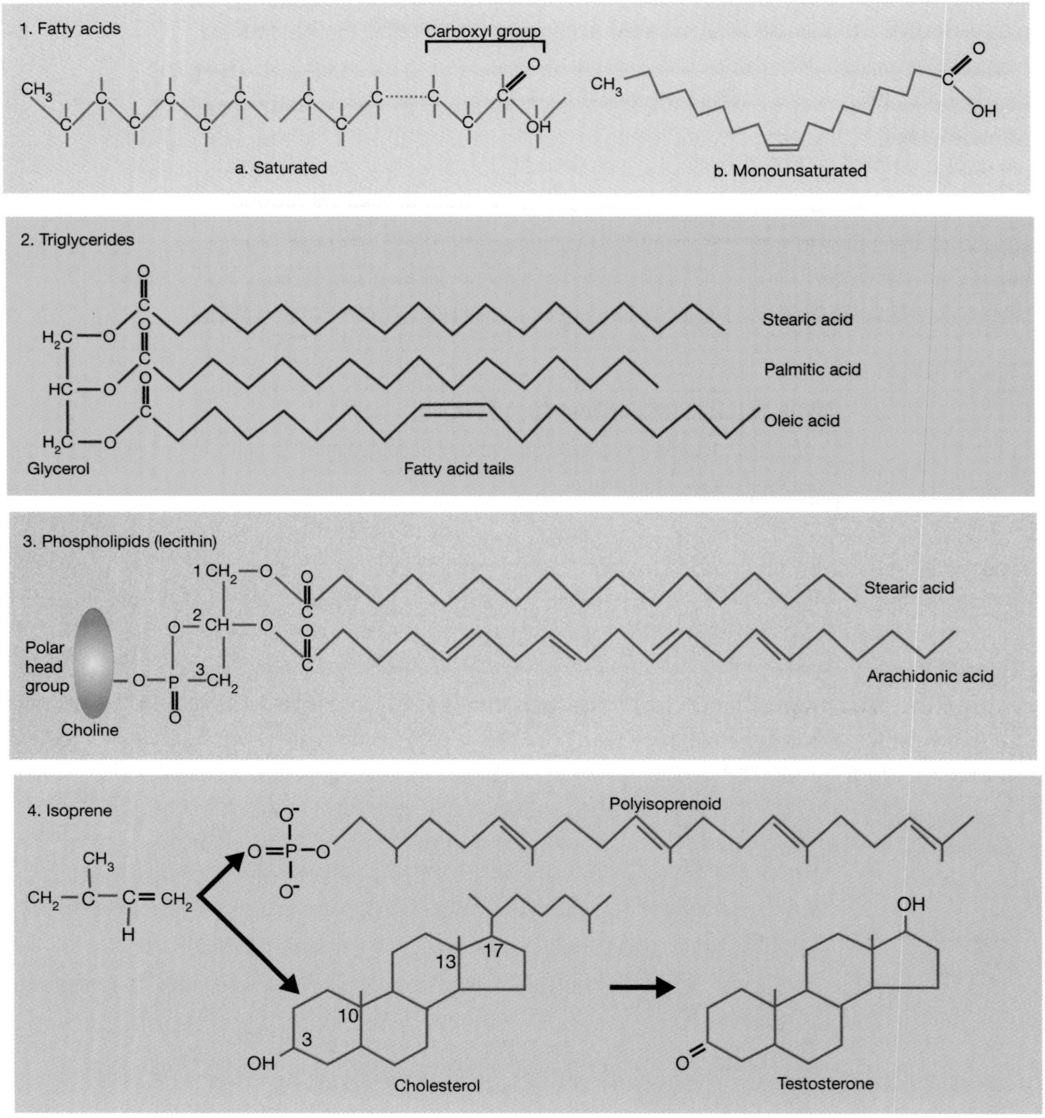

Figure 2-4
Structures of physiologically important fats and lipids

Reprinted with permission from Mahan, L.K., Escott-Stump, S., & Raymond, J.L. (2011). *Krause's Food and the Nutrition Care Process* (13th ed.). Philadelphia: W.B. Saunders Company.

Fatty acids, which are usually found linked to other molecules in nature, are long hydrocarbon chains with an even number of carbons and varying degrees of saturation with hydrogen. In nature, most fatty acids are found as part of triglycerides, which are formed by joining three fatty acids to a glycerol (carbon and hydrogen structure) backbone. Triglycerides are the chemical form in which most fat exists in food as well as in the body.

Unsaturated fatty acids contain one or more double bonds between carbon atoms, are typically liquid at room temperature, and are fairly unstable, which makes them susceptible to oxidative damage and a shortened shelf life. Monounsaturated fats contain one double bond between two carbons and may increase levels of **high-density lipoprotein (HDL),** which is known as the "good cholesterol" for its association with lowering plaque build-up within the arteries. Common sources include olive, canola, and peanut oils. Polyunsaturated fat contains a double bond between two or more sets of carbons. Sources include corn, safflower, and soybean oils, and cold-water fish (e.g. tuna, salmon, mackerel, and cod).

Essential fatty acids are a type of polyunsaturated fat that must be obtained from the diet. Unlike other fats, the body cannot produce omega-3 fatty acid (**linolenic acid**) or **omega-6 fatty acid** (**linoleic acid**). Omega-3 fatty acids come in three forms: alpha-linolenic acid (ALA), eicosapentaenoic acid (EPA), and docosahexanoic acid (DHA). ALA is the type of omega-3 found in plants. It can be converted to EPA and DHA in the body. DHA and EPA omega-3 fatty acids are naturally found in egg yolk (amounts vary depending on the chicken feed); some plant and nut oils like avocado, flaxseed, and walnut; and in cold-water fish and shellfish (e.g., crab, shrimp, and oyster). Overall, omega-3s reduce blood clotting, dilate blood vessels, and reduce inflammation. They are important for eye and brain development (and are especially important for a growing fetus in the late stages of pregnancy); act to reduce cholesterol and triglyceride levels; and may help to preserve brain function and reduce the risk of mental illness and attention deficit hyperactivity disorder (ADHD), though more research is needed to confirm these mental health benefits. Though omega-3 supplementation may provide many benefits and decrease risk factors for disease, research suggests that omega-3 supplementation does not decrease risk of all-cause mortality, cardiac death, sudden death, myocardial infarction, and **stroke** (Rizos et al., 2012).

Notably, most Americans tend not to get recommended amounts of omega-3 fatty acids. Though natural food sources are best, people who do not meet recommendations may benefit from supplementation or from fortified foods. In fact, the American Heart Association (AHA) recommends that, under the care of a physician, individuals with elevated triglycerides take a 2 to 4 gram DHA+EPA supplement (Miller et al., 2011).

While there is no established **Dietary Reference Intake (DRI)** for the optimal amount of EPA+DHA intake for the general population, the IOM has established an **Adequate Intake (AI)** for ALA, the precursor to EPA+DHA. The IOM (2002) considers 1.1 g per day of ALA to be the minimal amount necessary for normal growth and neural development. The IOM suggests that 10% of the needed ALA could come from EPA or DHA, which suggests a daily intake of about 100 mg per day. For reference, salmon, one of the highest omega-3 foods, contains 1,200 mg per 4 oz serving. Some expert panels have recommended much higher intakes of 250 and 500 mg per day due to the significant health benefits attributed to these fatty acids, and the low risk of complications such as bleeding, even at this higher range (Harris, 2010). Of note, while many products claim to be fortified with omega-3s, it is important for consumers to read the label. If the omega-3s are mostly ALA, they are unlikely to be optimally converted to EPA and DHA and likely have fewer of the health benefits.

Omega-6, which is generally consumed in abundance, is an essential fatty acid found in flaxseed, canola, and soybean oils and green leaves. Unlike omega-3s, which reduce inflammation, omega-6 fatty acids have been shown to contribute to inflammation and blood clotting. The balancing act between omega-6 and omega-3 is essential for maintaining normal circulation and other biological processes. In the past, scientists had hypothesized that reducing consumption of omega-6 fatty acids and increasing consumption of omega-3 fatty acids may lower chronic disease risk, but more recent research has shown that maintaining a high consumption of both omega-3 and omega-6 fatty acids has cardiovascular health benefits (Harris, 2010) (Table 2-1). The AHA

Table 2-1

Omega-3 and Omega-6 Content of Selected Foods

Fish and Shellfish (all servings 4 oz)	Total Omega-3 (mg)	Total Omega-6 (mg)
Salmon: Atlantic, Chinook, Coho	1,200–2,400	500
Anchovies, Herring, and Shad	2,300–2,400	90
Mackerel: Atlantic and Pacific	1,350–2,100	340
Tuna: Bluefin and Albacore	1,700	110
Sardines: Atlantic and Pacific	1,100–1,600	170
Trout: Freshwater	1,000–1,100	410
Tuna: White (Albacore) Canned	1,000	120
Salmon: Pink and Sockeye	700–900	450
Mussels: Blue	900	100
Oysters: Pacific	1,550	80
Pollock: Atlantic	600	50
Squid	750	10
Crab: Blue, King, Snow, Queen, and Dungeness	200–550	50–65
Tuna: Skipjack and Yellowfin	150–350	45–60
Flounder, Plaice, and Sole (Flatfish)	350	80
Clams	200–300	50
Nuts and Seeds (all servings 1 oz)		
Flax seeds	6,300	1,700
Chia seeds	4,900	1,600
Walnuts	2,500	10,700
Pistachios	700	3,700
Pecans	280	5,800
Almonds	200	3,400
Cashews	200	2,200
Peanuts	0	4,400

Table 2-1 (continued)		
Omega-3 and Omega-6 Content of Selected Foods		
Oils (all servings 1 tablespoon)		
Flaxseed oil	7,980	2,240
Walnut oil	1,400	7,195
Canola oil	1,300	2,840
Soybean oil	925	6,935
Olive oil	80	1,070
Sunflower oil	25	505
Palm oil	25	1,240
Sesame oil	40	5,615
Coconut oil	0	245
DHA Fortified Foods and Supplements		
DHA egg (1 egg)	100–150	650
Orange Juice (8 oz)	30	25
Milk, whole (8 oz)	30	290
Yogurt (4 oz)	15–30	0
Fish oil supplement (1 softgel)	590	varies

Note: DHA = Docosahexanoic acid

Sources: USDA Nutrient Database (http://ndb.nal.usda.gov/); Essential Fatty Acids Education Website of the National Institutes of Health (http://efaeducation.nih.gov/sig/esstable.html and http://efaeducation.nih.gov/)

recommends that Americans consume 5 to 10% of calories as omega-6 polyunsaturated fatty acids—that is about 12 g/day for women and 17 g/day for men (Harris et al., 2009).

Saturated fatty acids contain no double bonds between carbon atoms, are typically solid at room temperature, and are very stable, which gives them a long shelf life. Saturated fat comes in primarily four forms in the food supply: lauric acid, myristic acid, palmitic acid, and stearic acid. Animal fats such as red meat and full-fat dairy products contain mostly palmitic and stearic acids, while tropical vegetable oils such as palm kernel and coconut oils contain largely lauric and myristic acids. The different types of saturated fat induce different effects on cholesterol. When compared to other saturated fats, stearic acid exerts a beneficial effect on cholesterol [decreases **low-density lipoprotein (LDL)** cholesterol and decreases the ratio of total to HDL cholesterol]. However, when compared to unsaturated fats, stearic acid increases LDL, decreases HDL, and increases the ratio of total to HDL cholesterol (Hunter, Zhang, & Kris-Etherton, 2010). Lauric acid and myristic acid cause a much greater increase in total cholesterol than palmitic acid. Though lauric acid causes a large increase in cholesterol, the increase comes mostly from increasing the "good" HDL cholesterol (Kris-Etherton et al., 2007).

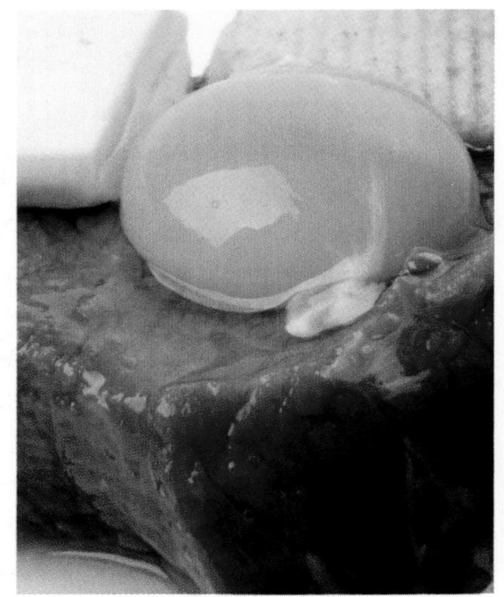

Because saturated fat increases levels of LDL cholesterol, which is referred to as the "bad" cholesterol due to its atherosclerotic properties, the AHA and the *Dietary Guidelines* have long advised consumers to limit saturated fat. However, a growing body of research seems to suggest that saturated fat in and of itself may not actually lead to increased risk of cardiovascular or cancer death.

Coconut Oil—The New "Health Food"?

Once maligned as a cholesterol-raising, artery-clogging, and waist-widening ingredient to be avoided, coconut oil has made a surprising comeback among health enthusiasts. While the science of nutrition has long been recognized as volatile and fluid (e.g., Are eggs healthy or not? Is soy good or bad? Should you use margarine or butter?), the rise of coconut oil from a demonized "bad" food to the purported "cure all" for a variety of health ailments is unexpected. The nutritional composition of coconut oil remains the same—namely about 90% saturated fat. So why the sudden change of heart?

The growing interest in coconut oil is due to at least two factors: (1) the scientific understanding of the effects of saturated fat (the main ingredient in coconut oil) on heart health has evolved and (2) a growing number of people who either avoid animal fats or are looking for a new flavor have discovered that coconut oil can transform a bland dish or baked product into a more tantalizing item, among its other purported benefits.

Evolving Science: Saturated Fat No Longer a Villain

The *2015-2020 Dietary Guidelines* and the AHA recommendations for optimal heart health both advise consumers to limit saturated fats, and to keep intake to less than 10% of total calories consumed. Physicians, nutritionists, and other health experts have long warned patients and clients of the risks of a diet that contains too much saturated fat—primarily, a sharp rise in LDL cholesterol.

Coconut oil is comprised mostly of the saturated fat lauric acid. Though lauric acid causes a large increase in cholesterol, the increase comes mostly from increasing the HDL cholesterol (Kris-Etherton et al., 2007). This differential elevation in "good" cholesterol (and thus a decrease in the total:HDL cholesterol ratio) is one reason that many health enthusiasts embrace coconut oil.

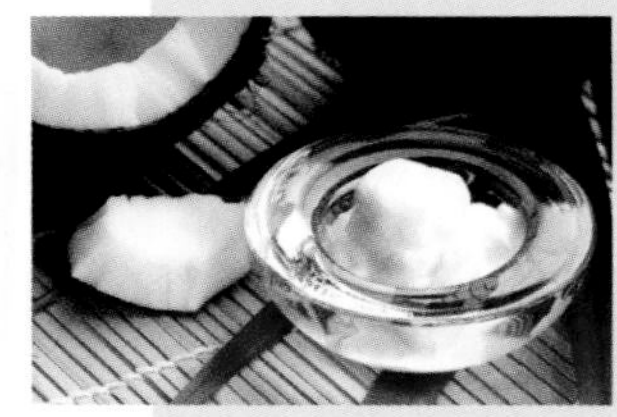

While coconut oil is mostly comprised of lauric acid, it does also contain other types of saturated fat that raise LDL cholesterol levels. However, a growing body of scientific evidence suggests that saturated fats may not be quite as bad as previously believed. A meta-analysis published in 2010 evaluated the findings of 21 studies that looked at the relationship between saturated fat intake and risk of coronary heart disease, stroke, and cardiovascular disease. The researchers found that even at the extremes of very low intake compared to very high intake of saturated fat, there was no difference in any of the studied health outcomes (Siri-Tarino et al., 2010). However, a pooled analysis of 11 studies found that when saturated fat is replaced with other types of fat (especially polyunsaturated fatty acids), cardiovascular disease risk decreases significantly (Jakobsen et al., 2009). These studies and others like them have provoked discussion and debate in the health and medical communities about the role of fat and health.

A description and summary of "The Great Fat Debate" was published as a series of short articles written by leading nutrition experts in the *Journal of the American Dietetic Association* (Zelman, 2011). Overall, the debate provided these key recommendations and take-away points:

- It is not the amount of fat intake, but rather the type of fat that is important for health. With that said, fat is more calorie-dense than carbohydrates and proteins and consumers should be careful to balance calories consumed with calories expended.
- The evidence against saturated fat is "not as strong as the dietary guidelines may have interpreted," but polyunsaturated (especially) and monounsaturated fats are clearly healthy.
- Saturated fats should not be viewed as "good for you," but a healthy, balanced diet can include saturated fats.
- Replacing saturated fat with polyunsaturated fat (like omega-3 and omega-6 fatty acids) is beneficial for overall health and cardiovascular disease risk reduction.
- **Trans fats** are unhealthy and should be avoided.
- Dietary fats are never purely one type of fat. Therefore, meal planning should focus on a balance of food types, rather than on specific nutrients.

What does all of this mean in the case for (or against) coconut oil? Virgin coconut oil may exert a modestly beneficial effect on blood lipids (through elevation of HDL cholesterol) and its regular consumption probably will not lead to harmful cardiovascular health outcomes. However, oils that are high in polyunsaturated acid (e.g., safflower, poppyseed, flaxseed, and grapeseed oils) and **monounsaturated fatty acid** (almond, avocado, and olive oils) probably provide greater health benefits than coconut oil. Note that partially hydrogenated coconut oil is detrimental to health due to its high **trans fatty acid** content.

Trans fat, listed as "partially hydrogenated" oil on a food ingredient list, results from a manufacturing process that makes unsaturated fat solid at room temperature with a goal of prolonging its shelf life. The process involves breaking the double bond of the unsaturated fat. The product is a heart-damaging fat that increases LDL cholesterol even more than saturated fat.

Legislation requiring food manufacturers to include the amount of trans fat on the nutrition label if it is more than 0.5 grams per serving has resulted in many processed foods that were once high in trans fat, such as chips, crackers, cakes, peanut butter, and margarine, to be made "trans-fat free." ACE Fitness Nutrition Specialists should advise their clients to look on the label's ingredients list for "partially hydrogenated" oil to determine if a food contains trans fat. If so, the food should be avoided.

Phospholipids such as lecithin and sphingomyelin are structurally similar to triglycerides, but the glycerol backbone is modified so that the molecule is water-soluble at one end and water-insoluble at the other end. Phospholipids play a critical role in maintaining cell-membrane structure and function. Lecithin is also a major component of HDL, which functions to remove cholesterol from cell membranes. Common food sources of lecithin include liver, egg yolks, soybeans, peanuts, legumes, spinach, wheat germ, and animal products.

Cholesterol, a fat-like, waxy, rigid four-ring steroid structure, plays an important role in cell-membrane function. It also helps to make bile acids (which are important for fat absorption), metabolize **fat-soluble vitamins** (A, D, E, and K), and make vitamin D and some steroid hormones, such as **estrogen** and **testosterone.** Saturated fat, once it is converted to cholesterol in the liver, is the main dietary cause of **hypercholesterolemia** (i.e., high blood levels of cholesterol), though high levels of cholesterol are also found in animal products such as egg yolks, meat, poultry, fish, and dairy products.

Too much cholesterol in the bloodstream causes problems. For cholesterol to get from the liver to the body's cells (in the case of endogenously produced cholesterol), or from the small intestine to the liver and adipose tissue (in the case of exogenously consumed cholesterol), it must be transported through the bloodstream. Because cholesterol is fat-soluble, it needs a water-soluble carrier protein to transport it. When the cholesterol combines with this protein en route to the body's cells, it becomes an LDL that when oxidized can attach to inner linings or walls of arteries, where it forms a plaque and may ultimately cause **atherosclerosis.** HDLs remove excess cholesterol from the arteries and carry it back to the liver, where it is excreted.

EXPAND YOUR KNOWLEDGE

Are Eggs Good or Bad?

Because of the always growing body of research, nutrition recommendations sometimes change. While this can be extremely frustrating for clients and the general public, it highlights the importance of health professionals, including ACE Fitness Nutrition Specialists, staying on top of the latest research and findings.

Historically, one of the most controversial foods has been the egg. Is it healthy or not? It used to be that eggs were well-known for their potential health harms given their high cholesterol content (there are 213 mg of cholesterol in one egg yolk. Then eggs were applauded for their high protein content and, more recently, for the notable amount of heart-healthy DHA omega-3 fatty acid in egg yolk (about 50 mg and eight times that in DHA-enriched eggs). At just about 15 cents each, eggs contain a load of nutrients at a very cheap price. But are they safe and healthy to eat?

A single egg has 70 calories, 6 grams of protein including all of the essential amino acids, 13 vitamins and minerals, and DHA omega-3 fatty acids. Few other foods could boast such a high nutritional density (Figure 2-5).

On the other hand, eggs also contain a high amount of cholesterol. However, dietary cholesterol is not very closely associated with elevated cholesterol levels in the body (that has more to do with saturated fat intake). In fact the *2015-2020 Dietary Guidelines for Americans* removed cholesterol as a nutrient to limit, while still noting that most foods high in cholesterol also tend to be high in saturated fat (with eggs as a notable exception). In addition to their cholesterol amounts, eggs also are a possible source of food-borne illness. Salmonella infection may be prevented most of the time with good food-handling techniques,

Nutrition Facts

1 Serving Per Container

Serving Size	**1 egg (50g)**
Amount Per Serving **Calories**	**70**
	% Daily Value*
Total Fat 3g	**7%**
Saturated Fat 1.5g	**8%**
Trans Fat 0g	
Cholesterol 215mg	**71%**
Sodium 65mg	**3%**
Total Carbohydrate Less than 1g	**0%**
Protein 6g	**10%**
Vitamin A	6%
Vitamin C	0%
Calcium	2%
Iron	4%

Not a significant source of Dietary Fiber or Sugars.

Figure 2-5
Egg nutrition label

including taking special care to fully cook eggs. That said, eggs pose a potential health risk, especially for the elderly and immune-suppressed people.

Ultimately, whether or not clients choose to include eggs in their daily diets will depend on taste preferences and their conclusions regarding the risks versus the benefits, but there is no doubt that eggs are an inexpensive source of a variety of nutrients.

DO THE MATH

Analyzing the Nutrition Label (see Figure 2-5)

1. If a client eats three eggs for breakfast, how many calories from saturated fat will he or she eat?
2. What percentage of total calories from an egg come from saturated fat?
3. How many calories from protein are contained in a single egg?

Answers:

1. 1.5 grams saturated fat x 9 calories per gram x 3 eggs = 40.5 calories
2. 1.5 grams saturated fat x 9 calories per gram = 13.5 calories from saturated fat per egg
   13.5 calories saturated fat/70 total calories per egg = 19% of calories from saturated fat
3. 6 grams of protein x 4 calories/gram of protein = 24 calories from protein

Metabolism and Storage

Fat consumed in the diet beyond what is immediately needed as an energy source is stored primarily as an energy reserve in adipose tissue, though it can also be used to replenish intramuscular triglyceride stores or remain in the bloodstream as free-floating fatty acids. Assuming 15% body fat, the average 176-pound (80-kg) young adult man stores about 26.4 lb (12 kg) of body fat. That translates to about 108,000 calories of fat (12,000 grams x 9 calories/gram). Most of this fat can be mobilized to provide energy to fuel exercise. Beyond serving as an energy source, fat also plays an essential role in thermal insulation, cushion for vital organs, nerve impulse conduction, and as a transport medium for fat-soluble vitamins.

ESSENTIALS OF DIGESTION AND ABSORPTION

In addition to the oxygen that enters the body through the lungs and is efficiently transported to the body's cells, the cells also need a constant supply of nutrients to provide energy and carry out basic metabolic functions. These nutrients can either come from storage (such as glycogen, stored fat, stored fat-soluble vitamins, or calcium stored in bones) or from breakdown of food through the **digestive system** (Figure 2-6). Some nutrients such as proteins and water-soluble vitamins are not effectively stored in the body and must be regularly obtained from foods to prevent deficiency.

The Digestive Pathway

The body has a remarkable ability to transform a food into its individual nutrients through the process of digestion. To understand this process, one can trace the digestive path of a half-cup serving of cottage cheese—a food that contains carbohydrate, protein, and fat as well as other micronutrients.

From the simple thought of eating to the sights and smell of food or drink, the body readies the digestive system. Through activation of the **parasympathetic nervous system,**

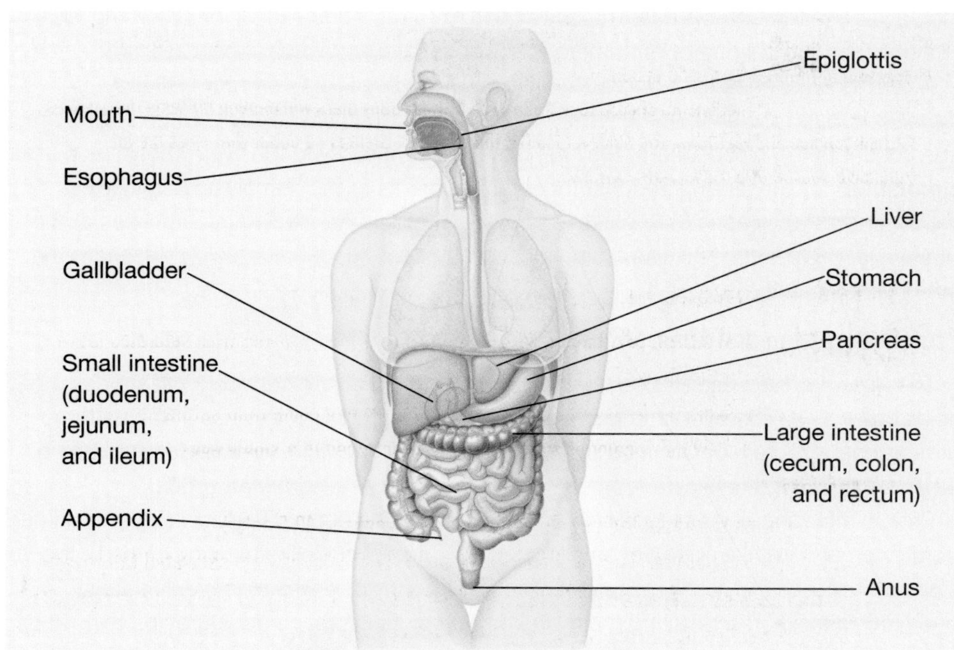

Figure 2-6
The digestive system

which is the part of the **autonomic nervous system** responsible for digestion, as soon as a liquid touches the tongue, salivary enzymes get ready to break it down to its individual nutrients. If the substance is a food instead of a drink, chewing the food also helps to activate the salivary enzymes. Digestion of the carbohydrate components of the cottage cheese begins in the saliva with release of the salivary enzyme *a*-amylase, which cleaves large polysaccharides into oligosaccharides and disaccharides. Chewing the cottage cheese breaks it down even more so that the salivary enzymes can come in contact with more of the surface area of the food.

With swallowing, the cottage cheese passes down the throat and into the **esophagus.** Muscles in the esophagus push the food through into the stomach in a wavelike motion called **peristalsis.** From here, each of the different macronutrient components of the cottage cheese is broken down differently.

Carbohydrate Digestion and Absorption

Partially digested carbohydrates (remember the salivary enzymes in the mouth begin the process of carbohydrate digestion) pass untouched through the stomach to the small intestine. The small intestine is the site of the majority of food digestion and absorption. With some help from pancreatic digestive juices and bile produced in the liver and stored in the **gallbladder,** the majority of food digestion occurs in the **duodenum,** the approximately 1-foot-long first portion of the small intestine. From there, the food, now called **chyme**, passes to the second and third portions of the small intestine, the **jejunum** and **ileum.** Together comprising about 20 feet of convoluted intestine, the jejunum and ileum are where the majority of food absorption occurs.

In the small intestine, **lactase** digests milk sugar, which is found in the cottage cheese, into its component parts—the monosaccharides glucose and galactose. (**Lactose intolerance** results from a deficiency in the enzyme lactase. This inability to break down lactose causes symptoms like cramps, bloating, diarrhea, and flatulence.) Other carbohydrates are broken down by various other pancreatic enzymes, including maltase, *a*-dextrinase, sucrose, and trehalase, into monosaccharides. The monosaccharides are then absorbed through the intestinal **brush border,** a membrane ideal for absorbing large amounts of nutrients due to its numerous tiny finger-like projections known as **villi.**

Nutrients cross the brush border in different ways depending on how well they dissolve in water (solubility), their size, and their relative concentration. Once sugars are absorbed into the bloodstream, they get fast-tracked directly to the liver (known as **portal circulation**) for processing and distribution of nutrients to the rest of the body. While the liver takes up much of the glucose from the bloodstream as well as almost all of the fructose and galactose, the remaining glucose is taken up by the body's cells under the influence of insulin.

Protein Digestion and Absorption

The goal of protein digestion is to break dietary protein down into individual amino acids that can be absorbed and later used by the body. Each protein has a unique three-dimensional structure determined by its amino-acid composition. In order for a protein to be digested, it must first lose its unique shape (a process called **denaturation**).

Protein digestion begins in the stomach. As soon as the body anticipates eating (whether from external cues like seeing or smelling food or internal cues like thinking of food), the stomach releases the hormone **gastrin.** The gastrin stimulates the stomach to release hydrochloric acid. The resulting rapid acidification of the stomach denatures proteins and triggers the activation of the enzyme **pepsin.** Pepsin breaks the peptide bonds between amino acids to shorten long protein complexes into shorter polypeptide chains. The stomach mixes and churns the food and releases the mixture in small quantities to the small intestine over the course of one to four hours. The pancreas then releases enzymes into the small intestine, which activate **trypsin,** an enzyme responsible for further breaking down proteins into single amino acids or amino acids joined in twos (dipeptides) or threes (tripeptides). The dipeptides and tripeptides are absorbed into the intestinal epithelial cells, cleaved into single amino acids, and passed to the bloodstream. Once absorbed into the bloodstream, the amino acids are transported to the liver.

For an amino acid to be of any use to the body, the liver first removes the amino acid nitrogen group through **deamination.** The nitrogen forms urea, which is then excreted in urine. Alternatively, in some cases the nitrogen can be transferred from one compound to another through **transamination.** In cases of an inadequate supply of carbohydrate or fat to fuel exercise, some deaminated amino acids derived from muscle proteins may be catabolized for energy, providing up to 10% of the total energy for exercise (Brooks, 1987).

Fat Digestion and Absorption

Lipid digestion begins in the mouth with the release of **lingual lipase,** which cleaves short- and medium-chain fatty acids. The **gastric lipase** released from the stomach further digests these fats. The mixing and churning of the **bolus** of food in the small intestine helps to break long-chain lipids into droplets to increase their surface area for digestion by pancreatic enzymes.

The presence of fat in the small intestine triggers the release of the hormone cholecystokinin (CCK). This hormone stimulates the release of **gastric inhibitory peptide** and **secretin,** which decrease gut movement and slow digestion. This explains why high-fat meals increase feelings of fullness compared with lower-fat meals. In the small intestine, bile acids emulsify the lipids, further increasing surface area so that pancreatic lipases can break the lipids into fatty acids, cholesterol, and lysolecithin. Products of lipid digestion and fat-soluble vitamins are carried by **micelles** to the absorptive surface of the intestinal cells, where they diffuse across the luminal membrane and are converted back into triglycerides, cholesterol, and phospholipids. While medium-chain triglycerides can pass directly into the portal circulation, the long-chain triglycerides join an apoprotein to form a **chylomicron.** These fats and fat-soluble vitamins are transferred into the **lymphatic system** and passed to the bloodstream through the thoracic duct, a large lymphatic vein that drains into the heart. The fatty acids contained within chylomicrons floating in the bloodstream can be delivered to working cells, where the enzyme **lipoprotein lipase** cleaves off the fatty acid. These fatty acids can be used in the metabolic process of fatty-acid oxidation to produce energy. Any fatty acids not immediately needed by the cells pass to the liver where they are repackaged and shuttled to the adipose tissue, where they are stored as fat.

Getting Rid of Waste

After the macronutrients and micronutrients have been digested and absorbed, all of the waste and indigestibles left over in the small intestine (such as fiber) are passed through the ileocecal valve to the 5-foot-long large intestine, where a few minerals and a significant amount of water are reabsorbed into blood. As more water gets reabsorbed, the waste passing through the colon portion of the large intestine gets harder until it is finally excreted as solid waste through the rectum and anus. Food can stay in the large intestine from hours to days. Total transit time from mouth to anus usually takes anywhere from 18 to 72 hours. Therefore, what is considered to be a "normal" frequency of bowel movements can range from three times daily to once every three days or more (Figure 2-7).

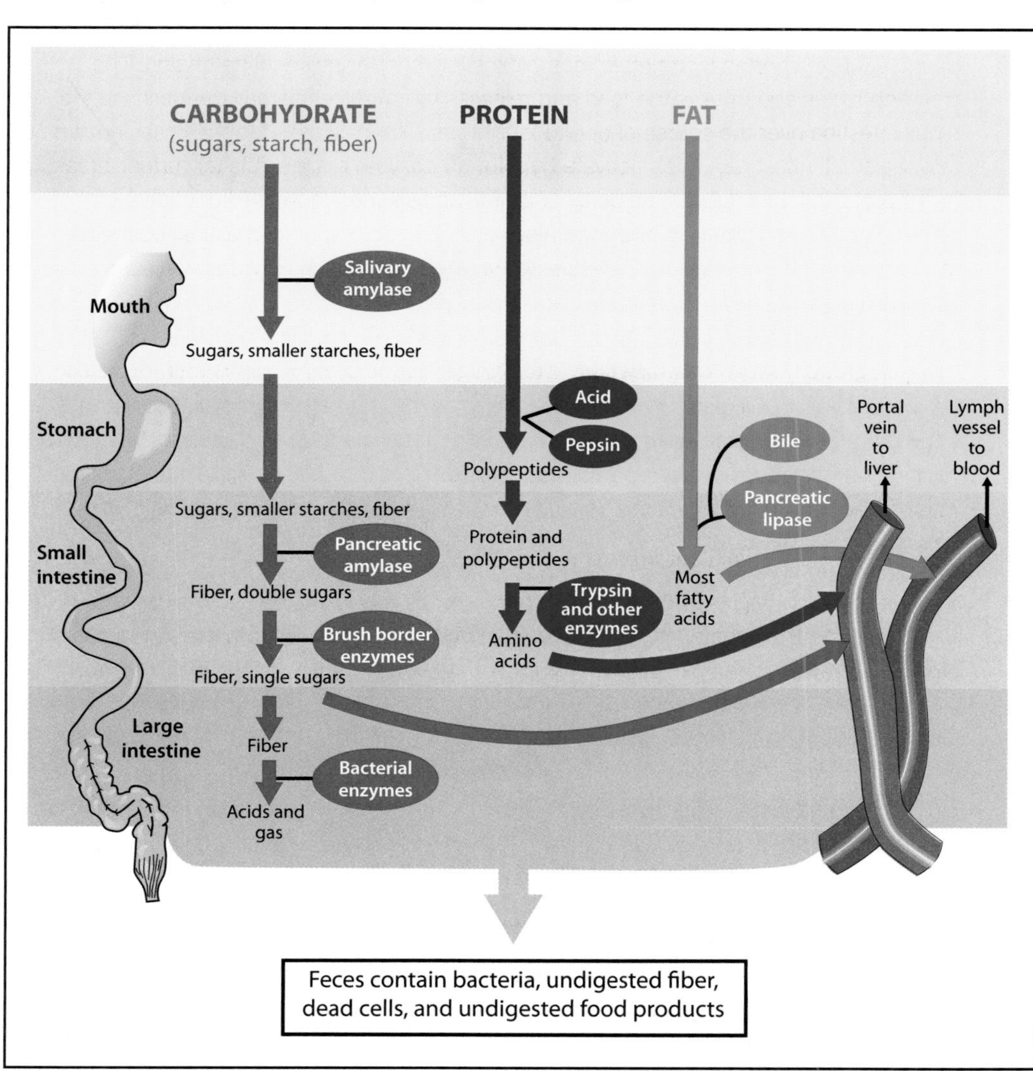

Figure 2-7
Summary of macronutrient digestion and absorption

Source: Adapted with permission from McArdle, W.D., Katch, F.I., & Katch, V.L. (2008). *Sports and Exercise Nutrition* (3rd ed.). Philadelphia: Lippincott Williams & Wilkins.

MICRONUTRIENTS

Micronutrients, by definition, are only needed in small amounts. The World Health Organization (WHO) refers to these nutrients as the "magic wands" that enable the body to produce enzymes, hormones, and other substances that are essential for proper growth and development" (WHO, 2010). When the body is deprived of micronutrients, the consequences are severe. But when the micronutrients are consumed in just the right amounts, they lead to optimal health and function.

Vitamins

Vitamins are organic (carbon-containing), non-caloric micronutrients that are essential for normal physiological function. Vitamins must be consumed through foods, with only three exceptions: vitamin K and biotin, which can be produced by normal intestinal flora (bacteria that live in the intestines and are critical for normal gastrointestinal function), and vitamin D, which can be self-produced with sun exposure. No "perfect" food contains all the vitamins in just the right amount. Instead, a variety of nutrient-dense foods must be consumed to ensure adequate vitamin intakes. Many foods (such as breads and cereals) are enriched or fortified with some nutrients to cut the risk of vitamin deficiency. And some foods contain inactive vitamins, which are called **provitamins.** The human body contains enzymes to convert these inactive vitamins into active vitamins.

Humans need 13 different vitamins, which are divided into two categories: water-

EXPAND YOUR KNOWLEDGE

What Are Nutrient-dense Foods?

Nutrient-dense foods and beverages provide vitamins, minerals, and other substances that may have positive health effects with relatively few calories. The term "nutrient-dense" indicates that the nutrients and other beneficial substances in a food have not been "diluted" by the addition of calories from added solid fats, added sugars, or added refined starches, or by the solid fats naturally present in the food. Nutrient-dense foods and beverages are lean or low in solid fats, and minimize or exclude added solid fats, sugars, starches, and sodium. Ideally, they also are in forms that retain naturally occurring components, such as dietary fiber. All vegetables, fruits, whole grains, seafood, eggs, beans and peas, unsalted nuts and seeds, fat-free and low-fat milk and milk products, and lean meats and poultry—when prepared without adding solid fats or sugars—are nutrient-dense foods. For most Americans, meeting nutrient needs within their calorie needs is an important goal for health. Eating recommended amounts from each food group in nutrient-dense forms is the best approach to achieving this goal and building a healthy eating pattern (USDA, 2010).

soluble vitamins (the B vitamins and vitamin C) and fat-soluble vitamins (vitamins A, D, E, and K). Choline—called a "quasi-vitamin" because it can be produced in the body, but also provides additional benefits through consumption of foods—plays a crucial role in **neurotransmitter** and platelet functions; may help prevent Alzheimer's disease (McDaniel, Maier, & Einstein, 2003) and fatty liver disease (Fischer et al., 2010); and is essential for normal fetal brain development (Zeisel & Niculescu, 2006). Table 2-2 includes the vitamin DRIs.

Water-soluble Vitamins

Thiamin, riboflavin, niacin, pantothenic acid, folate, vitamin B6, vitamin B12, biotin, and vitamin C are referred to as the water-soluble vitamins. Their solubility in water (which gives them similar absorption and distribution in the body) and their role as **cofactors** of enzymes involved in metabolism (i.e., without them, the enzyme will not work) are common

Table 2-2
Vitamin Facts

Vitamin	RDA/AI* Men†	RDA/AI* Women†	Best Sources	Functions
A (carotene)	**900 µg**	**700 µg**	Yellow or orange fruits and vegetables, green leafy vegetables, fortified oatmeal, liver, dairy products	Formation and maintenance of skin, hair, and mucous membranes; helps people see in dim light; bone and tooth growth
B1 (thiamin)	**1.2 mg**	**1.1 mg**	Fortified cereals and oatmeals, meats, rice and pasta, whole grains, liver	Helps the body release energy from carbohydrates during metabolism; growth and muscle tone
B2 (riboflavin)	**1.3 mg**	**1.1 mg**	Whole grains, green leafy vegetables, organ meats, milk, eggs	Helps the body release energy from protein, fat, and carbohydrates during metabolism
B6 (pyridoxine)	**1.3 mg**	**1.3 mg**	Fish, poultry, lean meats, bananas, prunes, dried beans, whole grains, avocados	Helps build body tissue and aids in metabolism of protein
B12 (cobalamin)	**2.4 µg**	**2.4 µg**	Meats, milk products, seafood	Aids cell development, functioning of the nervous system, and the metabolism of protein and fat
Biotin	30 µg	30 µg	Cereal/grain products, yeast, legumes, liver	Involved in metabolism of protein, fats, and carbohydrates
Choline	550 mg	425 mg	Milk, liver, eggs, peanuts	A precursor of acetylcholine; essential for liver function
Folate (folacin, folic acid)	**400 µg**	**400 µg‡**	Green leafy vegetables, organ meats, dried peas, beans, lentils	Aids in genetic material development; involved in red blood cell production
Niacin	**16 mg**	**14 mg**	Meat, poultry, fish, enriched cereals, peanuts, potatoes, dairy products, eggs	Involved in carbohydrate, protein, and fat metabolism
Pantothenic acid	5 mg	5 mg	Lean meats, whole grains, legumes, vegetables, fruits	Helps release energy from fats and vegetables
C (ascorbic acid)	**90 mg**	**75 mg**	Citrus fruits, berries, and vegetables—especially peppers	Essential for structure of bones, cartilage, muscle, and blood vessels; helps maintain capillaries and gums and aids in absorption of iron
D	15 µg	15 µg	Fortified milk, sunlight, fish, eggs, butter, fortified margarine	Aids in bone and tooth formation; helps maintain heart action and nervous system function
E	**15 mg**	**15 mg**	Fortified and multigrain cereals, nuts, wheat germ, vegetable oils, green leafy vegetables	Protects blood cells, body tissue, and essential fatty acids from destruction in the body
K	120 µg	90 µg	Green leafy vegetables, fruit, dairy, grain products	Essential for blood-clotting functions

* Recommended Dietary Allowances are presented in bold type; Adequate Intakes are presented in non-bolded type.

† RDAs and AIs given are for men aged 31–50 and nonpregnant, nonbreastfeeding women aged 31–50; mg = milligrams; µg = micrograms

‡ This is the amount women of childbearing age should obtain from supplements or fortified foods.

Reprinted with permission from *Dietary Reference Intakes* (various volumes). Copyright 1997, 1998, 2000, 2001 by the National Academy of Sciences. Courtesy of the National Academies Press, Washington, D.C.

traits. With the exception of vitamins B6 and B12, water-soluble vitamins cannot be stored in the body and are readily excreted in urine. This decreases the risk of toxicity from overconsumption and makes their regular intake a necessity.

Certain B vitamins—thiamin (vitamin B1), riboflavin (vitamin B2), niacin (vitamin B3), and pantothenic acid (vitamin B5)—are cofactors in energy metabolism. In other words, these vitamins are necessary to unlock the energy in food.

Thiamin

Thiamin is essential for carbohydrate metabolism. It also is thought to play a nonmetabolic role in nerve function. Signs of thiamin deficiency include decreased appetite, weight loss, and cardiac and neurologic irregularities that progress to beriberi—a constellation of symptoms that includes mental confusion, muscular wasting, swelling, decreased sensation in the feet and hands, a fast heart rate, and an enlarged heart. Thiamin deficiency is rare in the U.S. because of supplementation in rice and cereal products. Deficiency occasionally manifests in alcoholics, who are often malnourished and have impaired thiamin absorption. There have been no reports of adverse effects from too much thiamin.

Riboflavin

Riboflavin assists in carbohydrate, amino-acid, and lipid metabolism. It also helps with **antioxidant** protection through its role in reduction-oxidation (redox) reactions. Consumption of meat, dairy products, and green leafy vegetables helps prevent riboflavin deficiency, which causes eye problems, including sensitivity to light; excessive tearing, burning, and itching; and loss of vision, as well as soreness and burning of the mouth, tongue, and lips. No adverse effects have been reported from very high intakes of riboflavin.

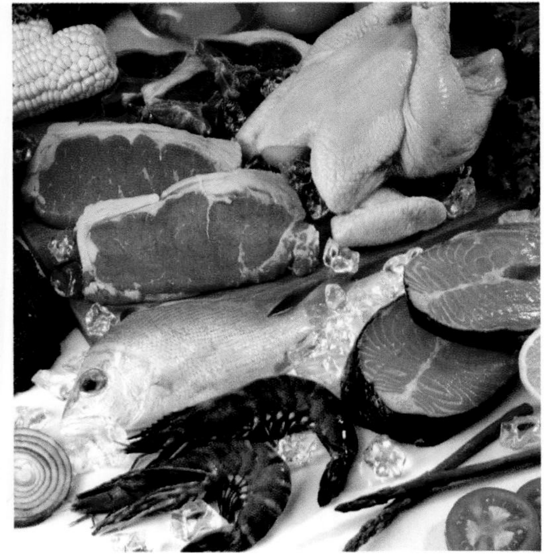

Niacin

Niacin acts as a cofactor for more than 200 enzymes involved in carbohydrate, amino-acid, and fatty-acid metabolism. Lean meats, poultry, fish, peanuts, and yeast contain ample amounts of niacin. Muscular weakness, anorexia, indigestion, and skin abnormalities are early signs of niacin deficiency and can cause the disease pellagra, which is characterized by the "three Ds": dermatitis (eczema), dementia, and diarrhea. Niacin intake above the tolerable upper intake level of 35 mg per day (or even less in certain individuals with chronic diseases such as liver dysfunction, diabetes, and cardiac disease) can cause flushing, nausea, vomiting, and, in extremely high doses, signs and symptoms of liver toxicity.

Pantothenic Acid

Panthothenic acid, which is present in all plant and animal tissues, forms an integral component of coenzyme A and acyl-carrier protein. These proteins are essential for metabolism of fatty acids, amino acids, and carbohydrates, as well as for normal protein function. Because this vitamin is ubiquitous, deficiency is rare. Massive doses of pantothenic acid may cause mild intestinal distress and diarrhea.

Vitamin B6

Vitamin B6 (pyridoxine) plays an important role in many bodily functions, including protein metabolism, red blood cell production, **glycogenolysis** (in which glycogen is broken down to glucose), conversion of the protein tryptophan to niacin, neurotransmitter formation, and immune-system function. Meats, whole-grain products, vegetables, and nuts contain high concentrations of vitamin B6, though bioavailability of the nutrient is highest in animal products. Deficiency leads to decreased neurologic and dermatologic function and weakened immunity. Excessive B6 intake can lead to sensory neuropathy and dermatological lesions.

Folate

Folate (vitamin B9; also known as **folic acid** in its supplement form) is named for its abundance in plant foliage (like green leafy vegetables). Folate plays a crucial role in the production of **deoxyribonucleic acid (DNA),** formation of red and white blood cells, formation of neurotransmitters, and metabolism of amino acids. Deficiency is relatively common, as folate is easily lost during cooking and food preparation, and also because most people do not eat enough green leafy vegetables. Folate deficiency early in pregnancy can be devastating for a developing fetus and can lead to neural tube defects such as spina bifida. For this reason, all women of childbearing age are advised to take a daily folate supplement. Deficiency also causes megaloblastic anemia, skins lesions, and poor growth. Notably, excessive consumption of folate can mask a vitamin B12 deficiency and impair zinc absorption.

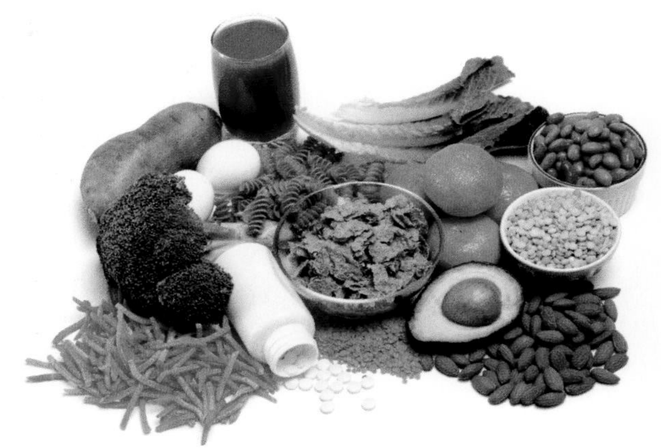

Vitamin B12

Vitamin B12 (cobalamin) is important for the normal function of cells of the gastrointestinal tract, bone marrow, and nervous tissue. The richest sources of vitamin B12 include clams and oysters, milk, eggs, cheese, muscle meats, fish, liver, and kidney. Long-time **vegans** are at risk for deficiency, as are the elderly, who tend to have a decreased ability to absorb the nutrient. Deficiency leads to megaloblastic anemia and neurologic dysfunction, in which neurons become demyelinated. This causes numbness, tingling, and burning of the feet, as well as stiffness and generalized weakness of the legs. Vitamin B12 poses very little risk of toxicity, even when consumed in large doses.

Biotin

Biotin (vitamin B7) is the ultimate "helper vitamin." Typically bound to protein, it carries around a carboxyl (-COOH) group, which it lends to any of four different enzymes that are important in various metabolic functions. Ultimately, biotin plays an important role in the metabolic functions of pantothenic acid, folic acid, and vitamin B12. The most important sources of biotin include milk, liver, egg yolk, and a few vegetables. Both deficiency and toxicity are uncommon.

Vitamin C

Vitamin C plays an important role as an antioxidant. Deficiency can result in scurvy (a deficiency disease that can cause dark purplish spots on the skin and spongy or bleeding gums). Vitamin C is also necessary to make collagen, a fibrous protein that is part of skin, bone, teeth, ligaments, and other connective structures. Vitamin C improves iron absorption, promotes resistance to infection, and helps with steroid, neurotransmitter, and hormone production. Citrus fruits and green leafy vegetables are excellent sources of vitamin C. Signs of deficiency include impaired wound healing, swelling, bleeding, and weakness in bones, cartilage, teeth, and connective tissues. Vitamin C intakes above the tolerable upper intake level of 2,000 mg per day may cause gastrointestinal distress and diarrhea.

Fat-soluble Vitamins

Vitamins A, D, E, and K are the fat-soluble vitamins and are often found in fat-containing foods. They are stored in the liver or adipose tissue until needed, and therefore are closely associated with fat. If fat absorption is impaired, so is fat-soluble-vitamin absorption. Unlike water-soluble vitamins, fat-soluble vitamins can be stored in the body for extended periods of time and eventually are excreted in feces. This storage capacity increases the risk of toxicity from overconsumption, but also decreases the risk of deficiency.

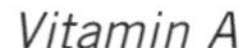

Vitamin A

Vitamin A and its provitamin beta-carotene are important for vision, growth, and development; the development and maintenance of epithelial tissue, including bones and teeth; immune function; and reproduction. Animal products, including liver, milk, and eggs, are rich in preformed vitamin A. Dark green leafy vegetables and yellow-orange vegetables and fruit contain lots of provitamin A carotenoids. (A good rule of thumb: The deeper the color, the higher the level of carotenoids.) Deficiency of vitamin A is the most common cause of blindness in the developing world. It begins with night blindness and progresses to poor growth and increased susceptibility to infection. Excess consumption, which overwhelms the capacity of the liver to store the vitamin (generally resulting from supplement misuse), leads to dryness and cracking of the skin and mucous membranes, headache, nausea and vomiting, and liver disease. Intake of more than 20,000 IU of vitamin A in pregnant women is associated with fetal malformations; pregnant women are advised to limit intake to less than 10,000 IU per day.

Vitamin D

Vitamin D is essential for calcium and phosphorus absorption and homeostasis. Vitamin D is referred to as the "sunshine vitamin," because small amounts of sunlight exposure (about 10 to 15 minutes twice a week) induce the body to make sufficient vitamin D from cholesterol. Fish liver oils provide an abundance of vitamin D. Smaller amounts are found in butter cream, egg yolk, and liver. Typically, Americans get the majority of their vitamin D intake from fortified milk. Regardless of the source, adequate vitamin D intake is critical. Without it, adults can develop **osteomalacia,** a condition in which the bones become weak and susceptible to pseudofractures, leading to muscular weakness and bone tenderness. This increases the risk of fracture, in particular of the wrist and pelvis. Low vitamin D intake may also play a role in the development of **osteoporosis** in postmenopausal women. Without vitamin D, children whose bones have not yet fully developed will experience impaired mineralization, which can lead to rickets and bowing of the legs. Too much vitamin D causes elevated calcium and phosphorus levels and may lead to headache, nausea, and eventually calcification of the kidney, heart, lungs, and the tympanic membrane of the ear, leading to deafness.

Vitamin D has been the subject of a high level of interest due to some research evidence suggesting that it may be a highly health-promoting vitamin and that the majority of people do not get enough of this vitamin. In response to this growing interest, the IOM completed a thorough evaluation of the evidence to date and released a report that concluded that the currently available data does not provide compelling evidence that vitamin D provides benefits beyond bone health, or that intakes higher than the DRIs provide any additional benefit (Slomski, 2011).

Vitamin E

Vitamin E, which is also known as alpha-tocopherol, plays a fundamental role in the metabolism of all cells. It may help protect against conditions related to oxidative stress, including aging, air pollution, arthritis, cancer, cardiovascular disease, cataracts, diabetes, and infection, though research remains contradictory and inconclusive. Vitamin

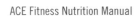

E is only synthesized by plants. The richest sources of vitamin E are polyunsaturated plant oils, wheat germ, whole grains, green leafy vegetables, nuts, and seeds. Vitamin E is easily destroyed by heat and oxygen. Therefore, its richest source, oils, should be stored in a cool, dark location. Vitamin E deficiency is rare in humans and tends to only occur in cases of fat malabsorption and transport problems. Toxicity is uncommon, though when present may decrease the absorption of other fat-soluble vitamins, impair bone mineralization, and lead to prolonged clotting times. This is especially relevant for individuals on anticlotting medication, such as coumadin.

Vitamin K

Vitamin K, which is produced by bacteria in the colon and present in large amounts in green, leafy vegetables (especially broccoli, cabbage, turnip greens, and dark lettuce), is important for blood clotting and maintenance of strong bones. Due to vitamin K's critical role in blood clotting, individuals on blood-thinning medications that interfere with vitamin K absorption need to carefully titrate (i.e., continually monitor and adjust the balance of) their vitamin K intake through diet under the supervision of a physician. Insufficient vitamin K intake can lead to hemorrhage, and potentially fatal anemia. Fortunately, vitamin K deficiency is rare, and usually only found in association with lipid malabsorption, destruction of intestinal flora (often due to chronic antibiotic therapy), and liver disease. Newborns are at risk for vitamin K deficiency, as the vitamin does not cross the **placenta** and is negligible in breast milk. For this reason, newborn infants routinely receive a vitamin K shot after birth to prevent (or slow) a rare problem of bleeding into the brain weeks after birth. Vitamin K also promotes blood clotting. Toxicity of vitamin K only occurs with excessive intake of the synthetic form, which is called menadione. At doses of about 1,000 times the **Recommended Dietary Allowance (RDA),** vitamin K can cause severe jaundice in infants and hemolytic anemia (i.e., the abnormal breakdown of red blood cells).

Minerals

With roles ranging from regulating enzyme activity and maintaining acid–base balance to assisting with strength and growth, minerals are critical for human life. Unlike vitamins, many minerals are found in the body as well as in food. The body's ability to use the minerals is dependent upon their bioavailability, or the degree to which the mineral can be absorbed by the body. Nearly all minerals, with the exception of iron, are absorbed in their free form—that is, in their ionic state unbound to organic molecules and complexes. When bound to a complex, the mineral is not bioavailable, and will be excreted in feces. Typically, minerals with high bioavailability (>40% absorption) include sodium, potassium, chloride, iodide, and fluoride. Minerals with low bioavailability (1 to 10% absorption) include iron, zinc, chromium, and manganese (bioavailability is 20 to 30% for heme iron). All other minerals, including calcium and magnesium, are of medium bioavailability (30 to 40% absorption).

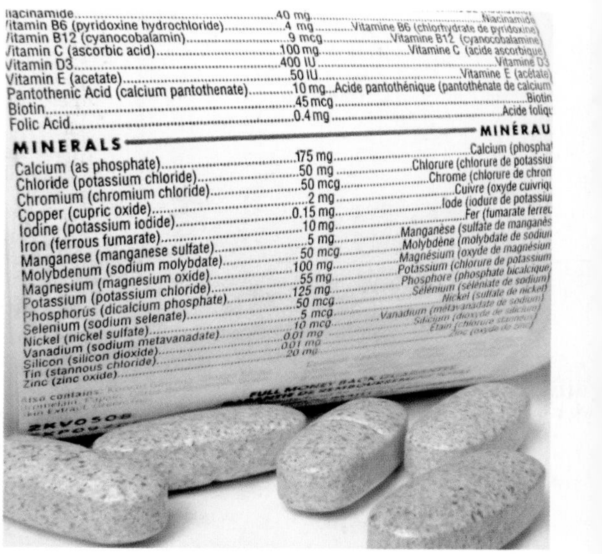

An important consideration when consuming minerals, and particularly when taking mineral supplements, is the possibility of mineral–mineral interactions. Minerals can interfere with the absorption of other minerals. For example, zinc absorption may be decreased through iron supplementation. Similarly, zinc excesses can decrease copper absorption. Too much calcium limits the absorption of manganese, zinc, and iron. When a mineral is not absorbed properly, a deficiency may develop.

Minerals are typically categorized as macrominerals (major elements) and microminerals (trace elements). Macrominerals include calcium, phosphorus, magnesium, sulfur, sodium, chloride, and potassium. Microminerals include iron, iodine, selenium, zinc, and various other minerals that do not have an established DRI, and will not be discussed in this chapter. Table 2-3 presents the DRIs for many minerals.

Table 2-3
Mineral Facts

Mineral	RDA/AI*		Best Sources	Functions
	Men†	Women†		
Calcium	1,000 mg	1,000 mg	Milk and milk products	Strong bones, teeth, muscle tissue; regulates heart beat, muscle action, and nerve function; blood clotting
Chromium	35 μg	25 μg	Corn oil, clams, whole-grain cereals, brewer's yeast	Glucose metabolism (energy); increases effectiveness of insulin
Copper	**900 μg**	**900 μg**	Oysters, nuts, organ meats, legumes	Formation of red blood cells; bone growth and health; works with vitamin C to form elastin
Fluoride	4 mg	3 mg	Fluorinated water, teas, marine fish	Stimulates bone formation; inhibits or even reverses dental caries
Iodine	**150 μg**	**150 μg**	Seafood, iodized salt	Component of hormone thyroxine, which controls metabolism
Iron	**8 mg**	**18 mg**	Meats, especially organ meats, legumes	Hemoglobin formation; improves blood quality; increases resistance to stress and disease
Magnesium	**420 mg**	**320 mg**	Nuts, green vegetables, whole grains	Acid/base balance; important in metabolism of carbohydrates, minerals, and sugar (glucose)
Manganese	2.3 mg	1.8 mg	Nuts, whole grains, vegetables, fruits	Enzyme activation; carbohydrate and fat production; sex hormone production; skeletal development
Molybdenum	**45 μg**	**45 μg**	Legumes, grain products, nuts	Functions as a cofactor for a limited number of enzymes in humans
Phosphorus	**700 mg**	**700 mg**	Fish, meat, poultry, eggs, grains	Bone development; important in protein, fat, and carbohydrate utilization
Potassium	4,700 mg	4,700 mg	Lean meat, vegetables, fruits	Fluid balance; controls activity of heart muscle, nervous system, and kidneys
Selenium	**55 μg**	**55 μg**	Seafood, organ meats, lean meats, grains	Protects body tissues against oxidative damage from radiation, pollution, and normal metabolic processing
Zinc	**11 mg**	**8 mg**	Lean meats, liver, eggs, seafood, whole grains	Involved in digestion and metabolism; important in development of reproductive system; aids in healing

* Recommended Dietary Allowances are presented in bold type; Adequate Intakes are presented in non-bolded type.

† RDAs and AIs given are for men aged 31–50 and nonpregnant, nonbreastfeeding women aged 31–50; mg = milligrams; μg = micrograms

Macrominerals (Bulk Elements)

By definition, macrominerals are essential for adults in amounts of 100 mg/day or more.

Calcium

Calcium is the most abundant mineral in the human body and serves various functions, including mineralization of the bones and teeth, muscle contraction, blood clotting, blood-pressure control, immunity, and possibly colon-cancer prevention (Mahan, Escott-Stump, & Raymond, 2011). Significant sources of calcium include milk products, small fish with bones, green leafy vegetables, and legumes. Most people in the U.S. do not consume the recommended amounts of calcium from food sources. To help counter this problem, calcium supplements are often used to increase intake. Calcium deficiency in childhood and adolescence can contribute to decreased peak bone mass and suboptimal bone strength. Calcium deficiency in adulthood, particularly in postmenopausal women, can lead to osteomalacia, **osteopenia,** and/or osteoporosis. Calcium toxicity, particularly when combined with vitamin D toxicity, can lead to hypercalcemia and calcification of soft tissues, particularly of the kidneys. High calcium intake also interferes with the absorption of other minerals, including iron, zinc, and manganese. Relatively common effects of excessive calcium intake include constipation and kidney stones.

Phosphorus

Phosphorus is the second most abundant mineral in the body (Mahan, Escott-Stump, & Raymond, 2011). Like calcium, phosphorus plays a role in mineralization of bones and teeth. Phosphorous also helps filter out waste in the kidneys and contributes to energy production in the body by participating in the breakdown of carbohydrates, protein, and fats. It also may help reduce muscle pain after a strenuous workout. Phosphorus is needed for the growth, maintenance, and repair of all tissues and cells, and for the production of the genetic building blocks, DNA and **ribonucleic acid (RNA).** Phosphorus is also needed to balance and metabolize other vitamins and minerals, including vitamin D, calcium, iodine, magnesium, and zinc. Animal products such as meat, fish, poultry, eggs, and milk are excellent sources of phosphorus. As a general rule, any food high in protein is also high in phosphorus. The outer coating of many grains contains phosphorus, but in the form of phytic acid, a bound form of phosphorus that is not bioavailable. The leavening process unbinds the phosphorus, making leavened breads a good source of the mineral. Phosphorus is also present in sodas. Deficiency of phosphorus is practically unheard of in the United States. In fact, most individuals consume much more than the DRI. People taking phosphate-binding medications may be at risk of deficiency, which can present with neuromuscular, skeletal, hematologic (blood), and renal abnormalities and may be deadly. Too much phosphorus intake interferes with calcium absorption and may lead to decreased bone mass and density.

Magnesium

Magnesium, which is present primarily in bone, muscle, soft tissue, and body fluids, is important for bone mineralization, protein production, muscle contraction, nerve conduction, enzyme function, and healthy teeth. Excellent food sources include nuts, legumes, whole grains, dark green leafy vegetables, and milk. In general, a diet high in vegetables and unrefined grains will include more than adequate amounts of magnesium. Unfortunately, most Americans eat a diet high in refined foods and meat and do not meet recommended magnesium intakes. High intakes of calcium, protein, vitamin D, and alcohol increase the body's magnesium requirements. Magnesium deficiency is very rare, but moderate depletion is fairly common, especially in the elderly. Magnesium depletion may contribute to many chronic illnesses and is associated with heart **arrhythmias** and **myocardial infarction.** Magnesium toxicity may prevent bone calcification, but toxicity is also very rare, even in cases of supplement overuse.

Sodium, Potassium, and Chloride

Known as **electrolytes**, these minerals exist as ions in the body and are extremely important for normal cellular function. All three electrolytes play at least four essential roles in the body: water balance and distribution, osmotic equilibrium [i.e., assuring that the negative ions (**anions**) balance with positive ions (**cations**) when electrolytes move in and out of cells], acid–base balance, and intracellular/extracellular differentials (i.e., assuring that the sodium and chloride stay mostly outside of the cell while potassium stays mostly inside the cell).

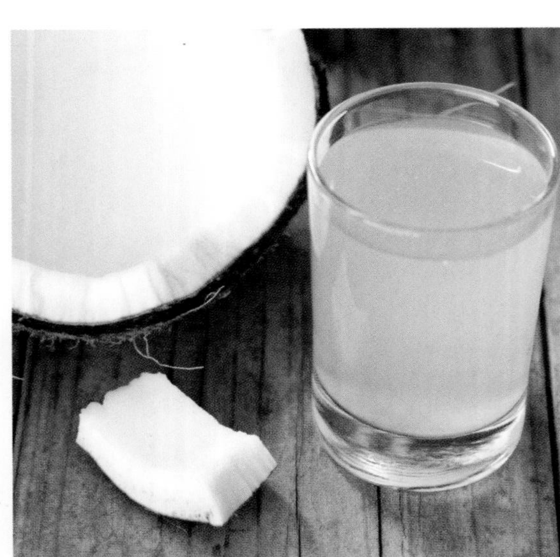

When electrolytes are out of balance, such as in a state of **dehydration** (leading to a high concentration of electrolytes) or **hyponatremia** (leading to a low concentration of electrolytes, namely sodium, resulting from overhydration), serious consequences may occur. Symptoms of dehydration include nausea, vomiting, dizziness, disorientation, weakness, irritability, headache, cramps, chills, and decreased performance. Symptoms of hyponatremia include nausea, vomiting, extreme fatigue, respiratory distress, dizziness, confusion, disorientation, coma, and seizures. In severe cases, both conditions can result in death. Electrolytes are excreted in urine, feces, and sweat. For more information on fluid and electrolyte balance related to exercise, see Chapter 4.

Generally, electrolyte deficiencies do not occur. In fact, sodium excess (and consequently, **hypertension**) is increasingly common given the typical American diet of highly processed and salty foods. *Note:* Hypertension related to sodium sensitivity has been more strongly linked to black and elderly populations (Champagne, 2006; Campese, 1994). Sodium excess may also contribute to osteoporosis, as high sodium increases calcium excretion. Potassium tends to be underconsumed, because most people do not consume enough fruits and vegetables. Insufficient potassium intake is linked to hypertension and osteoporosis.

Sulfur

Sulfur is an important component of many important bodily compounds, including two amino acids (cystine and methionine); three vitamins (thiamin, biotin, and pantothenic acid); and heparin, an anticoagulant found in the liver and other tissues. Meat, poultry, fish, eggs, dried beans, broccoli, and cauliflower are good food sources of the mineral. Sulfur deficiency is relatively uncommon and does not appear to cause any symptoms. Excess sulfur intake may lead to decreased bone mineralization, though sulfur toxicity is very rare.

Microminerals (Trace Elements)

Trace elements are found in minute amounts (less than 1 teaspoon) in the body. Despite the need for minimal doses of these minerals, they are critical for optimal growth, health, and development. RDAs have been established for only four trace elements: iron, iodine, selenium, and zinc.

Iron

Iron plays a very important role in normal human function. It is essential for the production of hemoglobin, the protein that carries inhaled oxygen from the lungs to the tissues, and myoglobin, the protein responsible for making oxygen available for muscle contraction. It also regulates cell growth and differentiation. Iron can be stored in the body for future use as the protein complex ferritin. Liver, oysters, seafood, kidney, heart, lean meat, poultry, and fish are excellent food sources, though many people use iron supplements to meet recommended intake amounts. Regardless of the source of iron intake, it is important to meet recommended intakes, as iron deficiency leads to fatigue, poor work performance, and decreased immunity. It is equally important to not exceed recommended intakes, as excess amounts can lead to accumulation of iron in the liver, causing toxicity, and sometimes even death.

Iodine

Iodine, a mineral stored in the thyroid gland and essential for normal growth and metabolism, is found naturally in seafood, though the most common source of iodine in the U.S. is iodized salt. Thanks to this fortification, iodine deficiency is rare in developed countries. However, in some developing countries, deficiency can cause goiter (enlargement of the thyroid gland) and impaired cognitive functioning in children of mothers who were iodine-deficient during pregnancy. Excessive iodine intake also causes goiter and, potentially, thyroid disease.

Selenium

Selenium, an important antioxidant found mostly in plant foods grown in selenium-rich soil, is needed only in small amounts for optimal function. A lack of this mineral may lead to heart disease, hypothyroidism, and a weakened immune system. Too much selenium can lead to a condition called selonosis, which is manifested as gastrointestinal distress, hair loss, white blotchy nails, garlic breath odor, fatigue, irritability, and nerve damage.

Zinc

Zinc is found in almost every cell and is the second most abundant trace element after iron. It stimulates the activity of enzymes, supports a healthy immune system, assists with wound healing, strengthens the senses (especially taste and smell), supports normal growth and development, and helps with DNA synthesis. Foods rich in zinc include meat, fish, poultry, milk products, and seafood such as oysters and other shellfish. Zinc deficiency causes delayed wound healing and immune-system dysfunction. Toxicity is rare in otherwise healthy individuals, although too much zinc as a result of overzealous supplementation can decrease healthy HDL cholesterol, interfere with copper absorption, and alter iron function [National Institutes of Health (NIH), 2011].

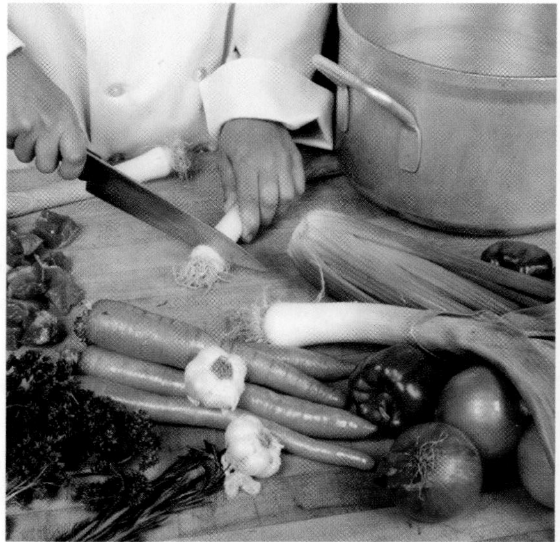

Antioxidants and Phytochemicals

Many of the vitamins and minerals already discussed, including vitamin C, beta-carotene, vitamin E, and selenium, function as antioxidants. Just as metal rusts over time when exposed to water and oxygen, cells are damaged from chronic oxygen exposure. This damage-causing process is called oxidation, and can set in motion various chemical reactions that at best cause aging and at worst cause cancer. Antioxidants function to prevent or repair oxidative damage. In the past, antioxidants were considered potent disease fighters. Subsequent research suggests that the agents not only fail to protect against disease, but also that, in excess, some of them may act to increase the risk of cancer, heart disease, and mortality in some individuals (Bjelakovic et al., 2007; Halliwell, 2007). Their true role in disease pathology has yet to be determined. What remains undisputed is that a diet high in fruits and vegetables is associated with a lower risk of developing chronic disease, such as heart disease, cancer, and possibly Alzheimer's disease. Their beneficial effects could be due to antioxidants, fiber, agents that stimulate the immune system, monounsaturated fatty acids, B vitamins, folic acid, or various other potential **phytochemicals**—substances in plants that are not necessarily required for normal functioning, but improve health and reduce the risk of disease. Therefore, it is important to emphasize a variety of plant foods in the diet and not rely on supplements. These plant-derived antioxidants and phytochemicals may work synergistically when consumed from whole plants and cannot be duplicated in a supplement.

Vitamin and Mineral Digestion, Absorption, and Metabolism

While vitamin and mineral absorption varies by nutrient, the majority of vitamin and mineral digestion and absorption occur in the small intestine.

Vitamin Digestion and Absorption

By the time they pass to the small intestine, most of the vitamins have been separated from the other food components. The vitamins pass unchanged primarily from the middle and lower portions of the small intestine (the jejunum and ileum) into the blood by passive diffusion. For the most part, water-soluble vitamins are absorbed in the jejunal portion of the small intestine and the fat-soluble vitamins in the ileal portion of the small intestine. However, vitamin K, vitamin B12, thiamin, and riboflavin can also be produced by bacteria in the large intestine, from which they are absorbed into the bloodstream.

Mineral Digestion and Absorption

Mineral digestion and absorption is considerably more complex than vitamin and water digestion and absorption. In the stomach, the digestive enzymes and stomach acids already have separated minerals from the other food components. The cations, or positively charged minerals (such as calcium, iron, zinc, and magnesium), dissolve into the acidic stomach chyme. As the dissolved minerals pass into the less acidic solution in the small intestine, the minerals form insoluble compounds with hydroxide molecules and protein carriers. These compounds are known as **chelation compounds.** For the most part, this phase of mineral digestion, referred to as the **intraluminal stage,** occurs in the uppermost portion of the small intestine, the duodenum. The small anions, or negatively charged minerals, are unaffected by pH and are easily digested and absorbed.

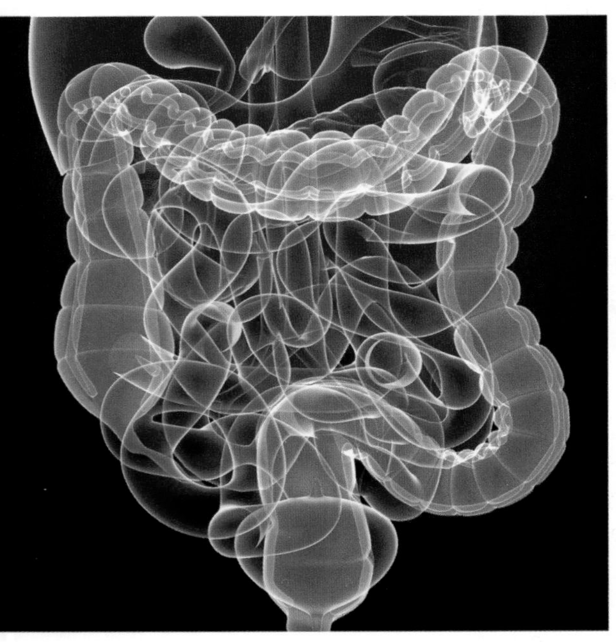

The negatively charged minerals pass across the border of the small intestine for absorption through **simple diffusion.** The positively charged minerals, formed into the chelation compounds, cross the small intestinal border through **facilitated diffusion** from high concentration to low concentration with a protein carrier that they attached to in order to cross the small intestinal border, and/or through **active transport** from low concentration to high concentration made possible through use of ATP. The method of transport depends on the concentration of the mineral on either side of the small intestinal border. This stage of absorption is referred to as the **translocation stage.**

Finally, once the mineral complex has crossed the small intestinal border, it arrives into the portal blood circulation, which will deliver it to the liver for processing and then distribution to the rest of the body. This is the **mobilization stage.** Some of the mineral complexes may not ultimately pass across the small intestinal border and instead may be sequestered within the absorptive cell for later use.

The bioavailability of the minerals depends on many factors. One factor is the presence or absence of other minerals. This is in large part due to the nonspecific nature of the carrier proteins required for facilitated diffusion and active transport. For example, high levels of iron and zinc may inhibit copper absorption, while high levels of copper may decrease iron and molybdenum absorption. Cobalt and iron compete and inhibit each other's absorption. Another factor involves the availability of the protein that binds with the mineral to form the chelation complex. For example, iron requires transferrin for absorption, while many other minerals require the nonspecific albumin protein carrier. In most cases, these protein carriers are undersaturated. However, if the mineral is consumed in excessive amounts, the mineral can overwhelm the carrier sites and lead to toxicity. Mineral absorption also can be impaired if minerals bind to free fatty acids in the intestinal lumen or if a mineral is present in very high concentrations, forming an unabsorbable precipitate (i.e., a formed solid within a solution).

While most minerals are digested and absorbed in the small intestine, the salts sodium and potassium are absorbed in the large intestine.

Micronutrient Metabolism

Once the vitamins and minerals are absorbed into the bloodstream, passed to the liver for processing, and then distributed to the rest of the blood, the metabolic activity and function of each micronutrient varies considerably, as described earlier in this section.

Vitamins, Minerals, and Weight Management

Though vitamins and minerals are calorie-free (and thus are not a source of energy), they are essential for optimal health. Given the body's demands for vitamins and minerals and the relative caloric restriction many clients may follow in an effort to lose weight, it is especially important for clients to adopt a nutrient-dense low-calorie eating plan. Not only should clients limit "empty calories" from nutrient-poor foods, but they should also pay special care to eat a balanced diet that includes all of the major food groups so as to ensure sufficient vitamin and mineral intake. Certain clients who restrict whole food groups or who have adopted a very restrictive eating plan should discuss the necessity of a daily multivitamin with their physician and/or **registered dietitian.**

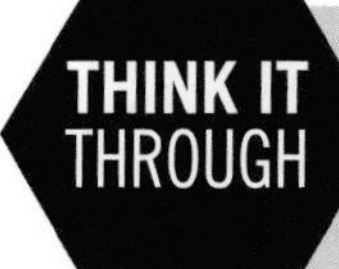

Many nutrition supplement products (including vitamins and minerals) are advertised as being necessary for good health for individuals who are on weight-loss programs. How would you respond to a client who asks you for specific recommendations on which supplements to take to ensure that he or she is getting adequate nutrients while working toward weight-loss goals?

WATER

When people think of nutrition, they often forget to think about water. Although it provides no calories and is inorganic in nature, it is as important as oxygen. Loss of only 20% of total body water could cause death. A 10% loss causes severe disorders (Figure 2-8). In general, adults can survive up to 10 days without water, while children can survive for up to five days (Mahan, Escott-Stump, & Raymond, 2011).

Water is the single largest component of the human body, making up approximately 50 to 70% of body weight. In other words, about 85 to 119 pounds (39 to 54 kg) of a 170-pound (77-kg) man is water weight. Physiologically, water has many important functions, including regulating body temperature, protecting vital organs, providing a driving force for nutrient absorption, serving as a medium for all biochemical reactions, and maintaining a high blood volume for optimal athletic performance. In fact, total body water weight is higher in athletes compared to nonathletes and tends to decrease with age due to diminishing muscle mass.

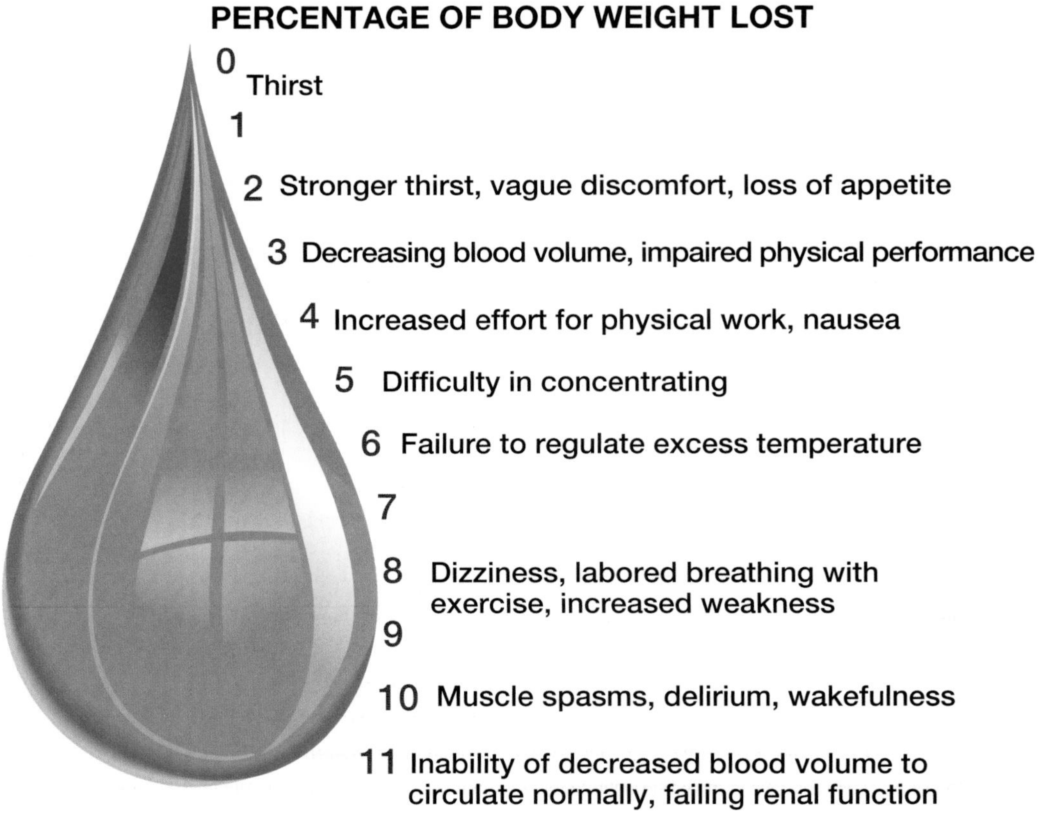

Figure 2-8
Adverse effects of dehydration

Reprinted with permission from Mahan, L.K., Escott-Stump, S., & Raymond, J.L. (2011). *Krause's Food and the Nutrition Care Process* (13th ed.). Philadelphia: W.B. Saunders Company.

PERCENTAGE OF BODY WEIGHT LOST

0 Thirst
1
2 Stronger thirst, vague discomfort, loss of appetite
3 Decreasing blood volume, impaired physical performance
4 Increased effort for physical work, nausea
5 Difficulty in concentrating
6 Failure to regulate excess temperature
7
8 Dizziness, labored breathing with exercise, increased weakness
9
10 Muscle spasms, delirium, wakefulness
11 Inability of decreased blood volume to circulate normally, failing renal function

Water volume can be influenced by a variety of factors, such as food and drink intake; sweat, urine, and feces excretion; metabolic production of small amounts of water; and losses of water that occur with breathing. These factors play an especially important role during exercise when metabolism is increased. The generated body heat is released through sweat, which is a solution of water, sodium, and other electrolytes.

If fluid intake is not increased to replenish the lost fluid, the body attempts to compensate by retaining more water and excreting more concentrated urine. Under these conditions, the person is said to be dehydrated. Severe dehydration can lead to **heat exhaustion** and eventually **heat stroke.** On the other hand, if people ingest excessive amounts of fluid to compensate for minimal amounts of water lost in sweat or excessive sodium loss in sweat with plain water replacement, they may become overloaded with fluid, a condition called hyponatremia. When the blood's water-to-sodium ratio is severely elevated, excess water can leak into brain tissue, leading to encephalopathy, or brain swelling.

Fortunately, the human body is well-equipped to withstand dramatic variations in fluid intake during exercise and at rest with little or no detrimental health effects. Most recreational exercisers will never suffer from serious hyponatremia or dehydration. The latest recommendations are to follow individualized hydration regimens and let thirst be the guide—if thirsty, drink water (Rodriguez, Di Marco, & Langley, 2009; Sawka et al., 2007). Exceptions include infants, vigorously exercising athletes, hospitalized patients, and the sick and elderly, who may have diminished thirst sensation. Because these individuals have higher water needs, they should be closely monitored.

Endurance Training and Hydration Status

Past headlines shared the unlikely but real tragedy of the 28-year-old novice Boston Marathon runner who suffered severe hyponatremia and later died en route to the hospital, as well as the story of the 24-year-old elite runner who collapsed from dehydration while exploring desolate trails in the Grand Canyon's summer heat without sufficient water. In all, a scattering of half-marathon and marathon deaths have drawn attention to the safety concerns of these endurance challenges.

Underlying heart conditions, dehydration, and overhydration (hyponatremia) most often are the causes of life-ending races in young athletes. Sadly, it turns out that not many runners are paying serious attention to hydration. In one study, a whopping 65% of the athletes studied were "not at all" concerned about keeping themselves hydrated (Brown et al., 2011). This nonchalance can come at a cost.

Drinking too little can lead to dehydration, which results from a sweat rate that exceeds fluid replenishment. Exercising at very high intensities, exercising in humid conditions, and low fluid intake all increase the likelihood of dehydration. Dehydration, along with high exercise intensity, hot and humid environmental conditions, poor fitness level, incomplete heat acclimatization, and a variety of other factors can all raise body temperature and together lead to heat stroke.

While dehydration is a serious concern, athletes should also be aware that drinking too much—out of fear of not drinking enough—could lead to hyponatremia, a less well-known and less understood but equally frightening condition characterized by a low blood sodium level. Exertional hyponatremia results from excessive intake of low-sodium fluids during prolonged endurance activities—that is, drinking a greater volume of fluid than the volume lost in sweat—and possibly, to a lesser extent, from inappropriate fluid retention.

A study of 488 Boston Marathon runners published in the *New England Journal of Medicine* found that 13% (22% of women and 8% of men) had hyponatremia, and 0.6% had critical hyponatremia, at the end of the race. Runners with hyponatremia were more likely to be of low **body mass index (BMI),** consume fluids at every mile (and more than 3 liters total throughout the race), finish the race in more than four hours, and gain weight during the run. The greatest predictor of hyponatremia was weight gain, which researchers attributed to excessive fluid intake (Almond et al., 2005). But hyponatremia is not limited to runners. Anyone exercising at a low to moderate intensity for an extended period of time (generally four hours or more) while consuming too much water can be at risk.

ENGINEERED FOODS, ALCOHOL, DRUGS, AND STIMULANTS

While nature has produced an abundance of nutrient-rich foods for human consumption, man has developed an ability to alter the natural form to create engineered foods, various alcoholic beverages, drugs, **stimulants,** and other compounds. Scientists have learned to process foods to make them taste better (though in general, the greater the processing, the lesser the nutritional value). Food manufacturers genetically modify produce to make a more perfect and abundant plant, and they develop products to help people lose weight or gain muscle. The processed-food industry is huge, with people spending billions of dollars each year to reap the promised benefits.

Some of these food products are considered **functional foods.** While various definitions exist, the Academy of Nutrition and Dietetics (A.N.D.), formerly the American Dietetic Association (ADA), considers a functional food to be any whole food or fortified, enriched, or enhanced food that has a potentially beneficial effect on human health beyond basic nutrition (ADA, 2009). Whole foods such as phytochemical-containing fruits and vegetables are functional foods, as are modified foods that have been fortified with nutrients or phytochemicals. Because functional foods may play a role in decreasing signs of aging, altering disease prevalence and progression, and providing various other benefits, the public is willing to pay more for these products. As a result, many manufacturers and various other companies and individuals are interested in profiting from these products.

At times, promises are made that are not backed by quality research or Food and Drug Administration (FDA) approval. ACE Fitness Nutrition Specialists play an important role in helping clients sift through quality products and hyped junk.

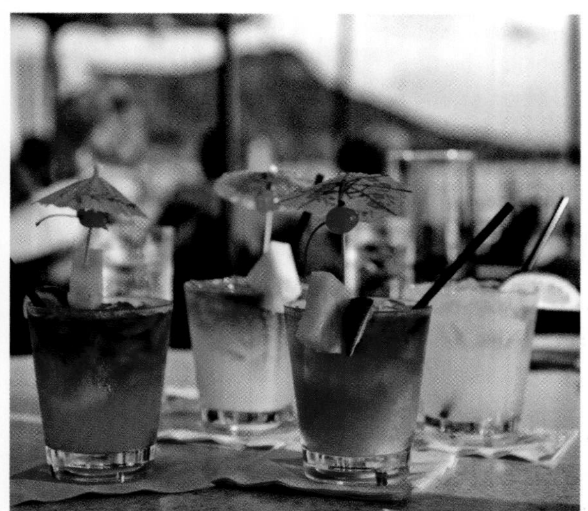

Clients also may be interested in learning how alcohol intake affects their weight-loss plans. Alcohol is a non-nutritive calorie-containing beverage (7 calories per gram). Moderate alcohol consumption provides many health benefits, such as increased HDL cholesterol and reduced risk for cardiovascular disease. However, too much alcohol may contribute to weight gain, regretful behavior, and serious accidents. In addition, alcohol use during pregnancy is linked to birth defects, and alcohol in excess can cause **cirrhosis** of the liver. Therefore, alcohol is best avoided altogether for those who are pregnant, cannot control intake, or take certain medications.

Herbal supplements, as well as legal and illicit drugs, have been used and abused in weight-loss efforts. While some herbs and other supplements may in fact have beneficial effects, consumers should purchase and use these products cautiously, as they are not regulated by the FDA. The **Dietary Supplement and Health Education Act (DSHEA)** dictates supplement production, marketing, and safety guidelines. The following are the highlights of the legislation. ACE Fitness Nutrition Specialists and their clients must be aware that savvy product manufacturers and marketing experts have found ingenious ways to get around some of the rules.

- A **dietary supplement** is defined as a product (other than tobacco) that functions to supplement the diet and contains one or more of the following ingredients: a vitamin, mineral, herb or other botanical, amino acid, a nutritional substance that increases total dietary intake, metabolite, constituent, or extract, or some combination of these ingredients.
- Safety standards provide that the Secretary of the Department of Health and Human Services may declare that a supplement poses imminent risk or hazard to public safety. A supplement is considered **adulterated** if it, or one of its ingredients, presents a "significant or unreasonable risk of illness or injury" when used as directed, or under normal conditions. It may also be considered adulterated if too little information is known about the risk of an unstudied ingredient.
- Retailers are allowed to display "third-party" materials that provide information about the health-related benefits of dietary supplements. DSHEA stipulates the guidelines that this literature must follow, including the fact that it must not be false or misleading and cannot promote a specific supplement brand.
- Supplement labels cannot include claims that the product diagnoses, prevents, mitigates, treats, or cures a specific disease. Instead, they may describe the supplement's effects on the "structure or function" of the body or the "well-being" achieved by consuming the substance. Unlike other health claims, these nutritional support statements are not approved by the FDA prior to marketing the supplement.
- Supplements must contain an ingredient label, including the name and quantity of each dietary ingredient. The label must also identify the product as a "dietary supplement" (FDA, 1995).

Many clients experiment with various herbs and supplements. The websites of the FDA (www.fda.gov) and the National Institutes of Health Office of Dietary Supplements (www.ods.od.nih.gov) provide reputable, up-to-date information about numerous supplements and herbs that ACE Fitness Nutrition Specialists can reference.

Caffeine

One supplement that warrants specific mention is caffeine. Caffeine is a ubiquitous stimulant found in coffee, tea, soft drinks, chocolate, and various other foods and drinks. Over 90% of Americans admit to regular caffeine use (Frary, Johnson, & Wang, 2005), and 20–30% consume a whopping 600 milligrams (equivalent to about 6 cups of coffee) or more each day (Armstrong et al., 2007).

Caffeine rapidly enters the bloodstream and within a short 40 to 60 minutes reaches all organs of the body, causing physiological changes that last for up to six hours (Table 2-4) (Keisler & Armsey, 2006). Due to its lipophilic, or "fat-loving," chemical structure, caffeine easily crosses the blood–brain barrier—the brain's security system aimed to prevent water-soluble toxins from damaging the all-important organ. To a nerve cell, caffeine resembles adenosine, a molecule that slows down the nervous system, dilates blood vessels, and allows sleep. The nerve's adenosine receptor cannot tell the difference between the two molecules, so caffeine and adenosine compete for receptor binding. When caffeine wins, the calming effects of adenosine are negated and an exaggerated stress response takes hold. The cell activity speeds up, the brain's blood vessels constrict, and neuron firing increases. The pituitary gland responds to the increased activity by sending a message to the adrenal glands to produce adrenaline (epinephrine), the "fight or flight" hormone. Pupils and breathing tubes dilate. Heart rate increases. Blood flow shunts to the muscles. Blood pressure rises. Muscles contract. The liver releases extra glucose into the bloodstream to fuel the fight or flight, thus sparing muscle glycogen stores (Keisler & Armsey, 2006).

Table 2-4
Physiological Effects of Caffeine by Organ System

Organ System	Effects
Central Nervous System	Increased alertness and mood Decreased pain and fatigue
Metabolism	Increased oxygen uptake, fat breakdown, and glycogen sparing
Endocrine System	Increased catecholamines, endorphins, and cortisol
Skeletal Muscle	Increased endurance Possible increased power and speed
Cardiovascular System	Increased heart rate, stroke volume, and blood pressure
Respiratory System	Increased respiratory rate
Kidneys	Increased urine production Possible increased loss of urinary electrolytes No change in 24-hour electrolyte or water balance
Temperature Regulation	No change in sweat rate, skin blood flow, or rectal (core) temperature

Reprinted with permission from Armstrong, L.E. et al. (2007). Caffeine, fluid-electrolyte balance, temperature regulation, and exercise-heat tolerance. *Exercise and Sports Science Reviews,* 35, 3, 135–140.

Research findings are clear: caffeine enhances athletic performance. Caffeine sustains duration, maximizes effort at 85% **$\dot{V}O_2$max** in cyclists, and quickens speed in an endurance event (Keisler & Armsey, 2006). Perceived exertion decreases and high-intensity efforts seem less taxing (Armstrong et al., 2007). Most research studying the ergogenic potential of caffeine has used dosages around 400 to 600 mg in capsule form, though benefits have been seen at doses as low as 250 mg (Keisler &Armsey, 2006).

The World Anti-Doping Agency (WADA) does not classify caffeine as a banned substance (www.wada-ama.org), while the National Collegiate Athletic Association (NCAA) allows intakes up to an approximately 800 mg dose, as measured by urine concentration of caffeine. There is a catch: performance-enhancing benefits of caffeine are stronger in nonusers (<50 mg/day) than regular users (>300 mg/day), as the brain adapts to chronic caffeine use by producing more adenosine receptors for adenosine binding. Caffeine's effects are lessened and the same dose produces fewer desirable physiological changes.

Some clients may also consider turning to caffeine to boost weight loss. The stimulant is a common ingredient in many weight-loss supplements. Caffeine may contribute to weight loss by suppressing appetite, increasing water loss (it is a **diuretic**), and potentially increasing resting metabolic rate. However, any effect on weight loss is likely to be small and the risks of caffeine overconsumption and dependence that could develop are greater than a small weight-loss benefit.

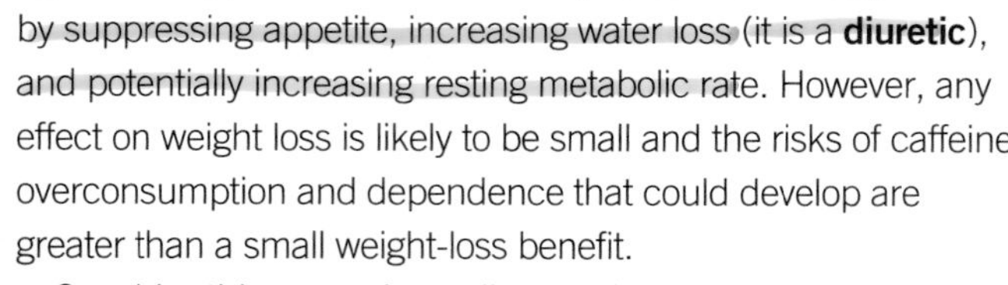

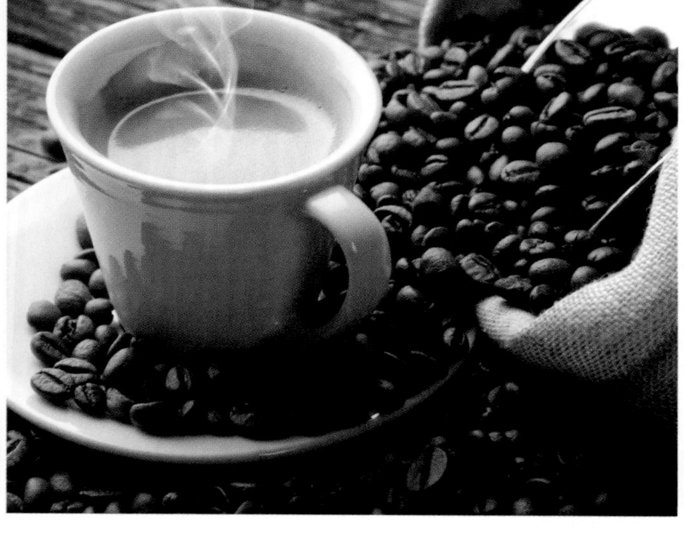

Consider this scenario: a client attributes increased performance and some weight loss to caffeine. But despite the same continued caffeine intake, the perceived benefits diminish. Having developed a tolerance to caffeine, the client consumes more caffeine. While the extra caffeine binds up the newly created adenosine receptors, the brain gets back to work increasing receptor production. As the dose continues to increase in pursuit of the invigorating caffeine jolt, risk of severe consequences multiply. *The U.S. News and World Report* reported that one teen spent the night in the pediatric intensive care unit after bingeing on caffeine pills and energy drinks to stay awake to play video games all night (Shute, 2007). A 19-year-old Connecticut man died of cardiac arrest from an overdose of 25 to 30 caffeine pills—the equivalent of about 30 cups of coffee (Shute, 2007). In addition to its toxicity at high doses, when combined with other substances like alcohol, ephedrine, or anti-inflammatory medications, even moderate caffeine use can be dangerous.

On top of tolerance, chronic caffeine use contributes to high blood pressure, high blood sugar, decreased bone density in women, jittery nerves, sleeplessness (Doheny, 2006), and for many, the dreaded withdrawal symptoms after a brief respite from the stimulant including headache, irritability, increased fatigue, drowsiness, decreased alertness, difficulty concentrating, and decreased energy and activity levels (Keisler & Armsey, 2006).

EXPAND YOUR KNOWLEDGE

Five-step Two-week Taper From Caffeine Use

The good news is that clients can moderate caffeine consumption to optimize its advantages and at the same time avert caffeine dependence and the ensuing withdrawal after a stint of quitting caffeine cold turkey. The following five-step two-week taper offers one way to get started:

- Choose a two week period of relative low stress. The taper may cause some tiredness—the key is to hit the sack, not the sodas. Aim for at least seven to eight hours of sleep each night.
- Tally daily caffeine intake from the first sip of coffee in the morning, to the lunch-time sodas, mid-afternoon energy drink, and evening tea. Remember to look beyond the nutrition label. The Center for Science in the Public Interest, a non-profit nutrition watchdog, and the American Medical Association have lobbied unsuccessfully for more than 10 years to convince the federal government to mandate caffeine information on nutrition labels. Sensing a possible shift in congress, many soda manufacturers now voluntarily include the caffeine content. But still, chances are that clients are going to have to search for the caffeine amounts

in their favorite foods and drinks. Table 2-5 lists caffeine amounts in some common sources.

- Substitute a caffeine-free beverage for one caffeinated beverage each day. Maintain this level of caffeine use for the week. The next week decrease by one more. Each week, decrease the total number of caffeinated beverages per day until total caffeine intake is less than 100 mg per day.
- Maintain a level of caffeine use less than or equal to 100 mg per day, the level below which dependency is unlikely to occur (Shapiro, 2007). Then try quitting cold turkey for three days. Research suggests withdrawal occurs around three days after quitting for new users and as quickly as 12 hours in regular users (Keisler & Armsey, 2006). The onset of a caffeine headache indicates the baseline dose is not low enough. Continue the taper to a 25 mg maintenance dose (Lu et al., 2007) or endure the headache and within a few days the caffeine habit will be history.
- Get out of crisis mode. Not every day, deadline, or life event should trigger the need for a caffeine boost to make it through. Choose wisely and carefully so that when the caffeine boost feels essential, the brain and body are prepared to give the maximal effect at the lowest possible dose.

Table 2-5
Caffeine Content of Popular Beverages

Substance	Caffeine per ounce (mg)
Coffee	13
Monster Energy Drink	10
Red Bull with caffeine	9
Full Throttle energy drink	9
Starbucks Mocha Frappucino	8
Iced Tea	6
Pepsi Max	6
Mountain Dew	5
Coca-Cola (regular or diet)	4
Dr. Pepper	3
Propel Invigorating Water	3
Sprite	0
Over-the-counter stimulants (e.g., NoDoz)	100 (per capsule)
Clif Shot: Strawberry, Mocha, Double Expresso	25, 50, 100 (per shot)

Sources: Caffeine content from product websites and www.energyfiend.com.

SUMMARY

An individual's health is at least partially determined by the nutrients he or she chooses to consume. While each nutrient plays a specific role in the body's well-being, it is the balance among these different nutrients that allows the body to function optimally. As such, a balanced and varied diet is the foundation for good health. ACE Fitness Nutrition Specialists should arm their clients with an understanding and appreciation of basic nutrition, digestion, and absorption to help them make proper choices and follow the path toward optimal health and well-being.

REFERENCES

Almond, C.S.D. et al. (2005). Hyponatremia among runners in the Boston Marathon. *New England Journal of Medicine,* 352, 1550–1556.

American Dietetic Association (2009). Position of the American Dietetic Association: Functional foods. *Journal of the American Dietetic Association,* 109, 735–746.

American Heart Association (2013). *Common Misconceptions About Cholesterol.* www.heart.org/HEARTORG/Conditions/Cholesterol/PreventionTreatmentofHighCholesterol/Common-Misconceptions-about-Cholesterol_UCM_305638_Article.jsp

Armstrong, L.E. et al. (2007). Caffeine, fluid-electrolyte balance, temperature regulation, and exercise-heat tolerance. *Exercise and Sports Science Reviews*, 35, 3, 135–140.

Bjelakovic, G. et al. (2007). Mortality in randomized trials of antioxidant supplements for primary and secondary prevention. *Journal of the American Medical Association,* 297, 842–857.

Brooks, G.A. (1987). Amino acid and protein metabolism during exercise and recovery. *Medicine & Science in Sports & Exercise,* 19, 5(suppl), S150–156.

Brown, S. et al. (2011). Lack of awareness of fluid needs among participants at a midwest marathon. *Sports Health: A Multidisciplinary Approach*, 3, 5, 451–454.

Campese, V. (1994). Salt sensitivity and hypertension: Renal and cardiovascular implications. *Hypertension,* 23, 531–550.

Champagne, C.M. (2006). Dietary interventions on blood pressure: The Dietary Approaches to Stop Hypertension (DASH) trials. *Nutrition Reviews,* 64, 2, S53–S56.

Doheny, K. (2006). Pros and Cons of the Caffeine Craze. *WebMD.* Retrieved November 9, 2011: www.webmd.com/diet/features/pros-and-cons-caffeine-craze?page=4

Duffey, K.J. & Popkin, B.M. (2008). High-fructose corn syrup: Is this what's for dinner? *American Journal of Clinical Nutrition,* 88(suppl),1722S–1732S.

Fischer, L.M. et al. (2010). Dietary choline requirements of women: Effects of estrogen and genetic variation. *American Journal of Clinical Nutrition,* 92, 1113–1119.

Food and Drug Administration (1995). *Dietary Supplement Health and Education Act of 1994.* www.cfsan.fda.gov/~dms/dietsupp.html

Frary, C.D., Johnson, R.K., & Wang, M.Q. (2005). Food sources and intakes of caffeine in the diets of persons in the United States. *Journal of the American Dietetic Association,* 105, 110–113.

Goyal, S.K., Samsher, & Goyal, R.K. (2010). Stevia (*Stevia rebaudiana)* a bio-sweetener: A review. *International Journal of Food Sciences and Nutrition,* 61, 1, 1–10.

Halliwell, B. (2007). Dietary polyphenols: Good, bad, or indifferent for your health? *Cardiovascular Research,* 73, 341–347.

Harris, W.S. (2010). Omega-6 and omega-3 fatty acids: Partners in prevention. *Current Opinions in Clinical Nutrition and Metabolic Care,* 13, 2, 125–129.

Harris, W.S. et al. (2009). Omega-6 fatty acids and risk for cardiovascular disease: A science advisory from the American Heart Association Nutrition Subcommittee of the Council on Nutrition, Physical Activity, and Metabolism; Council on Cardiovascular Nursing; and Council on Epidemiology and Prevention. *Circulation,* 119, 6, 902–990

Hunter, J.E., Zhang, J., & Kris-Etheron, P.M. (2010). Cardiovascular disease risk of dietary stearic acid compared with trans, other saturated, and unsaturated fatty acids: A systematic review. *American Journal of Clinical Nutrition*, 91, 1, 46–63.

Illian, T.G., Casey, J.C., & Bishop, P.A. (2011). Omega 3 chia seed loading as a means of carbohydrate loading. *Journal of Strength and Conditioning Research,* 25, 1, 61–65.

Institute of Medicine (2005). *Dietary Reference Intakes: Energy,Carbohydrates, Fiber, Fat, Fatty Acids,Cholesterol, Protein and Amino Acids.* Washington, D.C.: National Academies Press.

Institute of Medicine (2002). *Dietary Reference Intakes for Energy, Carbohydrate, Fiber, Fat, Fatty Acids, Cholesterol, Protein, and Amino Acids.* Washington, D.C.: The National Academies Press.

Jakobsen, M.U. et al. (2009). Major types of dietary fat and risk of coronary heart disease: A pooled analysis of 11 cohort studies. *American Journal of Clinical Nutrition*, 89, 5, 1425–1432.

Keisler, B.D. & Armsey, T.D. (2006). Caffeine as ergogenic acid. *Current Sports Medicine Reports*, 5, 215–219.

Kobylewski, S. & Eckhert, C.D (2008). *Toxicology of Rabaudioside A: A Review.* Retrieved June 14, 2011: www.cspinet.org/new/pdf/stevia-report_final-8-14-08.pdf

Kris-Etherton, P.M. et al. (2007). Position of the American Dietetic Association and Dietitians of Canada: Dietary fatty acids. *Journal of the American Dietetic Association*, 107, 9, 1599–1611.

Lappé, F.M. (1992). *Diet for a Small Planet.* New York: Ballantine Books.

Lu, Y.P. et al. (2007). Voluntary exercise together with oral caffeine markedly stimulates UVB light-induced apoptosis and decreases tissue fat in SKH-1 mice. *Proceedings of the National Academy of Sciences,*

104, 31, 12936–12941. Epub 2007 Jul 30.

Mahan, L.K., Escott-Stump, S., & Raymond, J.L. (2011). *Krause's Food Nutrition and Diet Therapy* (13th ed.). Philadelphia: W.B. Saunders Company.

Mattes, R.D. & Popkin, B.M. (2009). Nonnutritive sweetener consumption in humans: Effects on appetite and food intake and their putative mechanisms. *American Journal of Clinical Nutrition*, 89, 1, 1–14.

McArdle, W.D., Katch, F.I., & Katch, V.L.(2008). *Sports and Exercise Nutrition* (3rd ed.). Philadelphia: Lippincott Williams & Wilkins.

McDaniel, M.A., Maier, S.F., & Einstein, G.O. (2003). "Brain-specific" nutrients: A memory cure? *Nutrition*, 19, 957–975.

Miller, M. et al (2011). Triglycerides and cardiovascular disease: A scientific statement from the American Heart Association. *Circulation*, 123, 20, 2292–2333.

National Institutes of Health Office of Dietary Supplements (2011). *Dietary Supplement Fact Sheet: Zinc.* www.ods.od.nih.gov/factsheets/Zinc-QuickFacts/

Nieman, D.C. et al. (2009). Chia seed does not promote weight loss or alter disease risk factors in overweight adults. *Nutrition Research,* 29, 6, 414–418.

Nutrition Reviews (1975). Histidine: An essential amino acid for normal adults. *Nutrition Reviews,* 33, 200–202. DOI: 10.1111/j.1753-4887.1975.tbo5213.x

Rabobank Group (2009). *New Sweetener May Hit Sweet Spot in U.S. Market.* www.rabobank.com/content/news/news_archive/076-Newsweetenermayhitsweetspotin USmarket.jsp

Rizkalla, S.W. (2010). Health implications of fructose consumption: A review of recent data. *Nutrition and Metabolism (London),* 7, 82.

Rizos, E.C. et al. (2012). Association between omega-3 fatty acid supplementation and risk of major cardiovascular disease events: A systematic review and meta-analysis. *Journal of the American Medical Association,* 30, 10, 1024–1033.

Rodriguez, N.R., Di Marco, N.M., & Langley, S. (2009). Position of the American Dietetic Association, Dietitians of Canada, and the American College of Sports Medicine: Nutrition and athletic performance. *Journal of the American Dietetic Association,*109, 3, 509–527.

Sawka, M.N. et al. (2007). American College of Sports Medicine exercise and fluid replacement position stand. *Medicine & Science in Sports & Exercise,* 39, 2, 377–390.

Shapiro, R.E. (2007). Caffeine and headaches. *Neurological Science,* 28, S179–S183.

Shute, N. (2007). Over the limit? *U.S. News and World Report,* 142, 14, 60–68.

Sievenpiper, J.L. et al. (2012). Effect of fructose on body weight in controlled feeding trials: A systematic review and meta-analysis. *Annals of Internal Medicine,* 156, 4, 291–304.

Siri-Tarino, P.W. et al. (2010). Saturated fat, carbohydrate, and cardiovascular disease. *American Journal of Clinical Nutrition,* 91, 3, 502–509.

Slomski, A. (2011). IOM endorses Vitamin D, calcium only for bone health, dispels deficiency claims. *Journal of the American Medical Association,* 305, 5, 453–456.

Ulbricht, C. et al. (2009). Chia (Salvia hispanica): A systematic review by the Natural Standard Research Collaboration. *Review of Recent Clinical Trials,* 4, 3, 168–174.

U.S. Department of Agriculture (2015). *2015-2020 Dietary Guidelines for Americans* (8th ed.). www.health.gov/dietaryguidelines

Weihrauch, M.R. & Diehl, V. (2004). Artificial sweeteners: Do they bear a carcinogenic risk? *Annals of Oncology,* 15, 10, 1460–1465.

World Health Organization (2010). *Micronutrients.* www.who.int/nutrition/topics/micronutrients/en/index.html

Zeisel, S.H. & Niculescu, M.D. (2006). Perinatal choline influences brain structure and function. *Nutrition Reviews,* 64, 197–203.

Zelman, K. (2011). The great fat debate: A closer look at the controversy-questioning the validity of age-old dietary guidance. *Journal of the American Dietetic Association.* 111, 5, 655–658.

SUGGESTED READING

Academy of Nutrition and Dietetics (2012). Position of the Academy of Nutrition and Dietetics: Use of nutritive and nonnutritive sweeteners. *Academy of Nutrition and Dietetics,* 112, 5, 739–758.

Clark, N. (2008). *Nancy Clark's Sports Nutrition Guidebook.* Champaign, Ill.: Human Kinetics.

Institutes of Medicine (2005). *Dietary Reference Intakes.* www.iom.edu/CMS/3788/4574.aspx

National Institutes of Health, Office of Dietary Supplements: *Vitamin and Mineral Supplement Fact Sheets.* www.ods.od.nih.gov/Health_Information/Vitamin_and_Mineral_Supplement_Fact_Sheets.aspx

Rodriguez, N.R., DiMarco, N.M., & Langley, S. (2009). Position of the American Dietetic Association, Dietitians of Canada, and the American College of Sports Medicine: Nutrition and athletic performance. *Journal of the American Dietetic Association,*109, 3, 509–527.

U.S. Department of Agriculture (2015). *2015-2020 Dietary Guidelines for Americans* (8th ed.). www.health.gov/dietaryguidelines

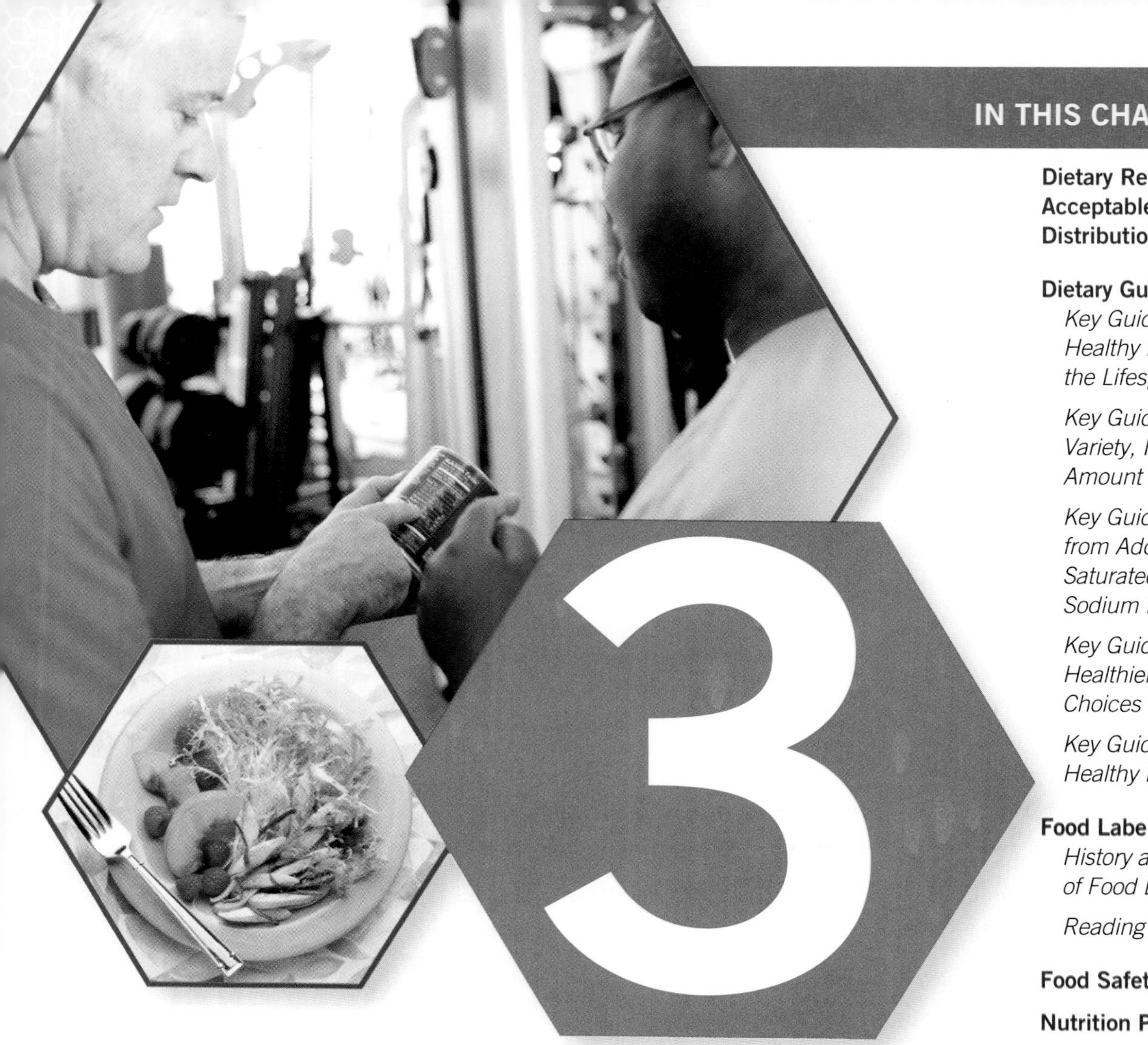

IN THIS CHAPTER

3

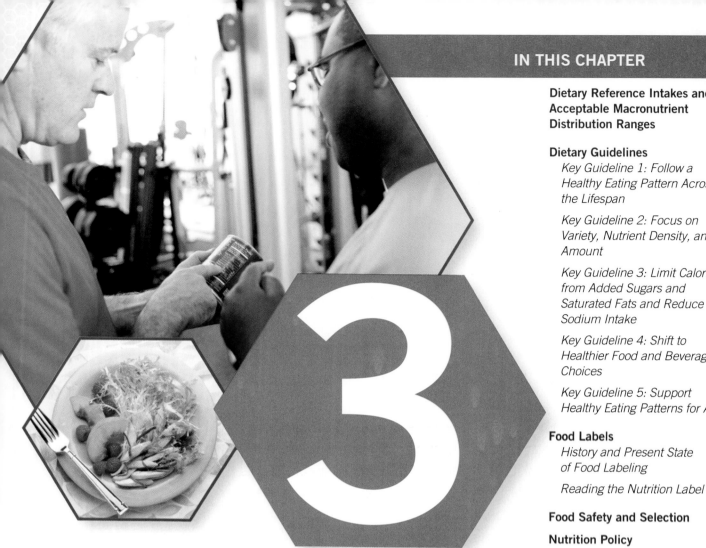

LEARNING OBJECTIVES

AFTER READING THIS CHAPTER, YOU WILL BE ABLE TO:

- DEFINE THE DIETARY REFERENCE INTAKES (DRIs) AND EXPLAIN HOW THEY ARE USED
- DESCRIBE THE ACCEPTABLE MACRONUTRIENT DENSITY RANGE (AMDR)
- OUTLINE THE NUTRITION INFORMATION CONTAINED WITHIN THE *2015-2020 DIETARY GUIDELINES FOR AMERICANS*
- USE THE *DIETARY GUIDELINES* TO DEVELOP NUTRITION EDUCATION TOOLS
- DESCRIBE THE MAJOR FEATURES OF MYPLATE AND EXPLAIN HOW TO ADVISE CLIENTS TO IMPLEMENT THE MYPLATE RECOMMENDATIONS
- EFFECTIVELY UTILIZE, INTERPRET, AND UNDERSTAND THE USDA'S SUPERTRACKER
- READ A NUTRITION LABEL AND EFFECTIVELY TEACH A CLIENT HOW TO DO THE SAME
- OUTLINE SEVERAL FOOD SAFETY PRINCIPLES
- DESCRIBE SEVERAL WAYS THAT FITNESS PROFESSIONALS CAN HELP SHAPE POLICY AND ADVOCATE FOR HEALTHIER LIFESTYLES

PRINCIPLES OF NUTRITION FOR THE HEALTH AND FITNESS **PROFESSIONAL**

By Natalie Digate Muth

Health and fitness professionals enjoy the rewarding opportunity to help clients not only improve their fitness but also adopt healthful nutrition habits. The federal government's *Dietary Guidelines for Americans* and its associated tools, including MyPlate and Supertracker, provide a foundation upon which professionals can help clients optimize their nutrition and overall health. In addition, use of these resources and tools provides health and fitness professionals an opportunity to incorporate nutrition into sessions with clients while staying within their **scope of practice.**

DIETARY REFERENCE INTAKES AND ACCEPTABLE MACRONUTRIENT DISTRIBUTION RANGES

In determining the types and amounts of foods to recommend, the *Dietary Guidelines* rely heavily on the latest scientific evidence as well as established reference intakes for specific **nutrients** for individuals across age and gender. In fact, much of the advice contained within the *2015-2020 Dietary Guidelines for Americans* (8th ed.) [U.S. Department of Agriculture (USDA), 2015] is based upon **Dietary Reference Intakes (DRIs)** published by the Institute of Medicine (IOM, 2006). DRI is a generic term used to refer to four types of reference values:

- **Recommended Dietary Allowance (RDA):** The level of intake of a nutrient that is adequate to meet the known needs of practically all healthy persons. If the level is at or above the RDA, then the client almost certainly consumes a sufficient amount (since the RDA covers 97 to 98% of the population).
- **Estimated Average Requirement (EAR):** An adequate intake in 50% of an age- and gender-specific group. If a person's intake falls well below the EAR, it is likely that person does not consume enough of the nutrient. If the level is between the EAR and the RDA, then it is likely the client consumes enough of the nutrient (50%+ likelihood).
- **Tolerable Upper Intake Level (UL):** The maximal intake that is unlikely to pose a risk of adverse health effects to almost all individuals in an age- and gender-specific group.

Comparing a person's usual intake of a nutrient to the UL helps to determine whether he or she is at risk of nutrient **toxicity.** The UL is set so that even the most sensitive people should not have an adverse response to a nutrient at intake levels near the UL. Thus, many people who have intakes above the UL may never experience a nutrient toxicity, though it is difficult to assess which clients may be most and least at risk for a nutrient overdose.

- **Adequate Intake (AI):** A recommended nutrient intake level that, based on research, appears to be sufficient for good health. If the nutrient in question has not been adequately studied and too little information is available to determine an EAR (a level good enough for 50% of the population), then it is also not possible to determine an RDA (a level good enough for 97 to 98% of the population). In these cases, the AI is published. If a client's intake is at or exceeds the AI, then it is very likely that he or she consumes enough of the nutrient to prevent deficiency. If intake is below the AI, then it is possible (but not certain) that the client is deficient in that nutrient.

DRIs for specific nutrients are available at www.nationalacademies.org. In addition, health and fitness professionals may access the DRI interactive calculator available at http://fnic.nal.usda.gov/fnic/interactiveDRI/ to determine recommended nutrient needs based on gender, age, height, weight, and activity level.

In addition to the DRIs, the IOM has established a range, known as the **Acceptable Macronutrient Distribution Range (AMDR),** for the percentage of calories that should come from **carbohydrates, protein,** and **fat** for both optimal health and reduction of chronic disease risk. While many weight-loss diets purport success based on variations from these recommendations, strong evidence supports that it is not the relative proportion of **macronutrients** that determines long-term weight-loss success, but rather calorie content and whether a person can maintain the intake over time.

Calorie needs, which form the basis for many nutrient needs, based on sex, age, and activity level are noted in Table 3-1, while overall nutritional goals by gender and age for macronutrients, **minerals,** and **vitamins** are shown in Table 3-2.

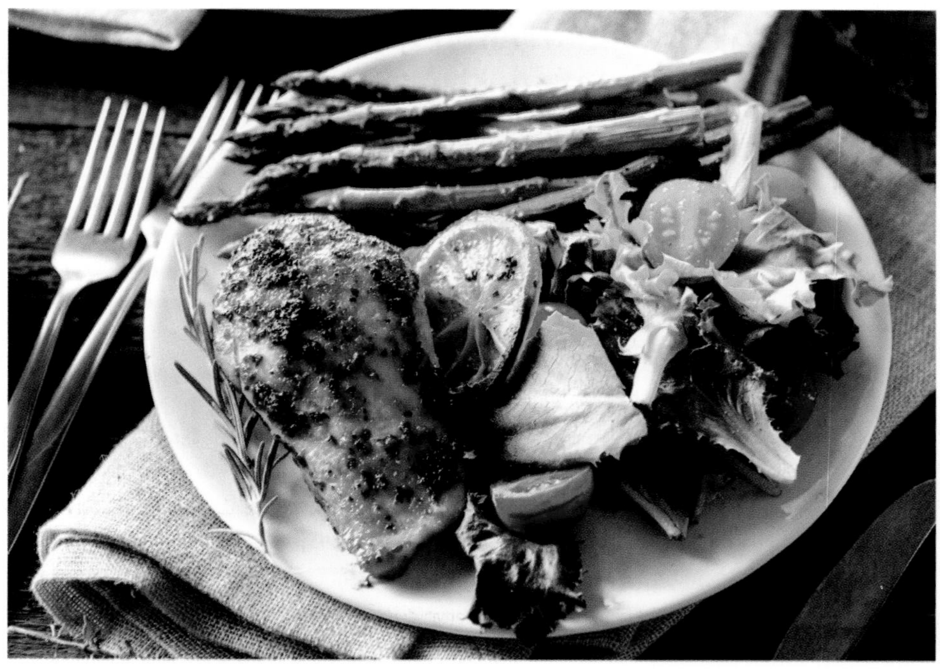

Table 3-1
Estimated Calorie Needs per Day, by Age, Sex, and Physical-activity Level

	MALES			FEMALES[D]		
AGE	SEDENTARY[A]	MODERATELY ACTIVE[B]	ACTIVE[C]	SEDENTARY[A]	MODERATELY ACTIVE[B]	ACTIVE[C]
2	1,000	1,000	1,000	1,000	1,000	1,000
3	1,000	1,400	1,400	1,000	1,200	1,400
4	1,200	1,400	1,600	1,200	1,400	1,400
5	1,200	1,400	1,600	1,200	1,400	1,600
6	1,400	1,600	1,800	1,200	1,400	1,600
7	1,400	1,600	1,800	1,200	1,600	1,800
8	1,400	1,600	2,000	1,400	1,600	1,800
9	1,600	1,800	2,000	1,400	1,600	1,800
10	1,600	1,800	2,200	1,400	1,800	2,000
11	1,800	2,000	2,200	1,600	1,800	2,000
12	1,800	2,200	2,400	1,600	2,000	2,200
13	2,000	2,200	2,600	1,600	2,000	2,200
14	2,000	2,400	2,800	1,800	2,000	2,400
15	2,200	2,600	3,000	1,800	2,000	2,400
16	2,400	2,800	3,200	1,800	2,000	2,400
17	2,400	2,800	3,200	1,800	2,000	2,400
18	2,400	2,800	3,200	1,800	2,000	2,400
19–20	2,600	2,800	3,000	2,000	2,200	2,400
21–25	2,400	2,800	3,000	2,000	2,200	2,400
26–30	2,400	2,600	3,000	1,800	2,000	2,400
31–35	2,400	2,600	3,000	1,800	2,000	2,200
36–40	2,400	2,600	2,800	1,800	2,000	2,200
41–45	2,200	2,600	2,800	1,800	2,000	2,200
46–50	2,200	2,400	2,800	1,800	2,000	2,200
51–55	2,200	2,400	2,800	1,600	1,800	2,200
56–60	2,200	2,400	2,600	1,600	1,800	2,200
61–65	2,000	2,400	2,600	1,600	1,800	2,000
66–70	2,000	2,200	2,600	1,600	1,800	2,000
71–75	2,000	2,200	2,600	1,600	1,800	2,000
76 and up	2,000	2,200	2,400	1,600	1,800	2,000

[A] Sedentary means a lifestyle that includes only the physical activity of independent living.

[B] Moderately Active means a lifestyle that includes physical activity equivalent to walking about 1.5 to 3 miles per day at 3 to 4 miles per hour, in addition to the activities of independent living.

[C] Active means a lifestyle that includes physical activity equivalent to walking more than 3 miles per day at 3 to 4 miles per hour, in addition to the activities of independent living.

[D] Estimates for females do not include women who are pregnant or breastfeeding.

Source: Institute of Medicine. Dietary Reference Intakes for Energy, Carbohydrate, Fiber, Fat, Fatty Acids, Cholesterol, Protein, and Amino Acids. Washington (DC): The National Academies Press; 2002.

Reprinted from United States Department of Agriculture (2015). *2015-2020 Dietary Guidelines for Americans* (8th ed.). www.health.gov/dietaryguidelines

Table 3-2
Daily Nutritional Goals for Age-Sex Groups Based on Dietary Reference Intakes and Dietary Guidelines Recommendations*

	SOURCE OF GOAL[A]	FEMALE 14–18	MALE 14–18	FEMALE 19–30	MALE 19–30	FEMALE 31–50	MALE 31–50	FEMALE 51+	MALE 51+
Calorie level(s) assessed		1,800	2,200, 2,800, 3,200	2,000	2,400, 2,600, 3,000	1,800	2,200	1,600	2,000
Macronutrients									
Protein, g	RDA	46	52	46	56	46	56	46	56
Protein, % kcal	AMDR	10-30	10–30	10–35	10–35	10–35	10–35	10–35	10–35
Carbohydrate, g	RDA	130	130	130	130	130	130	130	130
Carbohydrate, % kcal	AMDR	45–65	45–65	45–65	45–65	45–65	45–65	45–65	45–65
Dietary fiber, g	14g/1,000 kcal	25.2	30.8	28	33.6	25.2	30.8	22.4	28
Added sugars, % kcal	DGA	<10%	<10%	<10%	<10%	<10%	<10%	<10%	<10%
Total fat, % kcal	AMDR	25–35	25–35	20–35	20–35	20–35	20–35	20–35	20–35
Saturated fat, % kcal	DGA	<10%	<10%	<10%	<10%	<10%	<10%	<10%	<10%
Linoleic acid, g	AI	11	16	12	17	12	17	11	14
Linolenic acid, g	AI	1.1	1.6	1.1	1.6	1.1	1.6	1.1	1.6
Minerals									
Calcium, mg	RDA	1,300	1,300	1,000	1,000	1,000	1,000	1,200	1,000[B]
Iron, mg	RDA	15	11	18	8	18	8	8	8
Magnesium, mg	RDA	360	410	310	400	320	420	320	420
Phosphorus, mg	RDA	1,250	1,250	700	700	700	700	700	700
Potassium, mg	AI	4,700	4,700	4,700	4,700	4,700	4,700	4,700	4,700
Sodium, mg	UL	2,300	2,300	2,300	2,300	2,300	2,300	2,300	2,300
Zinc, mg	RDA	9	11	8	11	8	11	8	11
Copper, mcg	RDA	890	890	900	900	900	900	900	900
Manganese, mg	AI	1.6	2.2	1.8	2.3	1.8	2.3	1.8	2.3
Selenium, mcg	RDA	55	55	55	55	55	55	55	55
Vitamins									
Vitamin A, mg RAE	RDA	700	900	700	900	700	900	700	900
Vitamin E, mg AT	RDA	15	15	15	15	15	15	15	15
Vitamin D, IU	RDA	600	600	600	600	600	600	600[C]	600[C]
Vitamin C, mg	RDA	65	75	75	90	75	90	75	90
Thiamin, mg	RDA	1	1.2	1.1	1.2	1.1	1.2	1.1	1.2
Riboflavin, mg	RDA	1	1.3	1.1	1.3	1.1	1.3	1.1	1.3
Niacin, mg	RDA	14	16	14	16	14	16	14	16
Vitamin B6, mg	RDA	1.2	1.3	1.3	1.3	1.3	1.3	1.5	1.7
Vitamin B12, mcg	RDA	2.4	2.4	2.4	2.4	2.4	2.4	2.4	2.4
Choline, mg	AI	400	550	425	550	425	550	425	550
Vitamin K, mcg	AI	75	75	90	120	90	120	90	120
Folate, mcg DFE	RDA	400	400	400	400	400	400	400	400

* Refer to http://health.gov/dietaryguidelines/2015/guidelines/appendix-7/ for information about the needs for children and adolescents.

[A] RDA = Recommended Dietary Allowance; AI = Adequate Intake; UL = Tolerable Upper Intake Level; AMDR = Acceptable Macronutrient Distribution Range; DGA = *2015-2020 Dietary Guidelines* recommended limit; 14 g fiber per 1,000 kcal = basis for AI for fiber

[B] Calcium RDA for males ages 71+ years is 1,200 mg

[C] Vitamin D RDA for males and females ages 71+ years is 800 IU

Reprinted from United States Department of Agriculture (2015). *2015-2020 Dietary Guidelines for Americans* (8th ed.). www.health.gov/dietaryguidelines

DIETARY GUIDELINES

Every five years, a panel of nutrition experts from a variety of fields, such as dietetics, medicine, and public health, update the Dietary Guidelines through a rigorous process, including a review of the nutrition-related scientific literature and a series of meetings over several years. This committee of experts develops a report that is made available to the public and federal agencies for comment (the scientific report of the 2015 Dietary Guidelines Advisory Committee is available at www.health.gov/dietaryguidelines/2015-scientific-report/pdfs/scientific-report-of-the-2015-dietary-guidelines-advisory-committee.pdf). Ultimately, the report is reviewed and edited (sometimes heavily) before it is approved by Congress and becomes the federal government's official nutrition advice for Americans. Once published, the document is intended to be used by health professionals and government officials to develop educational materials and design and implement nutrition-related programs. It is within the scope of practice of the health and fitness professional to use and disseminate the information contained within the Dietary Guidelines, as well as its associated tools and resources.

Though the development of the *Dietary Guidelines* is influenced by political pressures, efforts are made to ultimately publish scientifically supported evidence for optimal nutrition for the generally healthy population. As such, the *Dietary Guidelines* generally reflect the best evidence on how to eat for optimal health for Americans aged two and older, including those at increased risk of chronic disease.

Most fitness professionals realize that sharing information contained within the *Dietary Guidelines* is within their scope of practice; however, few appreciate the quantity and depth of the nutrition information available to share with clients. Though the *Guidelines* do not typically reflect the latest nutrition trends and controversies, they do provide quality nutrition information supported by solid scientific evidence.

The major nutrition information, how it pertains to ACE Fitness Nutrition Specialists and other fitness professionals, and how fitness professionals can translate this information into programs, tip sheets, and value-added services for clients are described below. Readers are referred to www.health.gov/dietaryguidelines for a full review of the report.

The *2015-2020 Dietary Guidelines for Americans* offer five big-picture recommendations that are key to good nutrition. An overview of these five key recommendations, how they pertain to health and fitness professionals, and how you can best use this information to support clients in achieving their nutrition goals are provided here. In addition, readers are referred to www.health.gov/dietaryguidelines for a full review of the report.

THINK IT THROUGH

While each client is unique in his or her needs and goals, providing sound nutrition education is typically part of helping a client reach health- and fitness-related goals. How much time will you devote during your sessions to nutrition? What resources will you use to provide clients with the best information for their needs? Will you develop handouts with nutrition facts or will you provide nutrition-related website addresses? Think about how you can consistently deliver this content to your clientele so that it becomes a built-in part of the services you offer.

Key Guideline 1: Follow a Healthy Eating Pattern Across the Lifespan

All food and beverage choices matter. Choose a healthy eating pattern at an appropriate calorie level to help achieve and maintain a healthy body weight, support nutrient adequacy, and reduce the risk of chronic disease.

The *2015-2020 Dietary Guidelines for Americans* make a point to emphasize overall eating patterns more so than individual nutrients, recognizing that the overall nutritional value of a person's diet is more than "the sum of its parts."

The main components of a healthy eating pattern include:

- A variety of vegetables from five different groups—dark green, red and orange, legumes (beans and peas), starchy, and other
- Fruit
- Grains, primarily whole grains
- Fat-free or low-fat dairy, including milk yogurt, cheese, and/or fortified soy products
- A variety of foods rich in protein, including seafood, lean meats and poultry, eggs, legumes (beans and peas), nuts, seeds, and soy products
- Limited amounts of **saturated fats** and **trans fats** (less than 10% of calories), added sugars (<10% of calories), and sodium (less than 2,300 mg per day). If alcohol is consumed, it should be consumed in moderation, defined as up to one drink per day for women and two drinks per day for men.

The three types of healthy eating patterns discussed at most length in the *Dietary Guidelines* are the **Healthy U.S.-Style Eating Pattern,** the **Healthy Mediterranean-Style Eating Pattern,** and the **Healthy Vegetarian Eating Pattern**.

The Healthy U.S.-Style Eating Pattern is based on the types and proportions of foods Americans typically consume, but in nutrient-dense forms and appropriate amounts. It is designed to meet nutrient needs while not exceeding calorie requirements and while staying within limits for overconsumed dietary components.

The Healthy Mediterranean-Style Eating Pattern is adapted from the Healthy U.S.-Style Eating Pattern, modifying amounts recommended from some food groups to more closely reflect eating patterns that have been associated with positive health outcomes in studies of Mediterranean-Style diets. The Healthy Mediterranean-Style Eating Pattern contains more fruits and seafood and less dairy, meats, and poultry than does the Healthy U.S.-Style Eating Pattern. The pattern is similar to the Healthy U.S.-Style Eating Pattern in nutrient content, with the exception of providing less calcium and vitamin D.

The Healthy Vegetarian Eating Pattern is adapted from the Healthy U.S.-Style Pattern, modifying amounts recommended from some food groups to more closely reflect eating patterns reported by self-identified **vegetarians** in the National Health and Nutrition Examination Survey (NHANES). Based on a comparison of the food choices of these vegetarians to nonvegetarians in NHANES, amounts of soy products (particularly tofu and other processed soy products), legumes, nuts and seeds, and whole grains were increased, and meat, poultry, and seafood were eliminated. Dairy and eggs were included because they were consumed by the majority of these vegetarians. This pattern can be vegan if all dairy choices are comprised of fortified soy beverages (soy milk) or other plant-based dairy substitutes. This pattern is similar in meeting nutrient standards to the Healthy U.S.-Style Eating Pattern, but somewhat higher in calcium and **fiber** and lower in vitamin D.

Each of these patterns provides notable health benefits and can be consumed at varying calorie levels based on individual needs. They can also be adapted to meet cultural and personal preferences. In fact, moderate to strong evidence shows that these healthy eating patterns are associated with reduced risk of chronic diseases such as **cardiovascular disease, type 2 diabetes, obesity,** and some cancers (USDA, 2015). In all, the most important components of a healthy eating pattern include high intakes of vegetables and fruits and low intakes of processed meats and poultry, sugar-sweetened beverages (e.g., soda), and refined grains (e.g. processed "junk food" like chips). Table 3-3 provides a comparison of the Healthy U.S.-Style Eating Pattern, the Healthy Mediterranean-Style Eating Pattern, and the Healthy Vegetarian Eating Pattern.

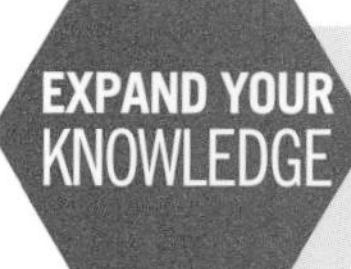

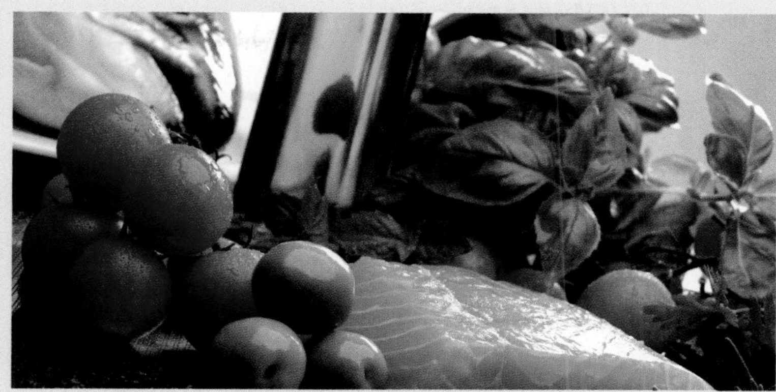

Does the Mediterranean Diet Increase Longevity?

The Greek island of Crete is famous for more than its stunning scenery and ancient roots. Fifty years ago, American scientist Ancel Keys, who himself lived to 100, attributed the exceptional longevity and miniscule rates of cardiovascular disease and cancer on the island to the "Cretan" Mediterranean diet—a diet rich in fruits, vegetables, legumes, whole grains, fish, and olive oil and moderate in red wine. Since then, a large body of research on the Mediterranean diet has accumulated, suggesting that adhering to a Mediterranean diet offers numerous benefits such as enhanced weight loss, heart health, and mental health, as well as a reduction in Alzheimer's disease, cancer, and Parkinson disease (Sofi et al., 2008). But is there enough evidence to support the assertion that adopting a Mediterranean diet may add years to your life?

Greek researchers from the University of Athens medical school set out to rigorously evaluate the assertion that adherence to a Mediterranean diet may improve longevity. They enrolled 22,043 adults in Greece who completed a comprehensive survey that included a food-frequency questionnaire aimed to evaluate how closely their current diet resembled the traditional Mediterranean diet. The researchers rated adherence to the Mediterranean diet on a nine-point scale that incorporated the diet's major features. They then checked up on the study participants 44 months later, during which 275 participants had died. A higher degree of adherence to the Mediterranean diet was associated with a lower likelihood of death from any cause as well as death from cardiovascular disease or cancer. Interestingly, associations between individual food groups within the Mediterranean diet and mortality were not significant. The authors concluded that adherence to the traditional Mediterranean diet is associated with a significant reduction in mortality and that greater adherence to a Mediterranean diet may be related to the increased longevity.

The authors evaluated adherence to a Mediterranean diet with a scale very similar to the one presented here. Fitness professionals can use this scale to assess how closely a client's typical diet resembles the Mediterranean diet. Clients get one point for each "yes." If they score 6 or higher, they are eating like they live in the Mediterranean.

	YES	NO
Vegetables (other than potatoes), 4 or more servings per day	❑	❑
Fruits, 4 or more servings per day	❑	❑
Whole grains, 2 or more servings per day	❑	❑
Beans (legumes), 2 or more servings per week	❑	❑
Nuts, 2 or more servings per week	❑	❑
Fish, 2 or more servings per week	❑	❑
Red and processed meat, 1 or fewer servings per day	❑	❑
Dairy foods, 1 or fewer servings per day	❑	❑
Alcohol, ½ to 1 drink per day for women, 1 to 2 for men	❑	❑

Source: Trichopoulou, A. et al. (2003). Adherence to a Mediterranean diet and survival in a Greek population. *New England Journal of Medicine,* 348, 2599–2608.

Table 3-3
Comparison of the Healthy U.S.-Style Eating Pattern, Healthy Mediterranean-Style Eating Plan, and the Healthy Vegetarian Eating Patterns at 2,000 Calories*

	U.S. Style	Mediterranean	Vegetarian
Food Group[A]	Daily amount[B] of food from each group (vegetable and protein food subgroup amounts are per week)		
Vegetables	2½ c-eq	2½ c-eq	2½ c-eq
Dark-green vegetables (c-eq/wk)	1½	1½	1½
Red and orange vegetables (c-eq/wk)	5½	5½	5½
Legumes (beans and peas) (c-eq/wk)	1½	1½	1½
Starchy vegetables (c-eq/wk)	5	5	5
Other vegetables (c-eq/wk)	4	4	4
Fruits	2 c-eq	2½ c-eq	2 c-eq
Grains	6 oz-eq	6 oz-eq	6½ oz-eq
Whole grains (oz-eq/day)	3	3	3½
Refined grains (oz-eq/day)	3	3	3
Dairy	3 c-eq	2 c-eq[C]	3 c-eq
Protein Foods	5½ oz-eq	6½ oz-eq	3½ oz-eq
Seafood (oz-eq/wk)	8	15[D]	—
Meats, poultry, eggs (oz-eq/wk)	26	26	—
Nuts, seeds, soy products (oz-eq/wk)	5	5	—
Eggs (oz-eq/wk)	—	—	3
Legumes (beans and peas) (oz-eq/wk)e	—	—	6
Soy products (oz-eq/wk)	—	—	8
Nuts and seeds (oz-eq/wk)	—	—	7
Oils	17 g	27 g	27g
Limits on Calories for Other Uses, calories (% of calories)f,g	110 (8%)	260 (13%)	290 (15%)

* For information on each Eating Pattern at various calorie levels, see Appendix 3 of the *Dietary Guidelines:* http://health.gov/dietaryguidelines/2015/guidelines/appendix-3/.

[A] For information on the foods in each group and subgroup, see Appendix 3 of the *Dietary Guidelines:* http://health.gov/dietaryguidelines/2015/guidelines/appendix-3/.

[B] For quantity equivalents for each food group, see Appendix 3 of the *Dietary Guidelines:* http://health.gov/dietaryguidelines/2015/guidelines/appendix-3/.

[C] In the Healthy Mediterranean-Style Eating Pattern, the amounts of dairy recommended for children and adolescents are as follows, regardless of the calorie level of the Pattern: For 2 year olds, 2 cup-eq per day; for 3 to 8 years olds, 2½ cup-eq per day; for 9 to 18 years olds, 3 cup-eq per day.

[D] The U.S. Food and Drug Administration (FDA) and the U.S. Environmental Protection Agency (EPA) provide joint guidance regarding seafood consumption for women who are pregnant or breastfeeding and young children. For more information, see the FDP or EPA websites: www.FDA.gov/fishadvice or www.EPA.gov/fishadvice.

[E] In the Healthy Vegetarian Eating Plan, about half of total legumes are shown as vegetables, in cup-eq, and half as protein foods, in oz-eq. Total legumes in this Pattern, in cup-eq, is the amount in the vegetable group plus the amount in the protein foods group (in oz-eq) divided by 4: for 2,000 calories, this equals 3 c-eq/wk.

[F] All foods are assumed to be in nutrient-dense forms, lean or low-fat and prepared without added fats, sugars, refined starches, or salt. If all food choices to meet food group recommendations are in nutrient-dense forms, a small number of calories remain within the overall calorie limit of the Pattern (i.e., limit on calories for other uses). The number of these calories depends on the overall calorie limit in the Pattern and the amounts of food from each food group required to meet nutritional goals. Calories up to the specified limit can be used for added sugars, added refined starches, solid fats, alcohol, or to eat more than the recommended amount of food in a food group. The overall eating Pattern also should not exceed the limits of less than 10% of calories from added sugars and less than 10% of calories from saturated fats. At most calorie levels, amounts that can be accommodated are less than these limits. For adults of legal drinking age who choose to drink alcohol, a limit of up to 1 drink per day for women and up to 2 drinks per day for men within limits on calories for other uses applies (see http://health.gov/dietaryguidelines/2015/guidelines/appendix-9/ for additional guidance); and calories from protein, carbohydrate, and total fats should be within the Acceptable Macronutrient Distribution Ranges (AMDRs).

[G] Values are rounded.

MyPlate

While the *Dietary Guidelines* describe these three types of eating patterns, many of the most robust tools available from the federal government to help translate recommendations into action are based on the Healthy U.S.-Style Eating Pattern. For example, the MyPlate recommendations aim to translate the *Dietary Guidelines* into a simple image that people can use to guide nutrition choices. MyPlate simplifies the government's nutrition messages into an easily understood and implemented graphic—a dinner plate divided into four sections: fruits, vegetables, protein, and grains, accompanied by a glass of nonfat milk (to represent calcium-rich foods) (Figure 3-1). The goal is to influence Americans to eat a more balanced diet by encouraging people to make half their plate vegetables and fruits. Free downloadable educational materials to share with clients are available on the MyPlate website (www.choosemyplate.gov).

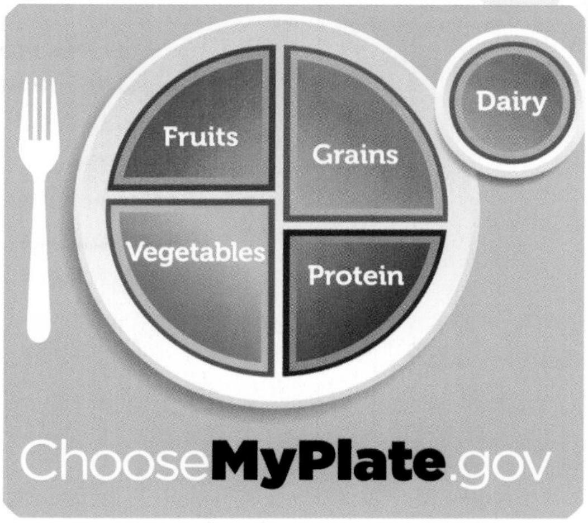

Figure 3-1
MyPlate

Supertracker and Body Weight Planner

While a health and fitness professional who is not a **registered dietitian (RD)** may not be qualified to analyze dietary logs, there are tools available to help track a client's intake and provide an analysis of dietary quality while staying within the scope of practice. For instance, the free USDA Supertracker tool is an excellent method to monitor intake. At www.supertracker.usda.gov, consumers can input their age, gender, height, weight, and physical-activity level to get an individualized eating plan to meet caloric needs. Within seconds, users are categorized into one of 12 different energy levels (from 1,000 to 3,200 calories per day) and are given the recommended number of **servings** to eat from each of the five food groups. The website also allows individuals to track nutrition intake and compare it to recommendations, track physical activity, monitor goals, and look up nutrition information for thousands of foods. Supertracker is also now available as an app. In addition, the Body Weight Planner, initially developed and validated by researchers at the Massachusetts Institute of Technology in partnership with the National Institutes of Health, is now available for widespread use at the Supertracker website (www.supertracker.usda.gov/bwp/).

As health and fitness professionals well know, the goal of a dietary intervention to decrease weight is to create a caloric deficit so that fewer calories are consumed than are expended. With about 3,500 calories in a pound of fat, a 500- to 1,000-calorie deficit each day through decreased food intake and increased physical activity leads to about a 1- to 2-pound (0.45 to 0.9 kg) weight loss per week, at least at first. While predicting weight loss based on the equation of 3,500 calories per pound is useful early on in weight loss, as an individual loses weight, metabolism (and thus energy expenditure) changes and the equation becomes less accurate and overpredicts weight loss.

The Body Weight Planner more accurately accounts for these metabolic changes. It approximates that for every 10-calorie decrease in intake, the average **overweight** adult will lose about 1 pound (0.45 kg), with half of the weight lost by one year and 95% of the weight change by three years (Hall et al., 2011). For example, a woman who decreased her daily caloric consumption from 2,200 calories to 2,000 calories would lose about 10 pounds (4.5 kg) within one year of the lowered caloric intake, and about 10 more pounds (4.5 kg) by the end of three years. If she had created a 500-kcal deficit each day, she would lose 25 pounds (11.4 kg) in the first year and about 25 more pounds (11.4 kg) by the end of three years.

Simply enter a client's age, gender, weight, height, current activity level, and goal weight, and the Body Weight Planner provides a roadmap for how to get there. Then, simply plug in the goal calorie level into Supertracker to get a meal plan and monitoring system to help guide the client toward attaining that goal.

Key Guideline 2: Focus on Variety, Nutrient Density, and Amount

To meet nutrient needs within calorie limits, choose a variety of nutrient-dense foods across and within all food groups in recommended amounts.

The *Dietary Guidelines* suggest that Americans are most likely to meet nutrient needs and manage weight by choosing nutrient-dense foods, which provide high levels of vitamins, minerals, and other nutrients that may have health benefits relative to caloric content. Categories of nutrient-dense foods include vegetables, fruits, grains, dairy, protein foods, and oils. Table 3-4 notes the function of various nutrients that are frequently referenced in discussion of the food groups.

Table 3-4
How Key Nutrients Contribute to Health

NUTRIENT	FUNCTION	SELECTED FOOD SOURCES
Macronutrient Subtypes		
Fiber	Increases feelings of fullness, promotes normal bowel function, and may help decrease risk of cardiovascular disease, obesity, and type 2 diabetes	Beans and peas, vegetables, fruits, whole grains, nuts
Omega-3 fatty acid (alpha-linolenic acid, docosahexanoic acid, eicosapentaenoic acid)	Reduces blood clotting, dilates blood vessels, reduces inflammation, reduces cholesterol and triglyceride levels; may help preserve brain function and reduce risk of mental illness and attention deficit hyperactivity disorder	Plant oils, egg yolk, tuna, salmon, mackerel, cod, crab, shrimp, oysters
Water-soluble Vitamins		
Thiamin (Vitamin B1)	Assists carbohydrate and amino acid metabolism and neural function	Enriched, fortified, or whole-grain products; fortified cereal
Riboflavin (Vitamin B2)	Assists in carbohydrate, amino acid, and fat metabolism	Milk products; bread products; fortified cereal; green leafy vegetables
Niacin (Vitamin B3)	Assists in carbohydrate, amino acid, and fat metabolism	Meat, fish, poultry; enriched and whole-grain breads and bread products; fortified cereal
Pantothenic acid (Vitamin B5)	Assists in carbohydrate, amino acid, and fat metabolism	Meat, mushrooms, avocados, broccoli, egg yolk, skim milk, sweet potatoes
Pyridoxine (Vitamin B6)	Assists in carbohydrate, amino acid, and fat metabolism; helps make neurotransmitters; may contribute to decreased cardiovascular risk by helping regulate homocysteine	Meat, fortified cereal, starchy vegetables, non-citrus fruits
Biotin (Vitamin B7)	Assists in carbohydrate, amino acid, and fat metabolism	Milk, liver, egg yolk
Folate (Vitamin B9)	Assists in amino acid metabolism; important for red and white blood cell formation and in the prevention of neural tube defects (such as spina bifida) in the developing fetus	Soybeans, oranges and orange juice, dark green leafy vegetables like spinach Many pregnant women do not meet the recommended folate intake of 400 µg per day. For this reason, the Centers for Disease Control and Prevention (2015) recommend that all women capable of becoming pregnant take a 400 µg folic acid supplement (the supplement form of folate) and that pregnant women take a vitamin containing 600 µg.
Cobalamin (Vitamin B12)	Assists in amino acid metabolism; important for gastrointestinal tract, bone marrow, and nervous system	Animal products including liver and kidney, milk, eggs, fish, cheese, muscle meat Vegetarians and older adults are at increased risk of vitamin B12 deficiency. These individuals should consume foods high in B12, such as cooked clams or foods fortified with vitamin B12, such as fortified cereals, or take B12 as a dietary supplement.
Choline	Important in metabolism and neurotransmitter synthesis	Milk, liver, egg, peanuts
Vitamin C	Antioxidant, enzyme cofactor, promotes resistance to infection	Citrus fruits (such as oranges, grapefruits, lemons, and limes), kiwi, strawberry, cantaloupe, peppers, broccoli, brussels sprouts, spinach, organ meats

Table 3-4 *(continued)*

NUTRIENT	FUNCTION	SELECTED FOOD SOURCES
Fat-soluble Vitamins		
Vitamin A	Vision, growth, immune function, reproduction, skin health	Liver, milk, eggs, cod, halibut, carrots, spinach, sweet potatoes, cantaloupe
Vitamin D	Helps reduce the risk of bone fractures and potentially provides myriad other health benefits, though that is currently under investigation and debate	Vitamin D is obtained from sunlight and fortified foods such as milk and some yogurts, cereals, orange juice, and soy products. Natural sources include certain fish (salmon, herring, mackerel, and tuna) and egg yolks.
Vitamin E	Antioxidant	Oils, nuts and seeds, green leafy vegetables
Vitamin K	Blood clotting	Green leafy vegetables (especially broccoli, cabbage, turnip greens, and dark lettuces)
Minerals		
Calcium	Bone health, nerve function, blood vessel constriction and dilation, and muscle contraction; children, adolescent girls, adult women, and adults older than 51 years old are at increased risk of negative effects of insufficient calcium intake	Milk and milk products are important sources of calcium. Those who do not consume milk products need to carefully plan calcium intake, recognizing that it is difficult to attain sufficient calcium from plant sources alone. Good sources of calcium include dairy products, fortified cereals and orange juice, soy and almond milk, sardines, and mustard spinach.
Chromium	Increases effects of insulin, restores glucose tolerance	Corn oil, clams, whole grain cereals, brewer's yeast
Copper	Formation of red blood cells; bone growth; skin health	Oysters, nuts, organ meats, legumes
Fluoride	Bone formation; prevents cavities	Fluorinated water, teas, marine fish
Iodine	Growth and metabolism	Iodized salt, seafood
Iron	Delivery of oxygen to cells, improves blood quality, increases resistance to stress and disease; many adolescent females and adult women in particular suffer from iron deficiency	Good sources of heme iron include lean meat, poultry, and seafood (especially clams, oysters, and mussels). Non-heme iron in plants such as beans, lentils, spinach, and iron-enriched foods are also acceptable sources of iron, though the iron is not as readily absorbed. Women who are pregnant should discuss iron supplementation with their obstetrician or other healthcare provider. Individuals with low iron levels should choose foods that supply heme iron, a type of iron more readily absorbed by the body. They should also consume iron in conjunction with foods that increase iron absorption such as vitamin C–rich foods.
Magnesium	Acid/base balance; carbohydrate and mineral metabolism	Seeds, nuts, legumes, unmilled cereal grains, dark green vegetables, milk
Manganese	Enzyme activation; carbohydrate and fat production; sex hormone production; skeletal development	Nuts, whole grains, vegetables, fruits
Phosphorus	Bone development; carbohydrate, protein, and fat utilization	Meat, poultry, fish, eggs
Potassium	Lowers blood pressure, decreases risk of kidney stones, and prevents bone loss	Fruits, vegetables, milk products
Selenium	Protect body tissues against oxidative damage from radiation, pollution, and normal metabolic processing	Brazil nuts, fish, clams, oysters, sunflower seeds
Zinc	Digestion and metabolism; important in development of reproductive systems; aids in healing	Lean meat, liver, eggs, seafood, whole grains

Figure 3-2
Vegetables

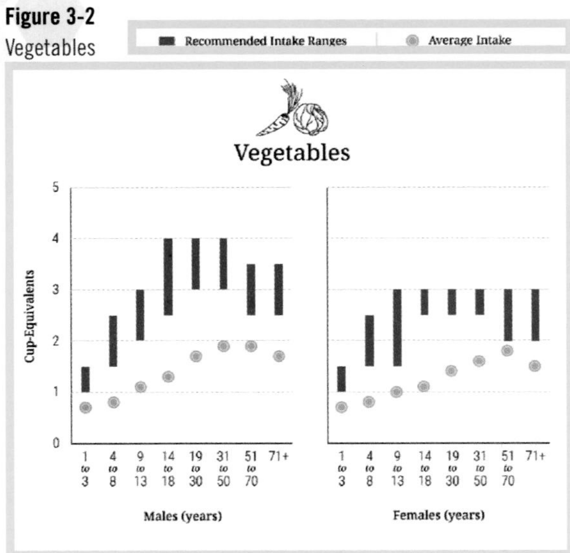

Figure 3-3
Fruits

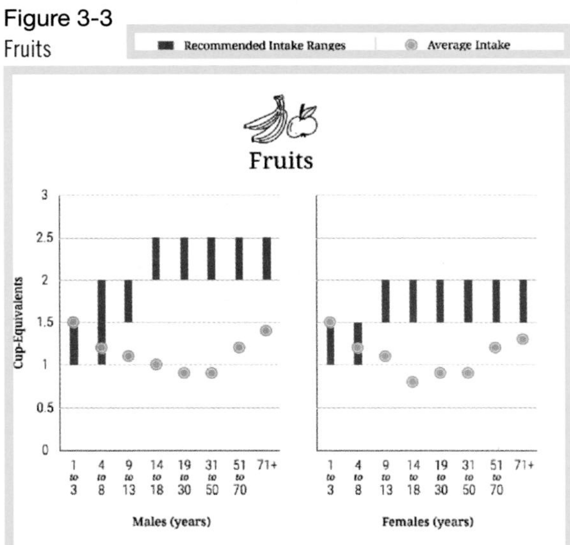

Figure 3-4
Grains

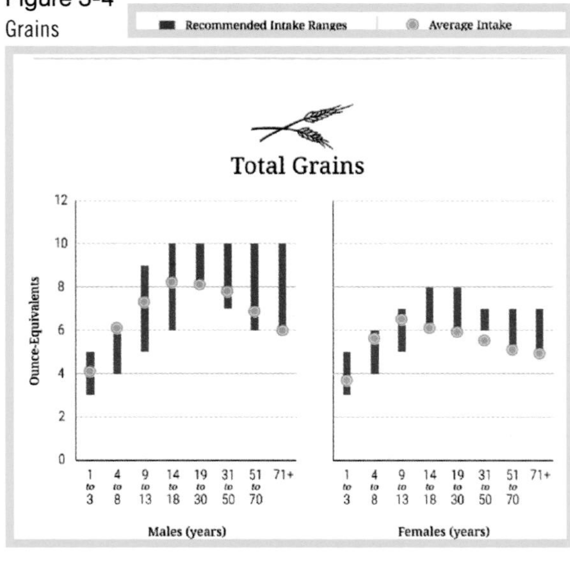

Vegetables

Vegetables are an important contributor to a healthy eating pattern. Vegetables are classified into five subgroups—dark green, red and orange, legumes (beans and peas), starchy, and other. While all subgroups are high in nutrients overall, some groups contain higher amounts of certain nutrients. For example, dark green vegetables are highest in vitamin K, while red and orange vegetables are high in vitamin A, legumes contain the most fiber, and starchy vegetables are highest in potassium. The *Dietary Guidelines* advise Americans to eat vegetables from all of the subgroups. Current vegetable intake compared to recommended intake is shown in Figure 3-2.

Fruits

Whole fruits, including fresh, frozen, canned, and dried forms, provide key nutrients, including dietary fiber, potassium, and vitamin C. Note that dried and canned fruits and fruit juices "count" as fruits, but are more calorie-dense than fresh and frozen fruits and thus should be consumed with attention to **portion** sizes. The *Dietary Guidelines* advise that no more than half of fruit should come from fruit juice and that juice that is less than 100% fruit is considered to be a "sugary drink" (and should be avoided, although the *Guidelines* come short of saying that directly, and instead note that added sugars can be accommodated as long as they do not exceed 10% of total calorie intake per day, while staying within calorie recommendations outlined in Table 3-1). Current fruit intake compared to recommended intake is shown in Figure 3-3.

Grains

Grains include foods such as rice, oatmeal, and popcorn, as well as products that contain grains like bread, cereals, crackers, and pasta. Grains can either be refined or whole grains. Refined grains are heavily processed and provide limited nutritional value (essentially, through processing, all of the nutrients are removed and then four B vitamins and **iron** are added back, thus creating "enriched grains"). Whole grains contain the entire grain kernel and provide health and nutritional value, including fiber, iron, zinc, manganese, folate, magnesium, copper, **thiamin, niacin,** vitamin B6, phosphorus, selenium, **riboflavin,** and vitamin A. Whole grains include foods such as brown rice, quinoa, and oats. The majority of grain consumption should come from whole grains. When choosing foods, it is easiest to identify whole-grain products by looking at the ingredient list on the nutrition label. "Whole grain" should be the first ingredient, or the second after water. Whole grains contain 16 grams of whole grain per 1 ounce-equivalent. Foods that are partly whole grain also can contribute to grain needs, and should contain at least 8 grams of whole grain per 1 ounce-equivalent. Examples of "1 ounce-equivalent" include a slice of bread, half a cup of pasta or rice, 1 cup of cereal, or one tortilla. Current grain intake compared to recommended intake is shown in Figure 3-4.

Dairy

The dairy group includes milk, yogurt, cheese, and fortified soy beverages. Dairy products are high in calcium, phosphorus, vitamin A, vitamin D (usually through fortification), riboflavin, vitamin B12, protein, potassium, zinc, choline, magnesium, and selenium. The *Dietary Guidelines* do not consider plant "milk," such as coconut, almond, rice, and hemp, as dairy because their overall nutritional value is not similar to dairy and soy milk, though they do contain calcium (Table 3-5).

Table 3-5
The Nutritional Value of Different Types of Milk

MILK	NUTRIENT HIGHLIGHTS (PER 8 OZ)	PROS	CONS
Cow's milk (conventional) (skim, 1%, 2%, whole)	80–150 calories 0–5 g saturated fat 8 g protein 30% calcium 20% vitamin D	Skim milk is low in calories and fat, and high in protein, calcium, and vitamin D. Go with skim or low-fat (1%) milk for kids over 2.	Lactose (problematic for some) High carbon footprint, though the industry is working to decrease
Organic cow's milk (skim, 1%, 2%, whole)	80–150 calories 0–5 g saturated fat 8 g protein 30% calcium 20% vitamin D	Same benefits as conventional milk with a smaller carbon footprint	Lactose (problematic for some) Expensive
Chocolate milk (1% low-fat)	150 calories 2 g saturated fat 8 g protein 29% calcium 18% vitamin D	More palatable than regular milk for some (especially appealing to kids)	11 grams added sugar per cup
Soy milk	100 calories 0.5 g saturated fat 7 g protein 29% calcium 16% vitamin D	Plant compounds may help decrease cholesterol	Too much soy could increase risk of breast cancer in premenopausal women
Almond milk	35 calories 0 g saturated fat 1 g protein 20% calcium 25% vitamin D	Lowest in calories; high in vitamin E and selenium	Highest in sodium (180 mg/8-ounce serving) Low in protein
Hemp milk	100 calories 0.5 g saturated fat 4 g protein 10% calcium (30% if fortified) 25% vitamin D	High in omega-3 fatty acids (900 mg per serving)	Relatively low in protein and calcium (unless fortified)
Oat milk	130–150 calories 0 g saturated fat 4 g protein 0% calcium (30% if fortified) 0% vitamin D	High in calcium and vitamin D, folic acid, fiber (2 g/serving)	High in calories and sugar; little to no calcium unless fortified
Coconut milk	80 calories 5 g saturated fat 1 g protein 1 0% calcium 30% vitamin D	Lowest in sodium; fairly low-calorie; fortified with vitamin B12 (especially important for vegans)	High in saturated fat Low in protein
Rice Milk	120 calories 0 g saturated fat 1 g protein 1% calcium (30% if fortified) 25% vitamin D	Naturally sweet taste; low risk of allergic reaction	Low in protein

People who do not eat dairy are advised to consume foods that contain nutrients generally obtained from dairy products. The *Dietary Guidelines* suggest that low-fat and fat-free dairy products may be preferable to higher-fat dairy products, as they have the same nutrients with fewer calories and saturated fat. This is somewhat controversial, as emerging research suggests that saturated fat may not be as harmful to health as previously believed.

The *Dietary Guidelines'* emphasis on milk products also has been a source of debate and controversy. While milk products are not necessary to meet nutrient needs, they do contain many nutrients, including calcium, vitamin D, and potassium—all nutrients consumed in inadequate amounts by much of the population. Moderate evidence suggests that milk intake improves bone health in children and adolescents and contributes to decreased risk of cardiovascular disease, type 2 diabetes, and **hypertension** in adults (USDA, 2015). The *Dietary Guidelines* suggest that adults should aim for 3 cups per day of milk, children older than three should consume 2.5 cups, and children ages two to three should consume 2 cups. However, the *Dietary Guidelines* also acknowledge that the Healthy Mediterranean-Style Eating Plan, which is low in dairy products, is comparable in nutritional value to the Healthy U.S.-Style Eating Plan. The current dairy intake compared to recommended intake recommended in the Healthy U.S.-Style Eating Pattern is shown in Figure 3-5.

Protein Foods

Protein foods include a diversity of foods from plant and animal sources, including the following subgroups: seafood; meats, poultry, and eggs; and nuts, seeds, and soy products. Legumes and peas also are considered protein foods in addition to being included in the vegetables group. Additionally, many dairy products are high in protein. Protein foods are high in nutrients, such as niacin, vitamin B12, vitamin B6, riboflavin, selenium, choline, phosphorus, zinc, copper, vitamin D, and vitamin E. Some subgroups contain higher levels of specific nutrients than others. For example, meat provides the most zinc; poultry the most niacin; seafood the most vitamin B12, vitamin D, and **omega-3 fatty acids**; eggs the most choline; seeds the most vitamin E; and meat, poultry, and seafood the most heme iron, which is better absorbed than plant sources of iron. Current protein intake compared to recommended intake is shown in Figure 3-6.

Due to the increasing evidence supporting the health benefits of seafood, the *Dietary Guidelines* recommend that adults consume 8 or more ounces of seafood per week [equivalent to about 250 mg per day of the omega-3 fatty acids eicosapentaenoic acid (EPA) and docosahexaenoic acid (DHA)], comprising about 20% of total recommended protein intake. Estimated EPA+DHA in various types of seafood are shown in Table 3-6. The *Dietary Guidelines* state that the benefit

Figure 3-5
Dairy

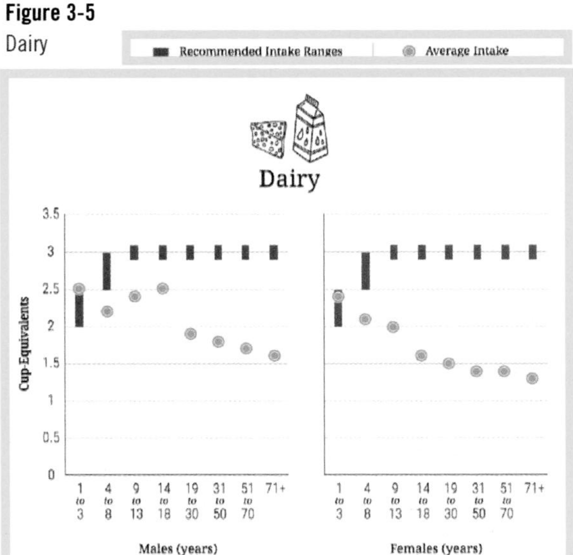

Figure 3-6
Protein foods

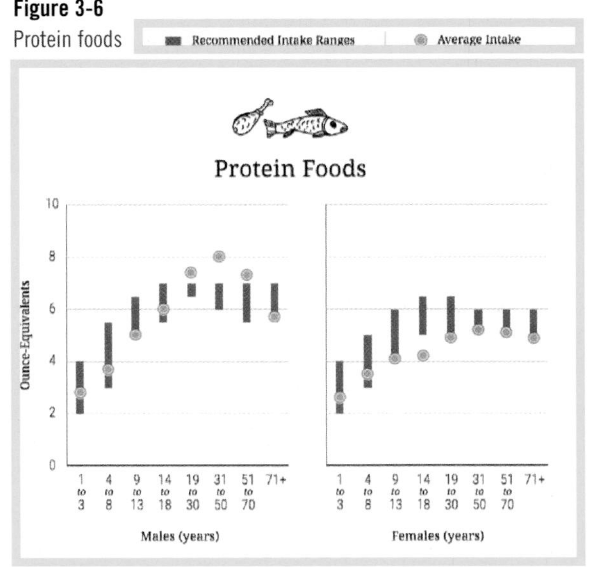

Table 3-6
Estimated EPA+DHA and Mercury Content in 4 Ounces of Selected Seafood Varieties

Common Seafood Varieties	EPA+DHA[a] mg/4 oz[b]	Mercury[c] μg/4 oz[d]
Salmon[†]: Atlantic*, Chinook*, Coho*	1,200–2,400	2
Anchovies*[,†], Herring*[,†], and Shad[†]	2,300–2,400	5–10
Mackerel: Atlantic and Pacific (not King)	1,350–2,100	8–13
Tuna: Bluefin*[,†] and Albacore[†]	1,700	54–58
Sardines[†]: Atlantic* and Pacific*	1,100–1,600	2
Oysters: Pacific[e,f]	1,550	2
Trout: Freshwater	1,000–1,100	11
Tuna: White (Albacore) canned	1,000	40
Mussels[†,f]: Blue*	900	NA
Salmon[†]: Pink* and Sockeye*	700–900	2
Squid	750	11
Pollock[†]: Atlantic* and Walleye*	600	6
Crab[f]: Blue[†], King*[,†], Snow[†], Queen*, and Dungeness*	200–550	9
Tuna: Skipjack and Yellowfin	150–350	31–49
Flounder*[,†], Plaice[†], and Sole*[,†] (Flatfish)	350	7
Clams[f]	200–300	0
Tuna: Light canned	150–300	13
Catfish	100–250	7
Cod[†]: Atlantic* and Pacific*	200	14
Scallops[†,f]: Bay* and Sea*	200	8
Haddock*[,†] and Hake[†]	200	2–5
Lobsters[f,g]: Northern*[,†] American[†]	200	47
Crayfish[f]	200	5
Tilapia	150	2
Shrimp[f]	100	0
Seafood varieties that should not be consumed by women who are pregnant or breastfeeding[h]		
Shark	1,250	151
Tilefish*: Gulf of Mexico[†,i]	1,000	219
Swordfish	1,000	147
Mackerel: King	450	110

[a] A total of 1,750 mg of Eicosapentaenoic (EPA) and Docosahexaenoic (DHA) per week represents an average of 250 mg per day, which is the goal amount to achieve at the recommended 8 ounces of seafood per week for the general public.

[b] EPA and DHA values are for cooked, edible portion rounded to the nearest 50 mg. Ranges are provided when values are comparable. Values are estimates.

[c] A total of 39 μg of mercury per week would reach the EPA reference dose limit (0.1 μg/kg/d) for a woman who is pregnant or breastfeeding and who weighs 124 pounds (56 kg).

[d] Mercury was measured as total mercury and/or methyl mercury. Mercury values of zero were below the level of detection. NA–Data not available. Values for mercury adjusted to reflect 4 ounce weight after cooking, assuming 25 percent moisture loss. Canned varieties not adjusted; mercury values gathered from cooked forms. Values are rounded to the nearest whole number. Ranges are provided when values are comparable. Values are estimates.

[e] Eastern oysters have approximately 500–550 mg of EPA+DHA per 4 ounces.

[f] Cooked by moist heat.

[g] Spiny Lobster has approximately 550 mg of EPA+DHA and 14 μg mercury per 4 ounces.

[h] Women who are pregnant or breastfeeding should also limit white (Albacore) Tuna to 6 ounces per week.

[i] Values are for Tilefish from the Gulf of Mexico; does not include Atlantic Tilefish, which have approximately 22 μg of mercury per 4 ounces.

*Seafood variety is included in EPA+DHA value(s) reported.

[†]Seafood variety is included in mercury value(s) reported.

Reprinted from U.S. Department of Agriculture (2010). *2010 Dietary Guidelines for Americans.* www.dietaryguidelines.gov

Sources: U.S. Department of Agriculture, Agricultural Research Service, Nutrient Data Laboratory (2010). *USDA National Nutrient Database for Standard Reference, Release 23.* Available at: www.ars.usda.gov/ba/bhnrc/ndl; U.S. Food and Drug Administration (2013). Mercury Levels in Commercial Fish and Shellfish. Available at: www.fda.gov/Food/FoodSafety/Product-Specificinformation/Seafood/FoodbornePathogensContaminants/Methylmercury/ucm115644.htm; Hall, R.A., Zook, E.G., & Meaburn, G.M. (1978). *National Marine Fisheries Service Survey of Trace Elements in the Fishery Resource.* Silver Spring, Md.: National Marine Fisheries Service; Environmental Protection Agency (2000). *The Occurrence of Mercury in the Fishery Resources of the Gulf of Mexico.* Washington, D.C.: Environmental Protection Agency.

of consuming high levels of omega-3 fatty acids contained in seafood outweighs the risks of increased mercury intake, though individuals should aim to consume a mix of different types of seafood to decrease mercury exposure. The benefits and recommended intake also hold true for pregnant and breastfeeding women. Pregnant women, however, should be especially cautious to choose seafood that is low in mercury and avoid tilefish, shark, swordfish, and king mackerel.

Oils

Oils are fats that contain a percentage of **monounsaturated fats** and **polyunsaturated fats** and are liquid at room temperature. Oils are not a food group; however, the *Dietary Guidelines* recognizes them as an important part of a healthy eating pattern because they contain essential **fatty acids** and vitamin E. Commonly consumed plant oils include canola, corn, olive, peanut, safflower, soybean, and sunflower oils. Oils are naturally present in olives, nuts, avocados, and seafood. Tropical plant oils such as coconut palm kernel and palm oil are not included in the oils category due to their high saturated fat content. Americans are advised to consume about 5 teaspoons of oil per day for a 2,000 calorie diet. The nutritional composition of commonly consumed oils is shown in Figure 3-7.

Figure 3-7
Oils

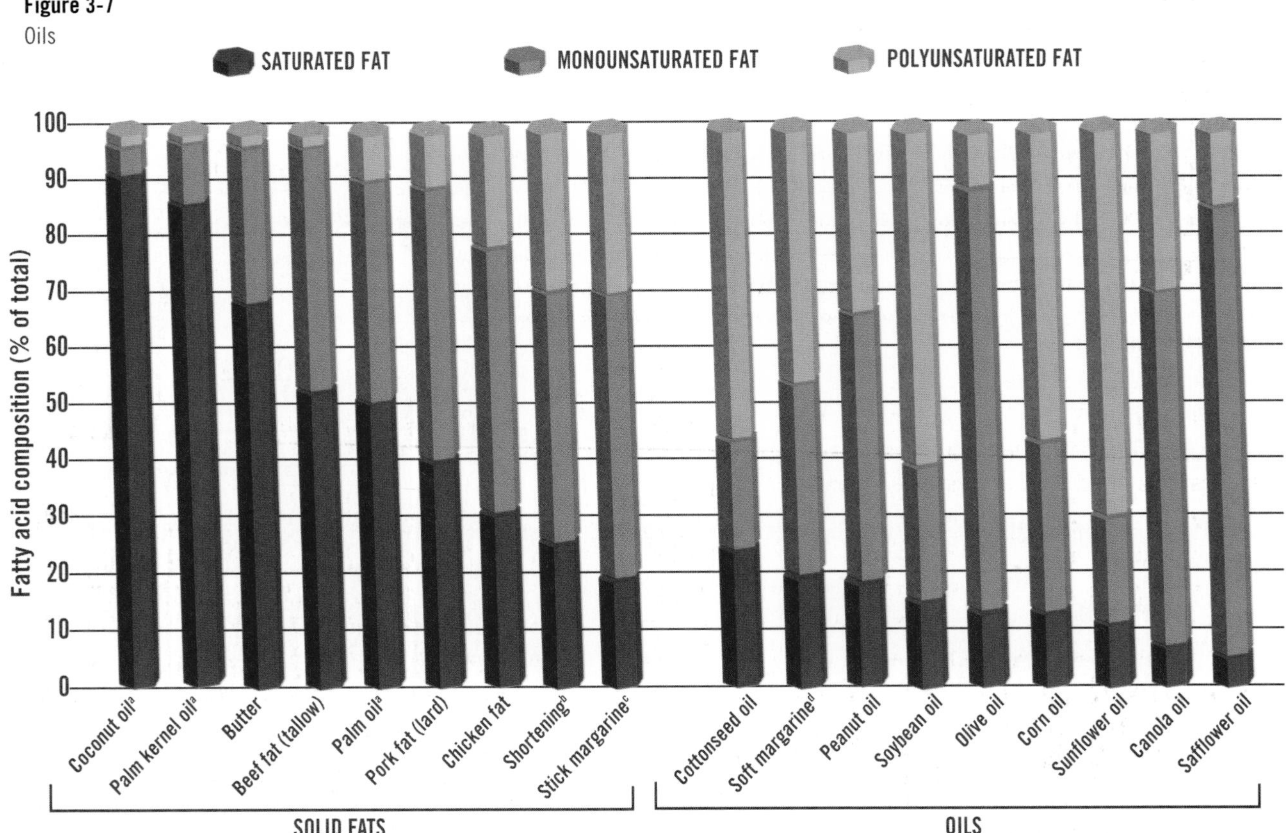

[a]Coconut oil, palm kernel oil, and palm oil are called oils because they come from plants. However, they are semi-solid at room temperature due to their high content of short-chain saturated fatty acids. They are considered solid fats for nutritional purposes.

[b]Partially hydrogenated vegetable oil shortening, which contains trans fats.

[c]Most stick margarines contain partially hydrogenated vegetable oil, a source of trans fats.

[d]The primary ingredient in soft margarine with no trans fat is liquid vegetable oil.

Reprinted from U.S. Department of Agriculture (2010). *2010 Dietary Guidelines for Americans.* www.health.gov/dietaryguidelines/2010

Source: U.S. Department of Agriculture, Agricultural Research Service, Nutrient Data Laboratory (2009). *USDA National Nutrient Database for Standard Reference.* www.ars.usda.gov/ba/bhnrc/ndl

Limits on Calories that Remain

The recommended food patterns are intended to meet nutritional needs while staying within calorie limits. For most people who follow the *Dietary Guidelines,* few calories will remain for "other purposes" (i.e., added sugars, added refined starches, solid fats, more than the recommended amounts of nutrient-dense foods, and alcohol).

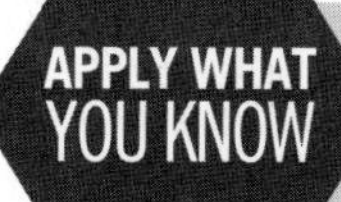

1. Record your nutritional intake for 2 weekdays and 1 weekend day in Supertracker.
2. Assess how your intake compares to the recommendations. Which food group recommendations are you meeting? Which are you exceeding? Where are you falling short?
3. What changes might you make to improve your nutrition? What are you already doing well?

Key Guideline 3: Limit Calories from Added Sugars and Saturated Fats and Reduce Sodium Intake

Consume an eating pattern low in added sugars, saturated fats, and sodium. Cut back on foods and beverages higher in these components to amounts that fit within healthy eating patterns.

The *Dietary Guidelines* urge Americans to pay attention to—and limit—consumption of foods with low to no nutritional value, especially those that are, or may be, harmful to health such as added sugars, saturated fat, and sodium. New to the *2015-2020 Dietary Guidelines* compared to previous editions, dietary **cholesterol** is no longer noted as a nutrient to limit, as it is likely not harmful to health for most people.

Added Sugars

Natural sugars include fruit sugar (**fructose**) and milk sugar (**lactose**). However, most sugars in the typical American diet are added sugars, which can come in many different forms (Table 3-7). While the body metabolizes natural and added sugars in the same way, most foods high in added sugars have very little nutritional value. These added sugars contribute about 270 calories or 13% of the total calories in the American diet. The most commonly consumed food products containing these added sugars are sugar-sweetened beverages and snacks and sweets. The *Dietary Guidelines* recommend that Americans consume no more than 10% of calories from added sugars, while staying within calorie limits. Non-caloric sweeteners may be used to reduce caloric intake in the short term, but their long-term value for helping to lose weight and maintain weight loss is still unclear. The primary sources of these added sugars for Americans ages 2 and older are shown in Figure 3-8.

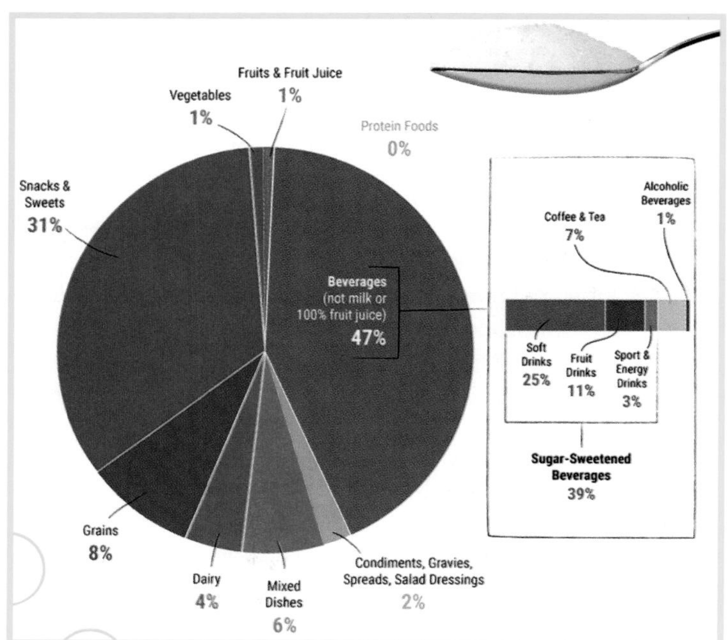

Figure 3-8
Food category sources of added sugars in the U.S. population ages 2 years and older

Table 3-7 The Many Ways To Say Sugar
Anhydrous dextrose
Brown sugar
Cane juice
Confectioner's powdered sugar
Corn sweetener
Corn syrup
Corn syrup solids
Crystal dextrose
Dextrin
Dextrose
Evaporated corn sweetener
Fructose
Fruit juice concentrate
Fruit nectar
Glucose
High-fructose corn syrup
Honey
Invert sugar
Lactose
Liquid fructose
Malt syrup
Maltose
Maple syrup
Molasses
Nectar
Pancake syrup
Raw sugar
Sucrose
Sugar
Sugar cane juice
Trehalose
Turbinado sugar
White granulated sugar

Saturated Fats

The types of fatty acids consumed play a more significant role in health than the amount of fat consumed. "Solid fats" include saturated fats and trans fats. A high intake of saturated fat is associated with increased total and **low-density lipoprotein (LDL)** cholesterol—both of which increase the risk of cardiovascular disease. The *Dietary Guidelines* recommend a diet containing <10% of total calories from saturated fat. Major sources of saturated fat for Americans include full-fat cheese, pizza, grain-based desserts, dairy-based desserts, fried foods, sausage, franks, bacon, and ribs. Evidence suggests that the health benefits are best when saturated fat is replaced with foods higher in polyunsaturated fats and monounsaturated fats, such as most types of vegetable oils. Salmon, tuna, and other fatty fish and many types of nuts and seeds, such as flaxseeds, are high in polyunsaturated fat. The scientific understanding of saturated fats continues to emerge, and there is debate whether or not saturated fats are as harmful to health as was previously believed. With that said, the *Dietary Guidelines* do not hedge and report that strong and consistent evidence shows that replacing saturated fats with polyunsaturated fats is associated with decreased total and LDL cholesterol and decreased risk of cardiovascular events such as heart attacks and cardiovascular disease–related deaths (USDA, 2015). The primary sources of saturated fat for Americans ages 2 and older are shown in Figure 3-9.

Figure 3-9
Food category sources of saturated fats in the U.S. population ages 2 years and older

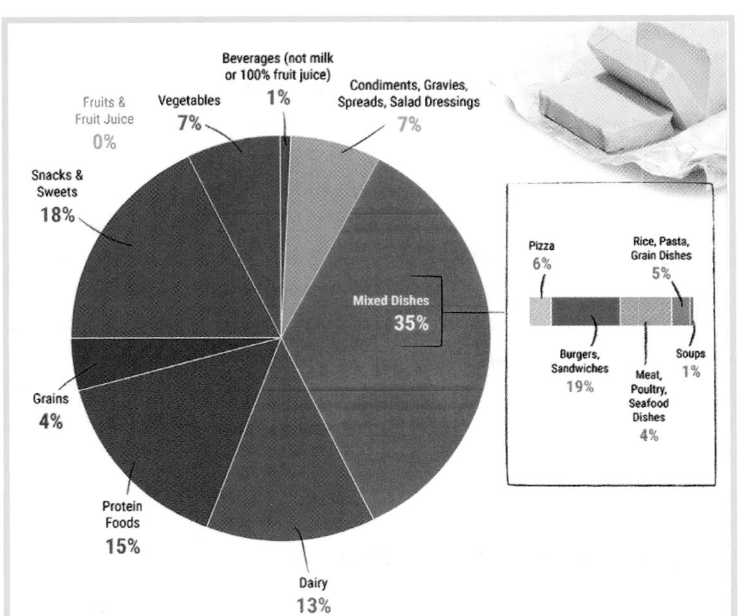

Trans Fats

Trans fats are found naturally in some foods ("ruminant trans fats"), but the majority of intake comes from processed foods ("artificial trans fats"). Artificial trans fats increase LDL cholesterol and contribute to increased cardiovascular disease risk. Trans fats are required by law to be listed on the food label, although foods that contain <0.5 grams of trans fat per serving are allowed to claim "0 grams" of trans fat. Consumers can identify these foods by looking on the ingredient list for the words "partially hydrogenated." Americans should consume as little artificial trans fats as possible.

Sodium and the Dietary Approaches to Stop Hypertension Eating Plan

Sodium intake is associated with blood pressure for most people. Maintaining a normal blood pressure decreases the risk of cardiovascular disease, **congestive heart failure,** and kidney disease. The estimated intake of sodium per day is 3,400 mg, far more than the recommended amount of <2,300 mg for lower-risk populations and 1,500 mg for higher-risk individuals (i.e., those who have **prehypertension** or hypertension—about 50% of adults). In fact, fewer than 15% of Americans meet sodium goals. This is at least in part due to the fact that sodium is ubiquitous in the food supply, especially in canned, processed, and restaurant-prepared dishes. Added table salt also contributes significantly to daily intake. The primary sources of sodium for Americans ages 2 and older are shown in Figure 3-10.

The health and fitness professional can help clients decrease sodium intake with the following advice:

- Read nutrition labels and pay attention to sodium content
- Consume more fresh foods and fewer processed foods
- Eat more home-prepared meals and add little table salt or sodium-containing seasonings
- When eating out, ask that salt not be added
- Reduce calorie intake (since most foods also contain sodium)

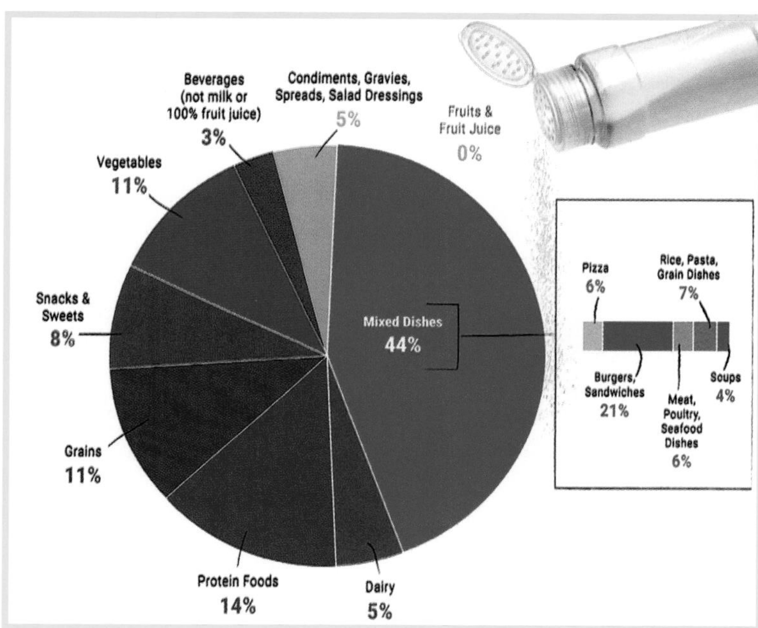

Figure 3-10
Food category sources of sodium in the U.S. population ages 2 years and older

In addition, individuals with hypertension are advised to follow the low-sodium **Dietary Approaches to Stop Hypertension (DASH) eating plan** to optimize health and decrease blood pressure. The DASH eating plan is low in saturated fat, cholesterol, and total fat. The staples are fruits, vegetables, and low-fat dairy products. Fish, poultry, nuts, and other unsaturated fats as well as whole grains are also encouraged. Consequently, it is rich in potassium, magnesium, calcium, protein, and fiber. Red meat, sweets, and sugar-containing beverages are very limited. Thus, it is low in saturated and total fat and cholesterol. The DASH eating plan recommends that men drink 2 or fewer and women drink 1 or fewer alcoholic beverages per day. One drink is equivalent to 12 ounces of beer, 5 ounces of wine, or 1.5 ounces of hard liquor. While developed to reduce blood pressure, the DASH eating plan can be adopted by anyone regardless of whether he or she has elevated blood pressure. In fact, some studies suggest that the eating plan may also reduce cardiovascular disease risk by lowering total cholesterol and LDL cholesterol in addition to lowering blood pressure (reviewed in Eckel et al., 2014). A breakdown of the DASH eating plan by calorie needs is shown in Table 3-8.

The DASH eating plan lowers **systolic blood pressure (SBP)** by about 5 to 6 mmHg and **diastolic blood pressure (DBP)** by 3 mmHg when compared to a typical American diet of the 1990s. This effect on blood pressure holds true across ages, gender, and ethnicity for individuals with blood

Table 3-8
DASH Eating Plan by Calorie Level

The number of daily servings in a food group vary depending on caloric needs[a]

Food Group[b]	1,200 calories	1,400 calories	1,600 calories	1,800 calories	2,000 calories	2,600 calories	3,100 calories	Serving Sizes
Grains	4–5	5–6	6	6	6–8	10–11	12–13	1 slice bread 1 oz dry cereal[c] ½ cup cooked rice, pasta, or cereal[c]
Vegetables	3–4	3–4	3–4	4–5	4–5	5–6	6	1 cup raw leafy vegetable ½ cup cut-up raw or cooked vegetable ½ cup vegetable juice
Fruits	3–4	4	4	4–5	4–5	5–6	6	1 medium fruit ¼ cup dried fruit ½ cup fresh, frozen, or canned fruit ½ cup fruit juice
Fat-free or low-fat milk and milk products	2–3	2–3	2–3	2–3	2–3	3	3–4	1 cup milk or yogurt 1½ oz cheese
Lean meats, poultry, and fish	3 or less	3–4 or less	3–4 or less	6 or less	6 or less	6 or less	6–9	1 oz cooked meats, poultry, or fish 1 egg
Nuts, seeds, and legumes	3 per week	3 per week	3–4 per week	4 per week	4–5 per week	1	1	⅓ cup or 1½ oz nuts 2 Tbsp peanut butter 2 Tbsp or ½ oz seeds ½ cup cooked legumes (dried beans, peas)
Fats and oils	1	1	2	2–3	2–3	3	4	1 tsp soft margarine 1 tsp vegetable oil 1 Tbsp mayonnaise 1 Tbsp salad dressing
Sweets and added sugars	3 or less per week	3 or less per week	3 or less per week	5 or less per week	5 or less per week	<2	<2	1 Tbsp sugar 1 Tbsp jelly or jam ½ cup sorbet, gelatin dessert 1 cup lemonade
Maximum sodium limit[d]	2,300 mg/day	2,300 mg/day	2,300 mg/day	2,300 mg/day	2,300 mg/day	2,300 mg/day	2,300 mg/day	

[a] The DASH eating patterns from 1,200 to 1,800 calories meet the nutritional needs of children 4 to 8 years old. Patterns from 1,600 to 3,100 calories meet the nutritional needs of children 9 years and older and adults. See Table 3-1 for estimated calorie needs per day by age, gender, and physical-activity level.

[b] Significance to DASH Eating Plan, selection notes, and examples of foods in each food group.

- Grains: Major sources of energy and fiber. Whole grains are recommended for most grain servings as a good source of fiber and nutrients. Examples: Whole-wheat bread and rolls; whole-wheat pasta, English muffin, pita bread, bagel, cereals; grits, oatmeal, brown rice; unsalted pretzels and popcorn.
- Vegetables: Rich sources of potassium, magnesium, and fiber. Examples: Broccoli, carrots, collards, green beans, green peas, kale, lima beans, potatoes, spinach, squash, sweet potatoes, tomatoes.
- Fruits: Important sources of potassium, magnesium, and fiber. Examples: Apples, apricots, bananas, dates, grapes, oranges, grapefruit, grapefruit juice, mangoes, melons, peaches, pineapples, raisins, strawberries, tangerines.
- Fat-free or low-fat milk and milk products: Major sources of calcium and protein. Examples: Fat-free milk or buttermilk; fat-free, low-fat, or reduced-fat cheese; fat-free/low-fat regular or frozen yogurt.
- Lean meats, poultry, and fish: Rich sources of protein and magnesium. Select only lean; trim away visible fats; broil, roast, or poach; remove skin from poultry. Since eggs are high in cholesterol, limit egg yolk intake to no more than four per week; two egg whites have the same protein content as 1 oz meat.
- Nuts, seeds, and legumes: Rich sources of energy, magnesium, protein, and fiber. Examples: Almonds, filberts, mixed nuts, peanuts, walnuts, sunflower seeds, peanut butter, kidney beans, lentils, split peas.
- Fats and oils: DASH study had 27 percent of calories as fat, including fat in or added to foods. Fat content changes serving amount for fats and oils. For example, 1 Tbsp regular salad dressing = one serving; 2 Tbsp low-fat dressing = one serving; 1 Tbsp fat-free dressing = zero servings. Examples: Soft margarine, vegetable oil (canola, corn, olive, safflower), low-fat mayonnaise, light salad dressing.
- Sweets and added sugars: Sweets should be low in fat. Examples: Fruit-flavored gelatin, fruit punch, hard candy, jelly, maple syrup, sorbet and ices, sugar.

[c] Serving sizes vary between ½ cup and 1¼ cups, depending on cereal type. Check product's Nutrition Facts label.

[d] The DASH Eating Plan consists of patterns with a sodium limit of 2,300 mg and 1,500 mg per day.

Reprinted from U.S. Department of Agriculture (2010). *2010 Dietary Guidelines for Americans.* www.dietaryguidelines.gov

pressures 120–159/80–95 mmHg (Eckel et al., 2014). Several variations of the DASH eating plan have been studied with even more pronounced results. For example, when 10% of calories from carbohydrates were replaced with an equal number of calories from protein or unsaturated fat, SBP decreased by an additional 1 mmHg compared to the standard eating plan in both hypertensive and nonhypertensive individuals. When looking at only hypertensive individuals, SBP decreases by 3 mmHg compared to the standard DASH eating plan (Eckel et al., 2014).

Note that certain populations, such as individuals participating in intensive physical activity in hot and humid environments, need sufficient sodium intake to replace sodium lost in fluid. The AI for sodium in people nine to 50 years old is 1,500 mg per day and the UL is 2,300 mg per day. Most athletes will meet sodium needs with a sodium intake within this range, although making recommendations regarding the timing and amount of sodium replacement is outside the scope of the *Dietary Guidelines*.

Key Guideline 4: Shift to Healthier Food and Beverage Choices

Choose nutrient-dense foods and beverages across and within all food groups in place of less healthy choices. Consider cultural and personal preferences to make these shifts easier to accomplish and maintain.

While the *Dietary Guidelines* advocate an overall healthy and balanced nutrition pattern that is low in added sugars and sodium, the reality is that most Americans eat nothing like the eating patterns recommended by the *Dietary Guidelines,* as shown in Figure 3-11. By making shifts in dietary patterns, Americans can achieve and maintain a healthy body weight, meet nutrient needs, and decrease the risk of chronic disease.

Overall, the *Dietary Guidelines* advise that Americans shift their eating patterns to:

- Consume more vegetables
- Consume more fruits
- Consume more whole grains, and fewer refined grains
- Consume more dairy products

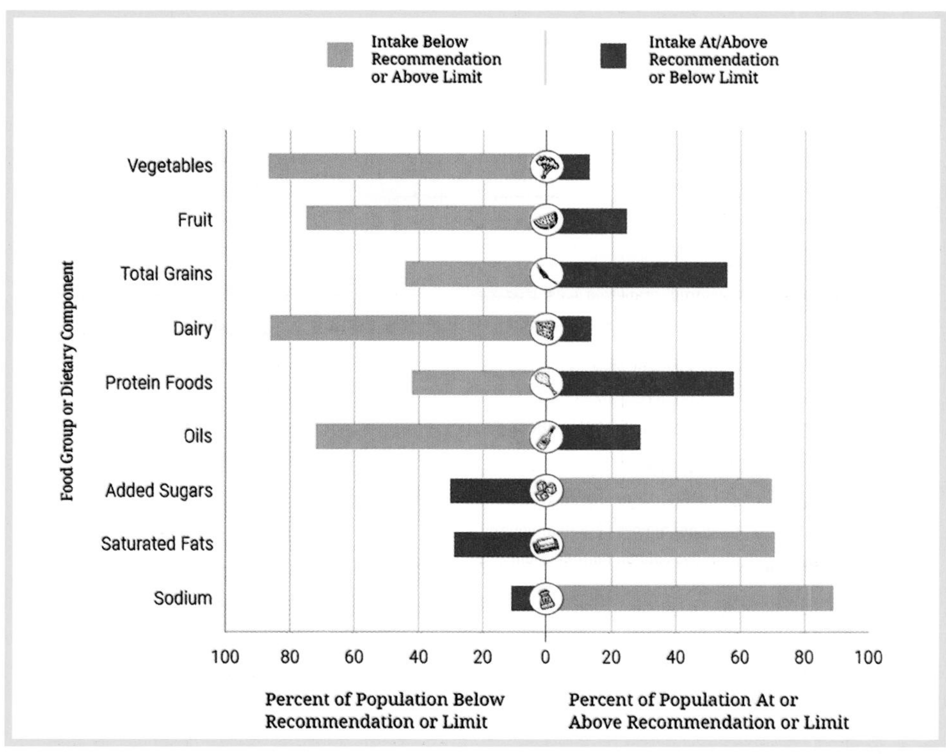

Figure 3-11
Dietary intakes compared to recommendations. Percent of the U.S. population ages 1 year and older who are below, at, or above each dietary goal or limit

- Increase variety in protein food choices and choose more nutrient-dense foods. That is, eat more seafood in place of meat, poultry, or eggs and use legumes or nuts and seeds in mixed dishes instead of some meat or poultry.
- Men and teenage boys should consume less protein, especially meat, poultry, and eggs
- Exchange solid fats for oils
- Reduce added sugar consumption to less than 10% of calories per day
- Reduce saturated fat intake to less than 10% of calories per day
- Reduce sodium intake

Examples of how these shifts might play out in a daily eating plan include:

- Shift from high-calorie snacks (such as tortilla chips with cheese dip) to nutrient-dense snacks (carrots with hummus dip)
- Shift from fruit products with added sugars (fruit-filled cereal bar) to whole fruit (apple)
- Shift from refined grains (white bread) to whole grains (whole-wheat bread)
- Shift from snacks with added sugars (chocolate bar with nuts) to unsalted snacks (unsalted cashews)
- Shift from solid fats (butter in a frying pan) to oils
- Shift from beverages with added sugars (soda) to no-sugar-added beverages (seltzer water)

The *Dietary Guidelines* also note that only 20% of Americans meet the *Physical Activity Guidelines for Americans* (U.S. Department of Health & Human Services, 2008) and 30% engage in no leisure-time physical activity (USDA, 2015). Most people would benefit from shifting screen time and sedentary activities toward increased activity and movement, even if for only 10 minutes at a time.

Key Guideline 5: Support Healthy Eating Patterns for All

Everyone has a role in helping create and support healthy eating patterns in multiple Settings nationwide, from home to school to work to communities.

The *Guidelines* charge all sectors of society to play an active role in the movement to make the United States healthier by developing coordinated partnerships, programs, and policies to support healthy eating. Food and activity behaviors are best viewed in the context of a **socio-ecological model.** The USDA (2015) describes this model as an approach that emphasizes the development of coordinated partnerships, programs, and policies to support healthy eating and active living. In this framework, interventions should extend well beyond providing traditional education to individuals and families about healthy choices, and should help build skills, reshape the environment, and reestablish social norms to facilitate individuals' healthy choices (Figure 3-12).

Health and fitness professionals can best "meet people where they are" to understand individual choices and motivators by paying particular attention to:

- *Food access:* Access to healthy, safe, and affordable food choices is influenced by several factors, including proximity to grocery stores, financial resources, transportation, and neighborhood resources such as average income and availability of public transportation.
- *Household food insecurity:* This occurs when access to nutritious and safe food is limited or uncertain. Food insecurity affects a family's ability to obtain food and make healthy choices and can worsen stress and chronic disease risk.
- *Acculturation:* Acculturation toward a typical American eating plan from what is often a more nutritious eating pattern of the home country. The recommended eating pattern is flexible to accommodate traditional and cultural foods. Individuals and families are encouraged to maintain the healthy eating patterns of their traditional eating and physical-activity patterns and avoid adopting less healthy behaviors (USDA, 2015).

The most effective interventions are multifaceted, using a combination of strategies to

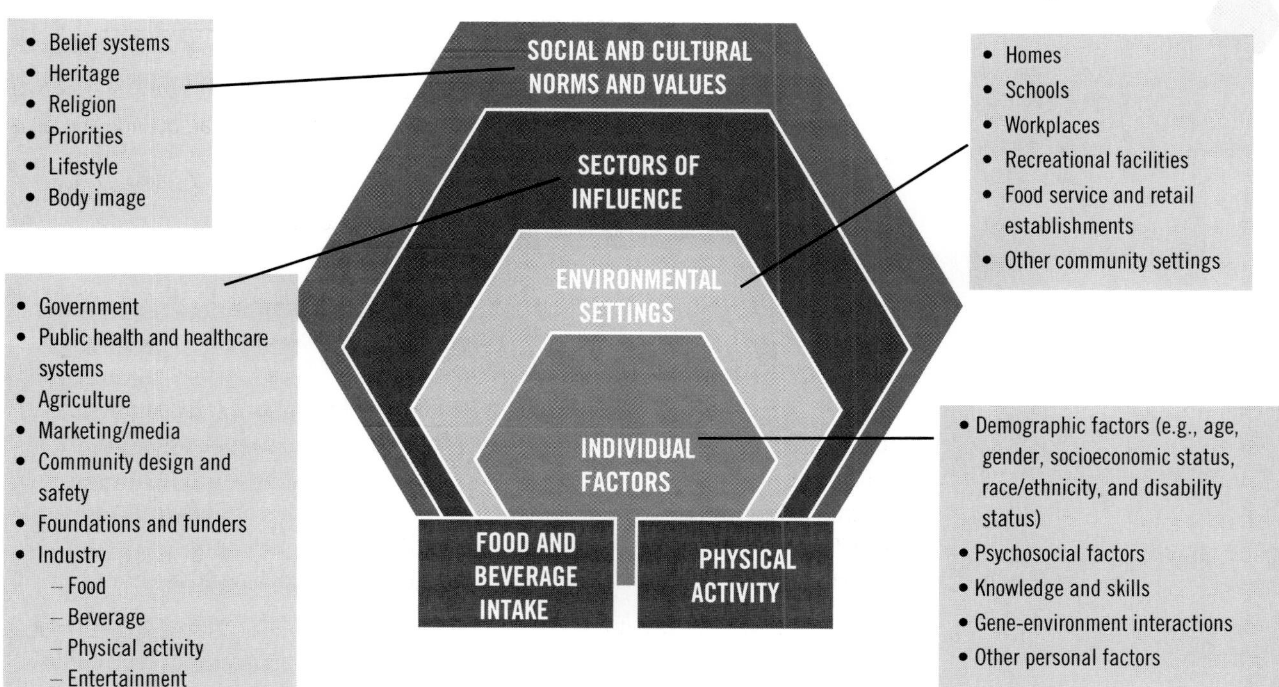

Figure 3-12
Socio-ecological model

impact behavior change, and also multilevel in that they function across the various aspects of the socio-ecological model. An impactful intervention might include a combination of changes across one or more of the below domains:

- *Home:* Develop skills in meal planning and cooking. Limit screen time at home and build in time for family physical activity.
- *School:* Commit to offering only healthy meals and snacks; provide nutrition labels and calorie and nutrient information in cafeterias; reach out to parents about making healthy changes at home; increase the amount and quality of nutrition education and school gardens; commit to support physical-activity programs, high-quality physical education, and active play.
- *Worksite:* Offer health and wellness programs, including nutritional counseling, active breaks, and flexible schedules that allow for physical activity and walking meetings. Provide stand-up desks to decrease sitting time.
- *Community:* Support shelters, food banks, farmers markets, community gardens, and walkable communities.
- *Food retail:* Reach out to consumers about making healthy changes; increase access to healthy and affordable food options.

Several specific strategies health and fitness professionals can employ to help clients make shifts in eating patterns to improve health and more closely resemble the recommended intakes include:

- Help individuals become more aware of the foods and beverages that make up their own or their family's eating patterns and identify areas where they can make small changes such as modifying recipes or food selections.
- Teach skills like gardening, cooking, meal planning, and label reading.
- Suggest ways that individuals can model healthy eating behaviors for friends and family.
- Develop plans to help clients limit screen time and time spent being sedentary and increase physical activity.

A Call to Action

Fitness Nutrition Specialists can play an important role in improving health, both within and outside of individual client encounters, taking into consideration a few guiding principles and action steps.

Guiding Principles	Action Steps	Role of the Fitness Professional
Ensure that all Americans have access to nutritious foods and opportunities for physical activity.	Create strategic plans to achieve *Dietary Guidelines* and *Physical Activity Guidelines* recommendations	Work with local like-minded health professionals to promote a healthier community
	Recognize health disparities and make efforts to ensure access to healthy food and physical activity for all people	Occasionally offer workshops and services in underserved communities
	Expand access to grocery stores, farmers markets, and other outlets for healthy foods	Be a local advocate supporting changes to the built environment
	Develop and expand agricultural practices to ensure availability of healthy food to all people	Advocate for increased access; support school lunch
	Increase food security by promoting nutrition assistance programs	Develop partnerships with local food banks and programs like the Women, Infants, and Children (WIC) program
Facilitate individual behavior change through environmental strategies	Empower individuals and families with improved nutrition literacy, gardening, and cooking skills to heighten enjoyment of preparing and consuming healthy foods	Organize cooking demonstrations Share nutrition handouts and information Participate in a community garden
	Initiate partnerships with food producers, suppliers, and retailers to promote nutritious foods	Build/engage in community partnerships
	Develop legislation, policies, and systems in key sectors, including healthcare, school, and recreation/fitness	Be part of community health collaboratives Offer after-school nutrition and activity programs Advocate for health-promoting policies
	Support future research to identify best practices to contribute to the adoption of healthy eating and physical activity	Stay abreast of the latest research pertaining to nutrition and activity
	Implement the U.S. National Physical Activity Plan to increase physical activity	Continue to promote and support physical activity

Guiding Principles	Action Steps	Role of the Fitness Professional
Set the stage for lifelong healthy eating, physical activity, and weight-management behaviors.	Ensure that all meals and snacks served and sold in schools and childcare are consistent with the *Dietary Guidelines*	Join a school health advisory committee Advocate for healthy snacks at children's after-school and extracurricular programs
	Provide comprehensive health, nutrition, and physical-education programs in educational settings. Place special emphasis on food-preparation skills, food safety, and lifelong physical activity	Expand fitness services to include children and adolescents. Include nutrition information
	Identify approaches for assessing and tracking children's body mass index for use by health professionals	Consider assessing body composition or referring children to their physician for a physical and body mass index measurement at the onset of programs
	Encourage physical activity in schools, childcare, and early childhood settings through physical education programs, recess, and support for a walk-to-school program	Volunteer at schools to promote physical activity Advocate
	Reduce children's screen time	Avoid TV in waiting rooms and lobbies at fitness facilities, especially in areas intended for children
	Develop and support effective policies to limit food and beverage marketing to children	Restrict access to advertisements to one's own children, promote media literacy
	Support children's programs that promote healthy nutrition and physical activity throughout the year	Get involved with youth nutrition and physical-activity programs

Source: U.S. Department of Agriculture (2010). *2010 Dietary Guidelines for Americans.* www.health.gov/dietaryguidelines/2010/

FOOD LABELS

For people to make healthy nutrition decisions, they first have to be able to understand which nutrients contribute to a healthy diet, and second, know which foods contain those nutrients. While the bulk of a healthy diet is made up of whole, unprocessed foods that do not carry food labels, there are processed or prepared foods (e.g., low-fat milk and milk products) that can be part of a healthy diet and do have food labels. The food label, a required component of nearly all packaged foods, can help people turn knowledge into action. It can also be a source of confusion and misunderstanding.

History and Present State of Food Labeling

It was not until the early 1970s, when consumers faced a boon in production of processed foods, that nutrition labels were included on packaged foods. As an increasing number of foods arrived on grocery store shelves, many of which made nutrition claims, the Food and Drug Administration (FDA) proposed regulations in 1972 to require food labels on packaged foods that added nutrients or made nutrition claims. The labels would be voluntary for foods without claims. The first nutrition labels contained basic nutrition information, including calories, protein, carbohydrate, and fat, as well as the RDA for protein and several vitamins and minerals. Inclusion of sodium, saturated fatty acids, and polyunsaturated fatty acids was optional (Food and Nutrition Board, 2010).

As more products arrived on shelves and consumers became increasingly interested in reviewing food labels, food manufacturers responded with a plethora of ambiguous claims touting nutritional value and health benefits, even though FDA regulations had long prohibited mention of disease or health on food labels. Though companies could not explicitly state or imply that a food's nutrient properties could help to prevent, cure, or treat any disease or symptom, ambiguous nutrition claims designed to catch consumers' attention (such as "extremely low in saturated fat") became commonplace. The FDA policy helped to protect consumers against potentially harmful claims. However, it also limited manufacturers' ability to advertise the benefits of foods that provided legitimate health benefits, such as foods that were high in fiber. In 1984, the National Cancer Institute and Kellogg's launched a food-labeling campaign on a high-fiber cereal box linking the high-fiber intake to a possible reduction in some cancers. In the absence of regulatory action, other food manufacturers followed suit, leading to a frenzy of nutrition and health claims on food labels (Food and Nutrition Board, 2010).

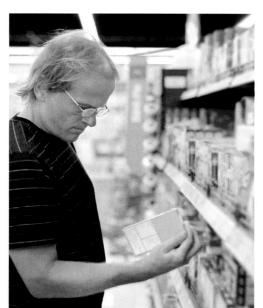

In 1990, congress passed the Nutrition Labeling and Education Act (NLEA), which gave the FDA the authority to require nutrition labeling on most food packages and specified the information and nutrients that must be included on the label. It also required specific criteria for approved health claims. The FDA's stated goal in developing the label criteria was to (1) minimize confusion, (2) help consumers choose healthier diets, and (3) provide an incentive to companies to improve the nutritional value of their products. The Nutrition Facts panel with which most of today's consumers are familiar was mandated in 1993. Though trans fats were not initially included on the nutrition label, their inclusion was required by 2003 if the product contained more than 0.5 grams of trans fat per serving. This regulation drastically decreased the amount of trans fats used in food production (Food and Nutrition Board, 2010).

Serving Sizes

The NLEA required that serving sizes reported on the nutrition label be based on "amounts customarily consumed" rather than recommended portion sizes or a standard amount, such as 100 grams. Though the FDA attempted to standardize serving sizes and ensure that similar products indicate servings in similar sizes, the serving sizes used on many foods continue to be a source of confusion. This is especially true for single-serving containers. FDA regulations allowed that, in certain cases, food manufacturers could choose whether or not to divide the contents into more than one serving. For example, a bag of chips that could reasonably be consumed in one sitting could be labeled as one serving or two servings. If consumers were not careful to review the number of "servings per container," they may mistakenly believe that the nutritional information on the label applied to the whole bag, rather than just half. In 2005, the FDA considered changing regulations so that nutrition information pertains to the entire package of a food that could reasonably be consumed in one sitting (Food and Nutrition Board, 2010). While this has long been under discussion, no significant changes have been made to date.

Health Claims

The issue of whether or not to allow health claims was also addressed by the NLEA. Claims that can be used on food and dietary supplement labels include **health claims, nutrient content claims,** and **structure/function claims.**

Health claims describe a relationship between a food or food component and the prevention or treatment of a disease or health-related condition. To be included on a nutrition label, health claims must be authorized by the FDA or be based on an authoritative statement of a scientific body of the federal government or the National Academies of Science, after notification to the FDA. A listing of currently allowed health claims is available at www.fda.gov/Food/GuidanceRegulation/GuidanceDocumentsRegulatoryInformation/LabelingNutrition/ucm064919.htm.

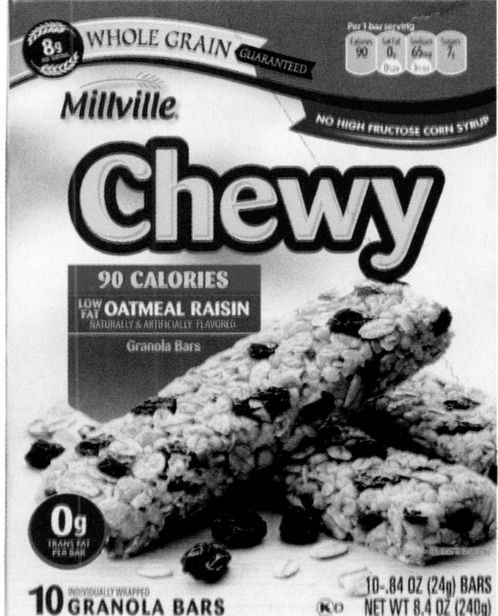

Qualified health claims are allowed on product labels if there is emerging evidence for a relationship between a food or food component and decreased risk of a disease or health condition, but the scientific evidence is not conclusive. The statement must include a qualifying statement saying that the evidence supporting the claim is limited.

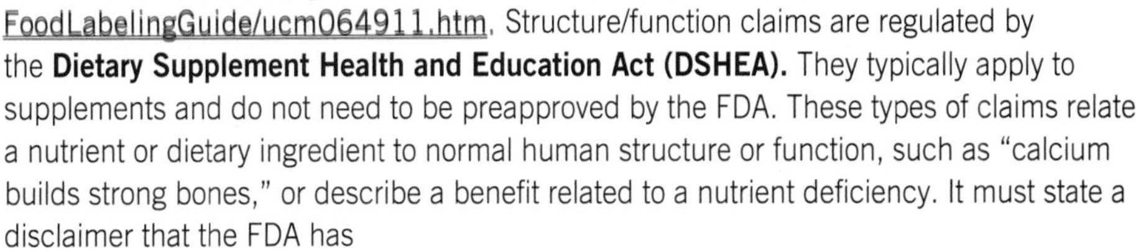

Nutrient content claims imply health benefits by describing the level of a nutrient in a product using terms like "free," "high," or "low," or compared to another product using terms like "more," "reduced," and "lite." A product can be labeled as "healthy" if it has "healthy" levels of total fat, saturated fat, cholesterol, and sodium. A listing of nutrient content claims is available at www.fda.gov/Food/GuidanceRegulation/GuidanceDocumentsRegulatoryInformation/LabelingNutrition/FoodLabelingGuide/ucm064911.htm. Structure/function claims are regulated by the **Dietary Supplement Health and Education Act (DSHEA).** They typically apply to supplements and do not need to be preapproved by the FDA. These types of claims relate a nutrient or dietary ingredient to normal human structure or function, such as "calcium builds strong bones," or describe a benefit related to a nutrient deficiency. It must state a disclaimer that the FDA has

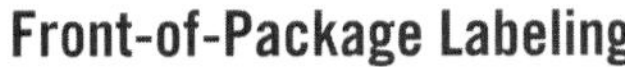

not evaluated the claim and that the supplement is not intended to treat, cure, or prevent any disease.

Front-of-Package Labeling

Since 1987, when the American Heart Association first developed the "Heart Guide Initiative" to tag foods that were the most heart healthy, organizations from PepsiCo and General Mills to grocery stores, nonprofits, and academic groups have implemented front-of-package (FOP) labeling to communicate with consumers. While intended to help consumers make healthier choices, the multiple and varied labels have been confusing and in many cases misleading. This issue came to public attention in 2009 when a popular sugar-sweetened cereal, along with macaroni and cheese, ice cream, and fruit roll-ups, were given a SmartChoice FOP label. In anticipation of potential regulation on FOP labeling systems, Congress mandated the IOM to develop a two-part report on FOP labeling. These reports were published in 2010 (www.nap.edu/catalog.php?record_id=12957) and 2011 (www.nationalacademies.org/hmd/Reports/2011/Front-of-Package-Nutrition-Rating-Systems-and-Symbols-Promoting-Healthier-Choices.aspx) (Food and Nutrition Board, 2011; Food and Nutrition Board, 2010). The IOM committee concluded that "It is time for a fundamental shift in strategy, a move away from systems that mostly provide nutrition information without clear guidance about its healthfulness, and toward one that encourages healthier food choices through simplicity, visual clarity, and the ability to convey meaning without written information. An FOP system should be standardized and it also should motivate food and beverage companies to reformulate their products to be healthier and encourage food retailers to prominently display products that meet this standard" (Food andNutrition Board, 2011).

The report advised a labeling system that is based on calories, saturated and trans fat, sugar, and salt. As of the time of this writing, no action has been taken.

Improvement and issues in food labels continues to be an ongoing process. In addition to considering FOP labeling, the FDA also has requested public input on increasing the prominence of calories on nutrition labels, amending serving-size regulations, and establishing new reference values.

EXPAND YOUR KNOWLEDGE

Highlights of New Proposed Rules for Food Labels

The FDA has issued two proposed approaches for new rules governing food labels. The first approach addresses new scientific information and design changes. The second addresses revised serving-size requirements, as well as criteria for labeling based on package size, among other issues. Major proposed changes can be grouped into three categories:

- Changes based on new nutrition science
- Updated serving size requirements and labeling for certain packages
- Refreshed design

For more information on these upcoming changes, visit the FDA's website: www.fda.gov/Food/GuidanceRegulation/GuidanceDocumentsRegulatoryInformation/LabelingNutrition/ucm387533.htm.

Reading the Nutrition Label

While the nutrition label provides a large amount of useful nutrition information, it can also be a source of confusion for many consumers. A health and fitness professional can play an important role in helping consumers effectively use the nutrition label to guide them in making healthy choices.

A Stepwise Approach

A health and fitness professional can advise individuals to dissect the food label (Figure 3-13) by taking a stepwise approach. Start from the top with the serving size and the number of servings per container. In general, serving sizes are standardized so that consumers can compare similar products. All of the nutrient amounts listed on the food label are for one serving, so it is important to determine how many servings are actually being consumed to accurately assess nutrient intake.

Serving Size
The label presents serving sizes as the amount that most people actually consume in a sitting. This is not necessarily the same as how much one should eat per serving. All of the nutrition information on the label is based on one serving. If you eat one-half of the serving size shown here, cut the nutrient and calorie values in half.

Total Fat
Fat is calorie-dense and, if consumed in large portions, can increase the risk of weight problems. While once vilified, most fat, in and of itself, is not bad.

Cholesterol
Many foods that are high in cholesterol are also high in saturated fat, which can contribute to heart disease. Dietary cholesterol itself likely does not cause health problems.

Sodium
You call it "salt," the label calls it "sodium." Either way, it may add up to high blood pressure in some people. So, keep your sodium intake low—less than 2,300 mg each day. (The American Heart Association recommends no more than 3,000 mg of sodium per day for healthy adults.)

Sugars
Too much sugar contributes to weight gain and increased risk of diseases like diabetes and fatty liver disease. Foods like fruits and dairy products contain natural sugars (fructose and lactose), but also may contain added sugars. It is best to consume no more than 10% of total calories from added sugar, or a total of 50 g per day based on a 2,000-calorie eating plan.

Vitamins and Minerals
Your goal here is 100% of each for the day. Don't count on one food to do it all. Let a combination of foods add up to a winning score.

Nutrition Facts

4 Servings Per Container
Serving Size **1/2 cup (114g)**

Amount Per Serving
Calories **90**

	% Daily Value*
Total Fat 3g	**5%**
Saturated Fat 0g	**0%**
Trans Fat 0g	**0%**
Cholesterol 0mg	**0%**
Sodium 300mg	**13%**
Total Carbohydrate 13g	**4%**
Dietary Fiber 3g	**12%**
Total Sugars 12g	
Includes 10g Added Sugars	**20%**
Protein 3g	
Vitamin D 2mcg	10%
Calcium 260mg	20%
Iron 8mg	45%
Potassium 235mg	6%

* The % Daily Value (DV) tells you how much a nutrient in a serving of food contributes to a daily diet. 2,000 calories a day is used for general nutrition advice.

Daily Value
Daily Values are listed based on a 2,000-calorie daily eating plan. Your calorie and nutrient needs may be a little bit more or less based on your age, sex, and activity level (see https://fnic.nal.usda.gov/fnic/interactiveDRI/). For saturated fat, sugars and added sugars, and sodium, choose foods with a low % Daily Value. For dietary fiber, vitamins, and minerals, your Daily Value goal is to reach 100% of each.

Ingredients: *This portion of the label lists all of the foods and additives contained in a product, in order from the most prevalent ingredient to the least.*

Allergens: *This portion of the label identifies which of the most common allergens may be present in the product.*

(More nutrients may be listed on some labels)

mg = milligrams (1,000 mg = 1 g)
g = grams (about 28 g = 1 ounce)

Calories
Are you trying to lose weight? Cut back a little on calories. Look here to see how a serving of the food adds to your daily total. A 5'4", 138-lb active woman needs about 2,200 calories each day. A 5'10", 174-lb active man needs about 2,900.

Saturated Fat
Saturated fat is part of the total fat in food. It is listed separately because it is an important player in raising blood cholesterol and your risk of heart disease. Eat less!

Trans Fat
Trans fat works a lot like saturated fat, except it is worse. This fat starts out as a liquid unsaturated fat, but then food manufacturers add some hydrogen to it, turning it into a solid saturated fat (that is what "partially hydrogenated" means when you see it in the food ingredients). They do this to increase the shelf-life of the product, but in the body the trans fat damages the blood vessels and contributes to increasing blood cholesterol and the risk of heart disease.

Total Carbohydrate
Carbohydrates are in foods like bread, potatoes, fruits, and vegetables, as well as processed foods. Carbohydrate is further broken down into dietary fiber and sugars. Consume foods high in fiber often and those high in sugars, especially added sugars, less often.

Dietary Fiber
Grandmother called it "roughage," but her advice to eat more is still up-to-date! That goes for both soluble and insoluble kinds of dietary fiber. Fruits, vegetables, whole-grain foods, beans, and peas are all good sources and can help reduce the risk of heart disease and cancer.

Protein
Most Americans get more than they need. Eat small servings of lean meat, fish, and poultry. Use skim or low-fat milk, yogurt, and cheese. Try vegetable proteins like beans, grains, and cereals.

Figure 3-13
Nutrition facts label

Next, consumers should look at the total calories. The total calories indicate how much energy a person gets from a particular food. Americans tend to consume too many calories, and too many calories from fat, without meeting daily nutrient requirements. This part of the nutrition label is the most important factor for weight control. In general, 40 calories per serving is considered low, 100 calories is moderate, and 400 or more calories is considered high [U.S. Food & Drug Administration (FDA), 2004].

The next two sections of the label note the nutrient content of the food product. Consumers should try to minimize intake of fat (especially saturated and trans fat), sugars, and sodium and aim to consume adequate amounts of fiber, as well as vitamins and minerals, especially vitamin A, vitamin C, calcium, and iron. The food label includes the total amount of sugars (natural and added). Though the label does not separately identify added sugars and specifies the amount of added sugars.

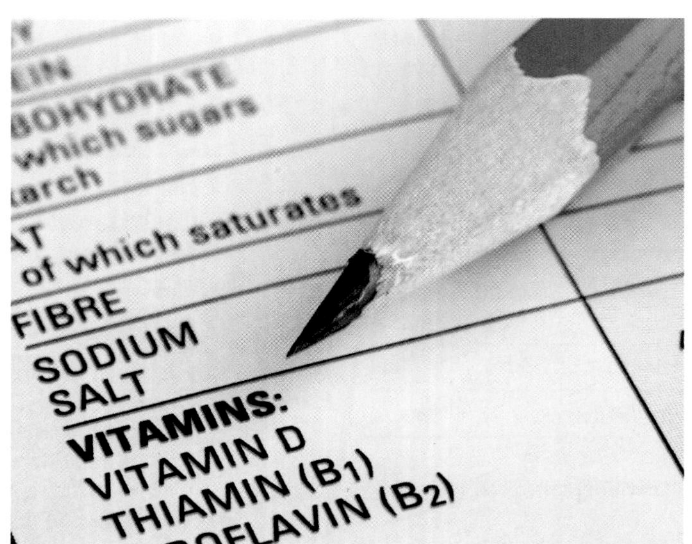

The **percent daily values (PDV)** are listed for key nutrients to make it easier to compare products (just make sure that the serving sizes are similar), evaluate nutrient content claims (does 1/3 reduced-sugar cereal really contain less carbohydrate than a similar cereal of a different brand?), and make informed dietary tradeoffs (e.g., balance consumption of a high-fat product for lunch with lower-fat products throughout the rest of the day). In general, 5% daily value or less is considered low, while 20% daily value or more is considered high (FDA, 2004).

The footnote at the bottom of the label reminds consumers that all PDV are based on a 2,000-calorie diet. Individuals who need more or fewer calories should adjust recommendations accordingly. For example, 3 grams of fat provides 5% of the recommended amount for someone on a 2,000-calorie diet, but 7% for someone on a 1,500-calorie diet. The footnote also includes daily values for nutrients to limit (total fat, saturated fat, trans fat, and sodium), recommended carbohydrate intake for a 2,000-calorie diet (60% of calories), and minimal fiber recommendations for 2,000- and 2,500-calorie diets, as well as total fat and cholesterol.

Legislation also requires food manufacturers to list all potential food **allergens** on food packaging. The most common food allergens are fish, shellfish, soybean, wheat, egg, milk, peanuts, and tree nuts. This information usually is included near the list of ingredients on the package. Clearly, this information is especially important to clients with food allergies. For clients who follow a gluten-free diet, this is also an easy way to identify if wheat is a product ingredient.

Carefully review the ingredients list. Note that the ingredient list is in decreasing order of substance weight in the product. That is, the ingredients that are listed first are the most abundant ingredients in the product. The ingredient list is useful to help identify whether or not the product contains trans fat, solid fats, added sugars, whole grains, and refined grains.

- *Trans fat:* Although trans fat is included in the "fat" section of the nutrition label, if the product contains <0.5 grams per serving, the manufacturer does not need to claim it. However, if a product contains "partially hydrogenated oils," then the product contains trans fat.
- *Solid fats:* If the ingredient list contains beef fat, butter, chicken fat, coconut oil, cream, hydrogenated oils, palm kernel oils, pork fat (lard), shortening, or stick margarine, then the product contains solid fats.

- *Added sugars:* Ingredients signifying added sugars are listed in Table 3-6. In many cases, products contain multiple forms of sugar.
- *Whole grains:* To be considered 100% whole grain, the product must contain all of the essential parts of the original kernel—the bran, germ, and endosperm. When choosing products, the whole grain should be the first or second ingredient. Examples of whole grains include brown rice, buckwheat, bulgur (cracked wheat), millet, oatmeal, popcorn, quinoa, rolled oats, whole-grain sorghum, whole-grain triticale, whole-grain barley, whole-grain corn, whole oats/oatmeal, whole rye, whole wheat, and wild rice.
- *Refined grains:* Refined grains are listed as "enriched." If the first ingredient is an enriched grain, then the product is not a whole grain. This is one way to understand whether or not a "wheat bread" is actually whole wheat or a refined product.

DO THE MATH

Nutrition Label Sample Problem

Using the nutrition label from Figure 3-13, determine (1) the number of calories per container; (2) the calories from carbohydrate, protein, and fat per serving; and (3) the percentage of calories from carbohydrate, protein, and fat.

- 90 calories per serving x 4 servings per container = 360 calories per container
- *Carbohydrate:* 13 grams carbohydrate per serving x 4 calories per gram = 52 calories per serving from carbohydrate

  Protein: 3 grams protein per serving x 4 calories per gram = 12 calories per serving from protein

  Fat: 3 grams fat per serving x 9 calories per gram = 27 calories per serving from fat

[*Note:* The nutrition label does these calculations for you and lists the calories from fat on the label. On this label, it states that the product contains the rounded number 30 calories from fat vs. the calculated 27 calories from fat. Also note that the total calories is 91 per the calculations but the label rounds to 90.]

- *Carbohydrate:* 52 calories from carbohydrate/91 calories = 57% carbohydrate

  Protein: 12 calories from protein/91 calories = 13% protein

  Fat: 27 calories from fat/91 calories = 30%

FOOD SAFETY AND SELECTION

An important but often underestimated key to healthy eating is to avoid foods contaminated with harmful bacteria, viruses, parasites, and other microorganisms. About one in six Americans, or 48 million people, become sick each year from foodborne illness, 128,000 are hospitalized, and approximately 3,000 die (Centers for Disease Control and Prevention, 2011). Special populations most at risk include pregnant women, infants and young children, older adults, and people who are immunocompromised. The majority of foodborne illnesses are preventable with a few simple precautions (Table 3-9). Refer to www.fightbac.org, www.foodsafety.gov, or www.cdc.gov/foodsafety for more information.

Advise clients to follow these tips while grocery shopping to reduce the risk of foodborne illness:

- Check produce for bruises, and feel and smell for ripeness.

- Look for a "sell-by" date for breads and baked goods, a "use-by" date on some packaged foods, an "expiration date" on yeast and baking powder, and a "packaged date" on canned and some packaged foods.
- Make sure packaged goods are not torn and cans are not dented, cracked, or bulging.
- Separate fish and poultry from other purchases by wrapping them separately in plastic bags.
- Pick up refrigerated and frozen foods last. Try to make sure all perishable items are refrigerated within one hour of purchase.

Table 3-9
Steps to Safe Food Handling

TO AVOID MICROBIAL FOODBORNE ILLNESS:
• Clean hands, food contact surfaces, and fruits and vegetables. Meat and poultry should not be washed or rinsed.
• Separate raw, cooked, and ready-to-eat foods while shopping, preparing, or storing foods.
• Cook foods to a safe temperature to kill microorganisms [bacteria grow most rapidly between the temperatures of 40 and 140° F (4 and 60° C)]. Pregnant women should eat only certain deli meats and frankfurters that have been reheated to steaming hot.
• Refrigerate perishable food promptly (within two hours) and defrost foods properly. Eat refrigerated leftovers within three or four days.
• Avoid raw (unpasteurized) milk or any products made from unpasteurized milk, raw or partially cooked eggs, or foods containing raw eggs, raw or undercooked meat and poultry, unpasteurized juice, and raw sprouts. This is especially important for infants and young children, pregnant women, older adults, and those who are immunocompromised.

Reprinted from United States Department of Agriculture (2015). *2015-2020 Dietary Guidelines for Americans* (8th ed.). www.health.gov/dietaryguidelines

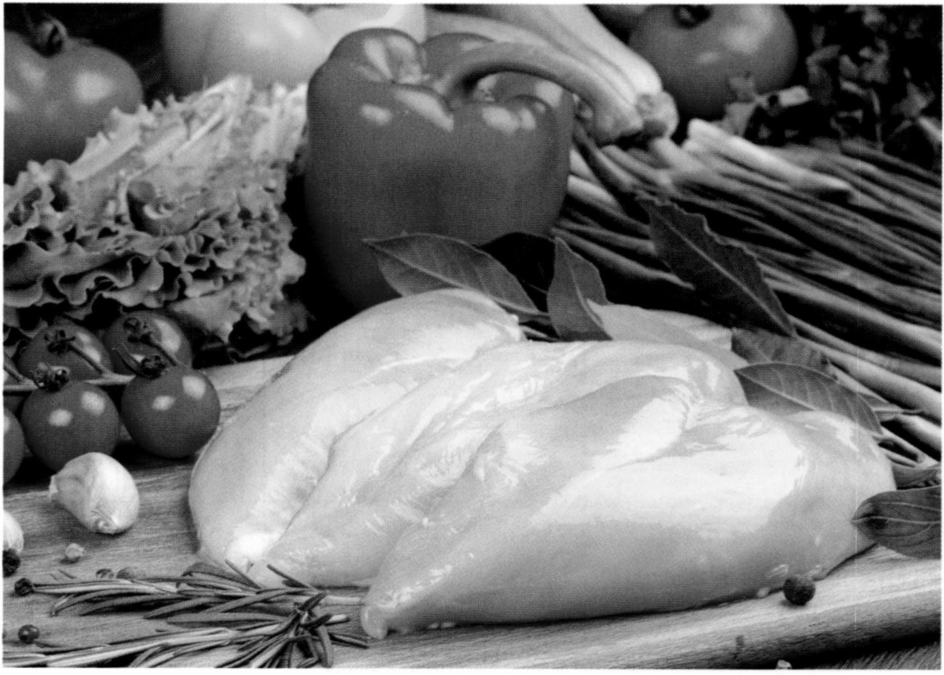

NUTRITION POLICY

Nutrition policy—from the *Dietary Guidelines* and MyPlate to ordinances and regulations that shape food choices and sales—play an important role in setting the stage for Americans to adopt a healthier lifestyle.

In an effort to improve nutrition and activity habits in Americans, countless health professionals, including nutrition and fitness experts, have focused on inspiring healthful change one individual at a time. Unfortunately, adherence to healthful eating habits and regular physical-activity programs has been poor. This is not necessarily due to a lack of willpower and motivation, but more so to an environment that discourages many health-promoting behaviors. Consider the following: there are 3,800 calories available in the food supply for each person daily (the average American needs only 2,350); most Americans eat at least one-third of their calories away from home; and 90% of Saturday morning cartoon food ads—watched by highly impressionable kids—are for sugar- and fat-laden junk food (Center for Science in the Public Interest, 2009). Modern conveniences such as remote controls, elevators, car washes, washing machines, leaf blowers, and drive-through windows reduce caloric expenditure for the average person by about 8,800 calories per month, which adds up to about 2.5 pounds of fat (Blair & Nichaman, 2002).

Several proposals have been suggested, and in some cases implemented, to help improve nutrition and physical-activity behaviors among Americans. A commentary published in the *Journal of the American Medical Association* outlined several policy strategies that may be effective in helping to reduce obesity rates and improve health (Gostin, 2007):

- *Taxation—Imposing higher taxes on calorie-dense and nutrient-poor foods might lower consumption of unhealthy foods and generate revenue to subsidize healthful foods.* Politicians have long debated whether adding an "obesity tax" on non-diet sodas and quasi-fruit drinks might generate tax revenue and decrease unhealthy habits.
- *Food prohibitions—Removing harmful ingredients from the food supply eliminates their health risk.* New York City was the first U.S. city to impose a trans-fat ban in all restaurants. Soon after, other cities and states followed suit. Now very few chain restaurants use trans fat. New York City also was the first to ban the sale of sugary beverages in containers larger than 16 ounces, though the legality of this ban is still being debated.

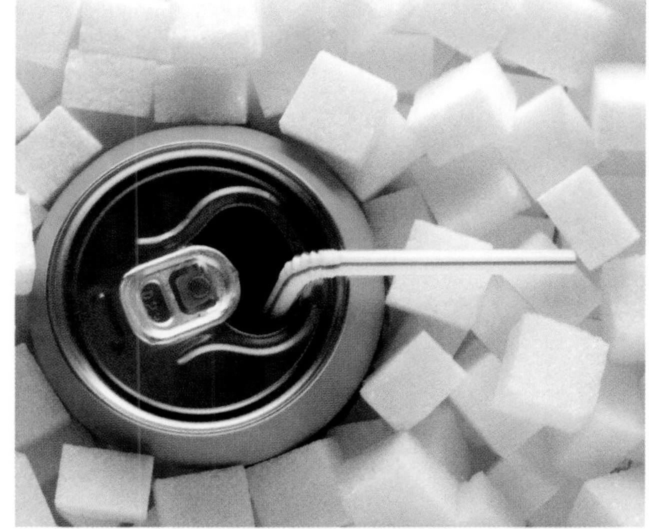

- *Regulation of food marketing to children and adolescents—Restricting food advertising during children's programs, counter-advertising to promote good nutrition and physical activity, limiting use of cartoon characters, and other regulations may help protect children who are unable to critically evaluate advertisements.* The role of food advertisements in the epidemic of childhood obesity has been well studied (U.S. Federal Trade Commission, 2013; Hingle & Kunkel, 2012). The charge to eliminate unhealthy food ads in children's programming has been a source of ongoing debate, with very little progress.
- *School policies—Many school districts already have removed vending machines, provided healthier menus, and offered more physical-activity opportunities for school children.* In 2012, the new school lunch requirements from the Healthy Hunger-Free Kids Act of 2010 were implemented, requiring increased fruits, vegetables, and whole

grains in the school lunch. Also in 2012, the school fitness standards were changed to reflect an emphasis on health rather than athletic performance. Ultimately, the task of getting the school nutrition and activity environment in line with the government recommendations for optimal health is underway but still incomplete.

- *The "built" environment—Zoning laws to limit the number of fast-food restaurants, expand recreational facilities, and encourage healthier lifestyles would increase the ability for people to live and play healthfully, especially in poor neighborhoods where access to parks and healthy foods is severely limited.* As zoning and development are under the jurisdiction of local governments, individual community members and leaders must act to change from an environment that fosters poor diet and inactivity to one that fosters a healthy lifestyle and sense of community. Many cities are paying increased attention to the "built environment" and ways to promote walking and biking.

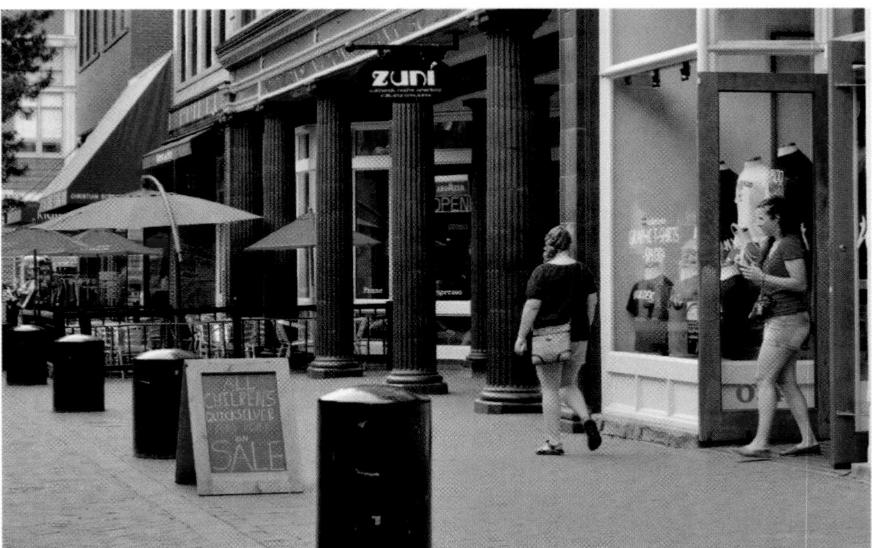

- *Disclosure—Restaurants and manufacturers could be required to disclose nutritional content and health warnings so that consumers may make more informed decisions.* The Affordable Care Act requires restaurants to provide calorie counts and nutritional information on restaurant menus and menu boards. Soon vending machines may also have to post this information.
- *Tort liability—Lawsuits against companies such as fast-food giants for selling "unreasonably hazardous" products might force companies to offer healthier alternatives and provide accurate information.* Legal and financial repercussions may also inspire some large food giants to be more discriminating in their health claims. Since 2002, the FDA has allowed "qualified health claims" (claims linking a food substance to prevention of a disease) on food labels for products that have a basis of scientific evidence to support the claim. While many food companies push the limits, several have received sanctioning letters from the FDA. Companies may also inappropriately use structure-function claims in promoting a food's benefits. For example, the Federal Trade Commission (FTC) sanctioned Kellogg's, first for claiming that Frosted Mini-Wheats™ was "clinically shown to improve kids' attentiveness by 20 percent" and then later for claiming that Rice Krispies cereal "now helps support your child's immunity." Increased authority of the FDA and FTC to regulate nutrition claims would go a long way in helping consumers to make more informed purchasing decisions.

- *Surveillance—Similar to how health departments monitor infectious disease, states could monitor chronic diseases such as diabetes.* New York City has led the way in adopting surveillance measures to monitor the health and nutrition status of its residents. The New York City Health and Nutrition Examination Survey (NYC HANES) randomly sampled NYC residents to undergo a physical examination, clinical and laboratory tests, and interview. Results revealed that the prevalence of **diabetes** and **prediabetes** is higher than expected, with more than one-third of New Yorkers with abnormal glucose levels. In an effort to further improve surveillance and management of diabetes, the New York City A1c Registry was started. The Registry collects hemoglobin A1c results (a measure of blood sugar control) from city laboratories, sends quarterly reports of patients' A1c level to their providers, and reminds patients to follow up with their providers.

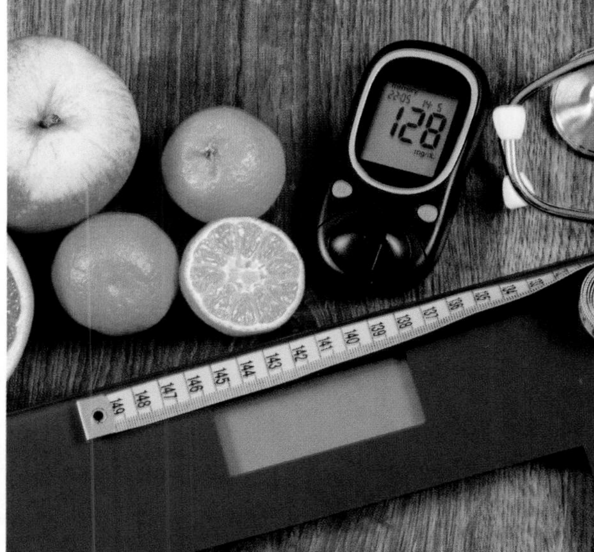

- *"Training" communities*—A commentary published in the *Journal of the American Medical Association* offers three strategies to better treat communities: consider individuals within the larger social, economic, and cultural context; form partnerships; and influence larger political and policy debates. Interventions that focus on changing physical-activity behavior through building, strengthening, and maintaining social networks within communities are highly effective in increasing physical activity and overall physical fitness (Task Force on Community Preventive Services, 2002).

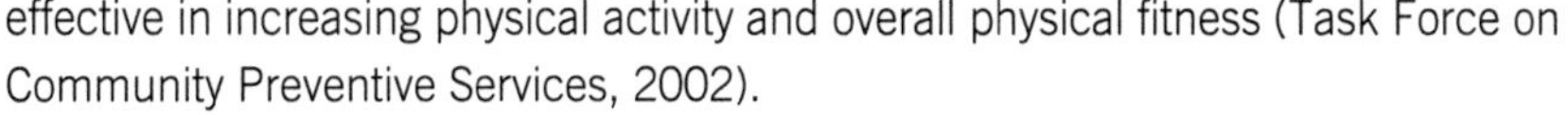

The ACE Fitness Nutrition Specialist is ideally positioned to inspire lasting improvements in health. Efforts that extend beyond working with individuals to incorporate social, community, environmental, and political change will go a long way in helping to make a physically active lifestyle the norm.

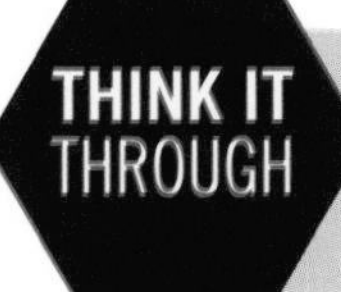

Do you have a strong desire to help shape the way nutrition policy is adopted and accepted by the American public? Based on what you have learned about how nutrition policy is developed, do you have any ideas that might influence social, community, environmental, or political change?

SUMMARY

State and federal governments play a large role in researching and understanding The major components of an optimal diet, promoting an optimal eating plan, developing food policy agendas, regulating the safety and quality of food available, and funding nutritional programs. A thorough understanding of state and federal dietary recommendations and policies offers the ACE Fitness Nutrition Specialist a basis from which to make general nutrition recommendations while staying within professional scope of practice.

While much of the buzz around nutrition often relates to individual ingredients or a proportion of calories from carbohydrates, proteins, and fats, the *Dietary Guidelines* emphasize a movement away from specific nutrients toward an overall healthy eating pattern based on food groups. Health and fitness professionals are ideally positioned not only to support and spread this message, but also to use the meal-planning tools and tips available, such as MyPlate and Supertracker, to help clients translate recommendations into real and practical nutrition changes.

Ultimately, by having a firm understanding of the *Dietary Guidelines* and its associated tools, health and fitness professionals can incorporate high-quality nutrition coaching based upon these resources into their work while simultaneously staying within scope of practice and maximizing impact.

REFERENCES

Blair, S.N. & Nichaman, M.Z. (2002). The public health problem of increasing prevalence rates of obesity and what should be done about it. *Mayo Clinic Proceedings,* 77, 2, 109–113.

Centers for Disease Control and Prevention (2015). *Folic Acid & Birth Defects.* www.cdc.gov/features/folicacidbenefits/index.html

Center for Science in the Public Interest (2009). *Why It's Hard to Eat Well and Be Active in America Today.* Retrieved October 27, 2012: www.cspinet.org/nutritionpolicy/food_advertising.html

Centers for Disease Control and Prevention (2011). *CDC Estimates of Foodborne Illness in the United States.* www.cdc.gov/foodborneburden/PDFs/FACTSHEET_A_FINDINGS_updated4-13.pdf

Eckel R.H. et al. (2014). 2013 AHA/ACC guideline on lifestyle management to reduce cardiovascular risk: A report of the American College of Cardiology/American Heart Association Task Force on Practice Guidelines. *Journal of the American College of Cardiology,* 63, 25 Pt B, 2960–2984.

Environmental Protection Agency (2000). *The Occurrence of Mercury in the Fishery Resources of the Gulf of Mexico.* Washington, D.C.: Environmental Protection Agency.

Food and Nutrition Board (2011). *Front-of-Package Nutrition Rating Systems and Symbols: Promoting Healthier Choices.* Washington, D.C.: National Academies Press.

Food and Nutrition Board (2010). *Examination of Front-of-Package Nutrition Rating Systems and Symbols: Phase 1 Report.* Washington, D.C.: National Academies Press.

Gostin, L.O. (2007). Law as a tool to facilitate healthier lifestyles and prevent obesity. *Journal of the American Medical Association,* 297, 1, 87–90.

Hall, K.D. et al. (2011). Quantification of the effect of energy imbalance on bodyweight. *Lancet,* 378, 9793, 826–837.

Hall, R.A., Zook, E.G., & Meaburn, G.M. (1978). *National Marine Fisheries Service Survey of Trace Elements in the Fishery Resource.* Silver Spring, Md.: National Marine Fisheries Service.

Hingle, M. & Kunkel, D. (2012). Childhood obesity and the media. *Pediatric Clinics of North America,* 59, 3, 677–692.

Institute of Medicine (2006). *Dietary Reference Intakes: The Essential Guide to Nutrient Requirements.* Washington, D.C.: National Academies Press.

Task Force on Community Preventive Services (2002). Recommendations to increase physical activity in communities. *American Journal of Preventive Medicine,* 22, 4S, 67–72.

Trichopoulou, A. et al. (2003). Adherence to a Mediterranean diet and survival in a Greek population. *New England Journal of Medicine,* 348, 2599–2608.

U.S. Department of Agriculture (2015). *2015-2020 Dietary Guidelines for Americans* (8th ed.) www.health.gov/dietaryguidelines

U.S. Department of Agriculture (2010). *2010 Dietary Guidelines for Americans.* www.health.gov/dietaryguidelines/2010/

U.S. Department of Agriculture, Agriculture Research Service and U.S. Department of Health and Human Services, Centers for Disease Control and Prevention (2010). *What We Eat in America.* www.ars.usda.gov/Services/docs.htm?docid=13793

Table 4-1
Estimating Portion Size

Food Group	Key Message	What Counts?	Looks Like …
Grains	Make half your grains whole.	1 oz equivalent = 1 slice of bread 1 cup of ready-to-eat cereal ½ cup cooked rice, pasta, or cooked cereal 5 whole-wheat crackers	CD cover A baseball ½ a baseball
Vegetables	Vary your veggies. Make half your plate fruits and vegetables.	1 cup = 1 cup of raw or cooked vegetable 2 cups of raw leafy salad greens 1 cup of vegetable juice	Baseball Softball
Fruits	Make half your plate fruits and vegetables.	1 cup = 1 cup raw fruit ½ cup dried fruit 1 cup 100% fruit juice	Tennis ball 2 golf balls
Milk	Switch to fat-free or low-fat (1%) milk.	1 cup = 1 cup of milk, yogurt, or soy milk 1.5 ounces of natural cheese or 2 ounces of processed cheese	Baseball 1½ 9-volt batteries
Protein Foods	Choose lean proteins.	1 ounce = 1 oz of meat, poultry, or fish ¼ cup cooked dry beans 1 egg 1 Tbsp peanut butter ½ oz nuts or seeds 2 Tbsp hummus	Deck of cards for lean meats (3 oz); checkbook = 3 oz fish ½ golf ball ½ of a Post-it® note Golf ball
Oils	Choose liquid oils and avoid solid fats.	3 tsp = 1 Tbsp vegetable oils ½ medium avocado 1 oz peanuts, mixed nuts, cashews, almonds, or sunflower seeds	Tip of thumb

For more specific amounts, please visit www.ChooseMyPlate.gov.

Carbohydrate Loading

Individuals training for long-distance endurance events lasting more than 90 minutes, such as a marathon or triathlon, may benefit from **carbohydrate loading** in the days or weeks prior to competition. Eating more carbohydrates helps muscles store more carbohydrates in the form of glycogen. If more glycogen is stored, it will take longer to deplete it during a prolonged workout. This effort to maximize available glycogen on competition day is the same reason that fitness professionals advise people to taper their workout duration as they approach an event. ACE Fitness Nutrition Specialists should warn clients who are carbohydrate loading that they may gain a few pounds because carbohydrates require water for storage. Those individuals who are serious about optimizing sports performance may consider a consultation with a Certified Specialist in Sports Dietetics (CSSD) (www.eatright.org) to help them adopt the most appropriate dietary plan and carbohydrate-loading regimen. The CSSD is a **registered dietitian (RD)** with additional board certification in sports dietetics.

While various carbohydrate-loading regimens exist, the following is a one-week sample plan:

- *Days 1–3:* Moderate-carbohydrate diet (50% of calories)
- *Days 4–6:* High-carbohydrate diet (80% of calories). This equates to about 4.5 grams of carbohydrate per pound (0.45 kg) of body weight. For a 170-lb (77.2-kg) man, that is 765 grams, or a whopping 3,000 calories from carbohydrates per day.
- *Day 7—Competitive event:* Pre-event meal (typically dinner the night before the event) with >80% of calories from carbohydrates. This equates to more than 4.5 grams of carbohydrate per pound (0.45 kg) of body weight.

The ACE Fitness Nutrition Specialist should feel comfortable explaining the purpose of carbohydrate loading and sharing basic information about different regimens that may be used; however, it is important not to advise or recommend that a client adopt a specific meal plan.

THINK IT THROUGH

One of your regular clients, Jamie, is a physically active college student. She performs the following workouts consistently each week:

- Running on a treadmill at 70% heart-rate reserve for 30 minutes on Monday, Wednesday, and Friday
- Lifting weights at a moderate intensity for all the major muscle groups on Tuesday, Thursday, and Saturday

One of Jamie's friends is a marathon runner who recently underwent a carbohydrate loading program to prepare for a race. While Jamie has no desire to run in endurance competitions, she is curious about the potential for carbohydrate loading to help her with her current training program. What would your advice to Jamie be regarding carbohydrate loading for the type of training program in which she currently engages?

Glycemic Index

As far as refueling goes, not all carbohydrates are created equal. Historically, much debate has centered on whether consumption of **simple** or **complex carbohydrates** is better for athletic performance. The role of a particular carbohydrate in athletic performance may be better determined by its **glycemic index (GI)** than its structure. GI ranks carbohydrates based on their blood glucose response. High-GI foods break down rapidly, causing a large glucose spike; low-GI foods are digested more slowly and cause a smaller glucose increase. **Glycemic load (GL)** accounts for GI as well as the amount of carbohydrate being consumed (GL = GI x grams of carbohydrate/100).

The role of GI in exercise performance has been a source of ongoing research for the past two decades. Initial studies suggested that a low-GI diet prior to exercise improves performance. While this still seems to be true, further research found that this benefit is negated as soon as a carbohydrate-containing sports drink, gel, or bar is consumed during an exercise session (O'Reilly, Wong, & Chen, 2010). It seems logical that a high-GI diet would be more effective at repleting glycogen stores after exercise. After all, carbohydrates with a high GI are more rapidly absorbed and more quickly release sugar into the bloodstream (Table 4-2). Thus, they should be more effective at replenishing energy stores than low-GI foods, which are broken down more slowly and take longer to release sugar into the bloodstream. While an early body of research supported this supposition, more recent studies have found that low-GI foods eaten before exercise may contribute to increased performance by increasing the availability of nonessential **fatty acids** during an exercise session (Stevenson et al., 2009; Trenell et al., 2008). Overall, despite years of research on the glycemic index and endurance performance, the jury is still out as to how GI affects performance. In regards to overall health, several high-quality studies suggest that a low-GI eating plan may be better for weight loss and improvement in **cholesterol** levels (Thomas, Elliott, & Baur, 2007) and for people with diabetes (Thomas & Elliott, 2009).

Table 4-2
Glycemic Index (GI) of Various Foods

High GI ≥70	Medium GI 56–69	Low GI ≤55
White bread	Rye bread	Pumpernickel bread
Corn Flakes	Shredded Wheat	All Bran
Graham crackers	Ice cream	Plain yogurt
Dried fruit	Blueberries	Strawberries
Instant white rice	Refined pasta	Oatmeal

Protein and Sports Nutrition

While low-carbohydrate/high-protein diets, such as the Atkins and South Beach plans, are no longer the hottest trend, "high-protein" diets [eating plans on the higher end of the **Acceptable Macronutrient Distribution Range (AMDR)** for protein of 10 to 35% of calories] seem to be just as good as, if not better than, high-carbohydrate diets for weight loss and health benefits (Gardner et al., 2007; Dansinger et al., 2005; Foster et al., 2003). A high-protein diet can even help to optimize athletic performance (and muscle strengthening) due to the important role of protein in both endurance and resistance-training exercise. The two modes of exercise stimulate muscle protein synthesis, which is further enhanced if protein is consumed around the time of the physical activity. Eating protein immediately after exercising helps in the repair and synthesis of muscle proteins. Protein intake during exercise probably does not offer any additional performance benefit if sufficient amounts of carbohydrate—the body's preferred energy source—are consumed. However, for endurance athletes who need to consume adequate calories to fuel extended training sessions, or for any exerciser striving to lose weight, protein can help preserve lean muscle mass and ensure that most weight loss comes from fat rather than lean tissue.

The average person requires 0.8 to 1.0 g/kg of body weight of protein per day (0.4 to 0.5 g/lb). Athletes need anywhere from 1.2 to 1.7 g/kg (0.5 to 0.8 g/lb) depending on gender, age, and type and intensity of the exercise (less for endurance athletes and more for strength-trained athletes) (Rodriguez, Di Marco, & Langley, 2009). Clients can ensure adequate protein consumption if recommendations are based on the AMDR of 10 to 35% of daily energy intake [Institute of Medicine (IOM), 2005]. Table 4-3 shows the total protein intake at various levels of energy intake within the AMDR for protein. Recommended protein intakes are best met through diet, though many athletes do turn to **whey**- or **casein**-based protein powders and other supplements to boost protein intake.

Several factors come into play when choosing the "best" type of protein from food, including protein quality, health benefits, dietary restrictions, cost, convenience, and taste. While no one type of protein is best for everyone, keep these considerations in mind:

- *Protein quality varies.* Similar to lean meats, poultry, and fish, whey, casein, egg, soy, and chia contain all of the **essential amino acids** in amounts proportional to

Table 4-3				
Protein Intake (grams) at Various Levels of Energy Intake				
Energy intake (kcal/d)	**Low-protein diet (<10% kcal)**	**Average diet (~15% kcal)**	**High-protein diet (≥20% kcal)**	**Very-high protein diet (≥30% kcal)**
1,200	30	45	60	90
2,000	50	75	100	150
3,000	75	112	150	225

Note: Each gram of protein contains 4 calories.

Reprinted with permission from the American Heart Association, Inc.; St. Jeor, S.T. et al. (2001). Dietary protein and weight reduction: A statement for healthcare professionals from the nutrition committee of the Council on Nutrition, Physical Activity, and Metabolism of the American Heart Association. *Circulation,* 104, 1869–1874.

need and are easily digested and absorbed. Fruits, vegetables, grains, and nuts are incomplete proteins and must be combined over the day to ensure adequate intake of each of the essential amino acids (Figure 4-2).

- *Different types of proteins are better at different times.* Many athletes consume the milk proteins whey and casein in an effort to maximize muscle building. Whey protein—the liquid remaining after milk has been curdled and strained—is rapidly digested, resulting in a short burst of **amino acids** into the bloodstream. Whey is known for its ability to stimulate muscle protein synthesis, even more so than casein and soy. Casein—the protein that gives milk its white color and accounts for the majority of milk protein—is slowly digested, resulting in a more prolonged release of amino acids lasting up to hours. If the goal is for amino acids to be readily available for muscle regeneration immediately following a workout, an athlete may consider timing protein intake accordingly to best maximize muscle building and repair. (For example, in theory, consuming casein-based proteins prior to exercise and whey-based proteins during and immediately following exercise may enhance skeletal muscle protein synthesis, though the efficacy of this approach has not been confirmed.) In any case, the ACE Fitness Nutrition Specialist should feel comfortable sharing credible information with clients, but should not recommend or advise clients to follow a specific diet regimen or take supplements.

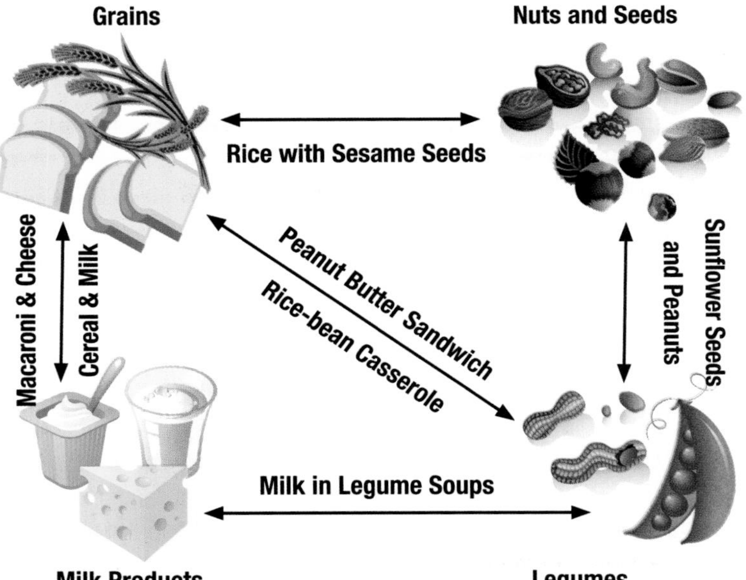

Figure 4-2
Protein complementarity chart

Adapted with permission from Lappé, F.M. (1992). *Diet for a Small Planet.* New York: Ballantine Books.

- *More is not always better.* Total daily protein intake should not be excessive. Protein consumption beyond recommended amounts is unlikely to result in further muscle gains because the body has a limited capacity to use amino acids to build muscle. Most studies suggest that there is a threshold effect of 1.6 to 1.7 g/kg protein (Rosenbloom & Coleman, 2012). Beyond that amount, there is no further increase in skeletal muscle protein synthesis. In fact, consumption of protein beyond 1.6 to 1.7 g/kg promotes increased amino acid **catabolism** and protein oxidation, and may provide excess caloric intake that is stored as fat (Moore et al., 2009).

Ultimately, the science is still evolving regarding the best amounts, mechanisms, and methods of protein intake. However, it seems that when combined with regular exercise and an overall healthy lifestyle, an appropriate amount of protein can help clients gain muscle, lose weight, and improve health.

Fats and Sports Nutrition

Fat is an important source of energy, fat-soluble vitamins, and **essential fatty acids.** Athletes should consume a comparable proportion of food from fat as the general population—that is, 20 to 35% of total calories. There is no evidence for performance benefit from a very low-fat diet (<15% of total calories) or from a high-fat diet (Rodriguez, Di Marco, & Langley, 2009). A complete discussion of the role of fat in maintaining optimal health and fat's impact on blood lipids is presented in Chapter 2.

Fueling Before, During, and After Exercise

Physically active individuals need the right types and amounts of food before, during, and after exercise to maximize the amount of energy available to fuel optimal performance and minimize the amount of gastrointestinal distress. Sports nutrition strategies should address three exercise stages: pre-exercise, during exercise, and post-exercise (Figure 4-3).

Pre-exercise

The two main goals of a pre-exercise exercise snack are to (1) optimize glucose availability and glycogen stores and (2) provide the fuel needed for exercise performance. Keeping this in mind, in the days up to a week before a strenuous endurance effort, an athlete should consider what nutritional strategies might set the stage for optimal performance. For example, an individual preparing for a long endurance event might consider the pros and cons of carbohydrate loading. On the day of the event or an important

Figure 4-3
Sports nutrition strategies

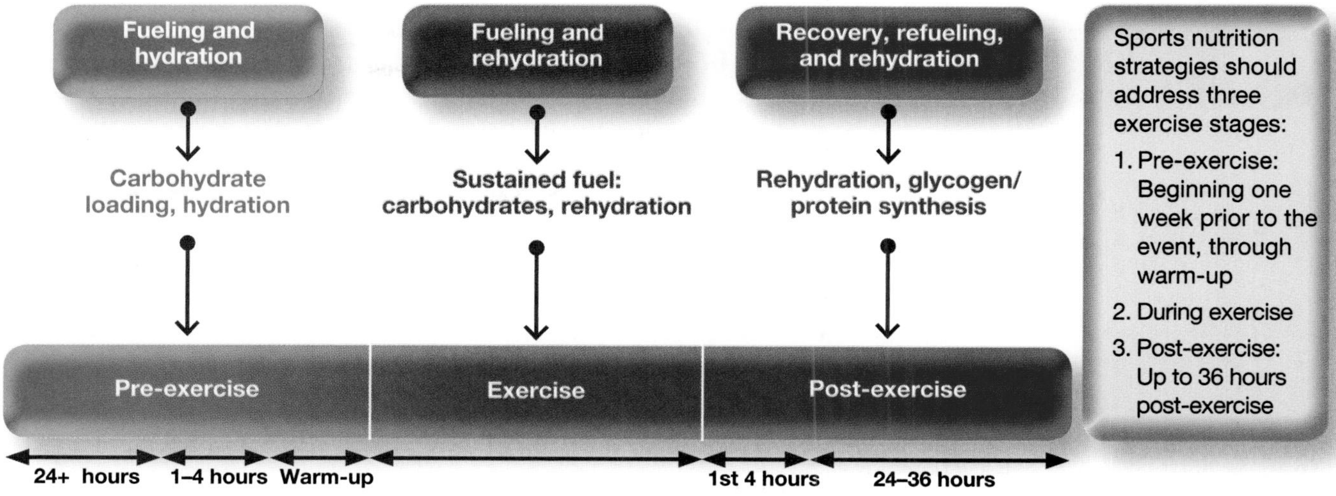

training session, the athlete should aim to eat a meal about four to six hours prior to the workout to minimize gastrointestinal distress and optimize performance. Four hours after eating, the food will already have been digested and absorbed; now liver and muscle glycogen levels are increased. To translate this into an everyday, practical recommendation, athletes who work out in the early afternoon should be certain to eat a wholesome carbohydrate-rich breakfast. Those who exercise in the early morning may benefit from a carbohydrate-rich snack before going to bed.

Some research also suggests that eating a relatively small carbohydrate- and protein-containing snack (e.g., 50 grams of carbohydrate and 5 to 10 grams of protein) 30 to 60 minutes before exercise helps increase glucose availability near the end of the workout and helps to decrease exercise-induced protein catabolism (Kreider et al., 2010). The exact timing and size of the snack for peak performance will vary by athlete and type of exercise. As a general rule, athletes should try out any snacks or drinks with practice sessions prior to relying on them to help optimize athletic performance during competition. In general, a pre-exercise meal or snack should be:

- Relatively high in carbohydrate to maximize blood glucose availability
- Relatively low in fat and **fiber** to minimize gastrointestinal distress and facilitate **gastric emptying**
- Moderate in protein
- Well-tolerated by the individual

Fueling During Exercise

The goal of during-exercise fueling is to provide the body with the essential nutrients needed by muscle cells and to maintain optimal blood glucose levels. During a prolonged endurance effort, such as a marathon, an athlete is at risk of "hitting the wall"—a phenomenon often occurring around mile 20 of a marathon race. This is when extreme fatigue sets in due to drained carbohydrate stores. But, there are gradations on the physical demands of exercise based on the duration of the exercise session. Exercise lasting less than one hour can be adequately fueled with existing glucose and glycogen stores. No additional carbohydrate-containing drinks or foods are necessary. When exercise lasts longer than one hour, blood glucose levels begin to dwindle. After one to three hours of continuous moderate-intensity exercise (65 to 80% $\dot{V}O_2max$), muscle glycogen stores may become depleted. If no glucose is consumed, the blood glucose levels drop, resulting in further depletion of muscle and liver glycogen stores. When this happens, regardless of the athlete's mental toughness or desire to maintain intensity, performance falters.

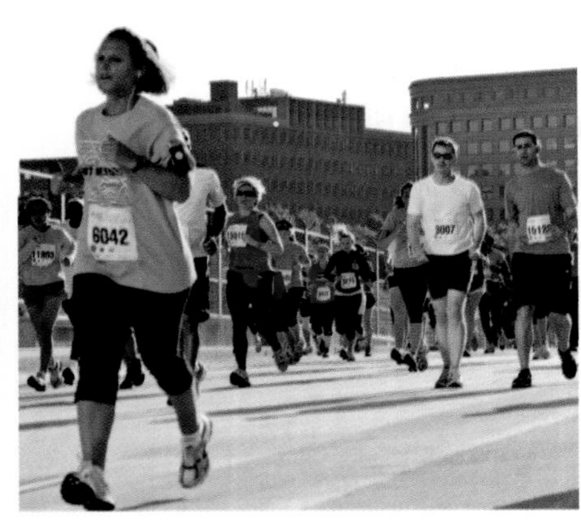

To maintain a ready energy supply during a prolonged, moderate-to-vigorous, continuous exercise session (>60 minutes), athletes should consume glucose-containing beverages and snacks. Athletes should consume 30 to 60 grams of carbohydrate per hour of training (Rodriguez, Di Marco, & Langley, 2009). This is especially important for prolonged exercise and exercise in extreme heat, cold, or high altitude; for athletes who did not consume adequate amounts of food or drink prior to the training session; and for athletes who did not carbohydrate load or who restricted energy intake for weight loss.

Carbohydrate consumption during prolonged exercise should begin shortly after the initiation of the exercise. The carbohydrate will be more effective if the 30 to 60 grams per hour are consumed in small amounts in 15- to 20-minute intervals rather than as a large **bolus** after two hours of exercise (Rodriguez, Di Marco, & Langley, 2009). Some experts believe that adding protein to carbohydrate during exercise will help to improve performance, but to date the evidence is inconclusive.

Post-exercise Replenishment

The main goal of post-exercise fueling is to replenish glycogen stores and facilitate muscle repair. The average client training at moderate intensities every few days does not need any aggressive post-exercise replenishment. Normal dietary practices following exercise will facilitate recovery within 24 to 48 hours. But athletes following vigorous training regimens, especially those who will participate in multiple training sessions in a single day (e.g., triathletes or athletes participating in training camp for a team sport), benefit from strategic refueling. Studies show that the best post-workout meals include mostly carbohydrates accompanied by some protein (Kreider et al., 2010). Refueling should begin within 30 minutes after exercise and be followed by a high-carbohydrate meal within two hours (Kreider et al., 2010). The carbohydrates replenish the used-up energy that is normally stored as glycogen in muscle and liver. The protein helps to rebuild the muscles that were fatigued with exercise. A carbohydrate intake of 1.5 g/kg of body weight in the first 30 minutes after exercise and then every two hours for four to six hours is recommended (Rodriguez, Di Marco, & Langley, 2009). After that, the athlete can resume his or her typical, balanced diet. Of course, the amount of refueling necessary depends on the intensity and duration of the training session. A long-duration, low-intensity workout may not require such vigorous replenishment.

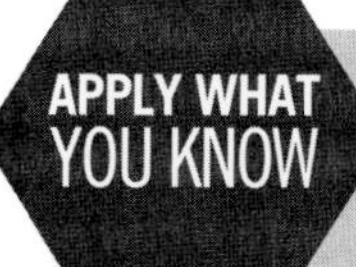

Post-workout Snack and Meal Ideas

In the several hours following a prolonged and strenuous workout, consuming snacks and meals high in carbohydrate with some protein can set the stage for optimal glycogen replenishment and subsequent performance. Here are a few snack and meal ideas that fit the bill:

- *Snack 1:* In the first several minutes after exercise consume 16 oz of Gatorade™ or other sports drink, a power gel such as a Clif Shot™ or GU™, and a medium banana. This quickly begins to replenish muscle carbohydrate stores. *Carbohydrates: 73 g; Protein: 1 g; Calories: 290*
- *Snack 2:* After cooling down and showering, grab another quick snack such as 12 oz of orange juice and ¼ cup of raisins. *Carbohydrates: 70 g; Protein 3 g; Calories: 295*
- *Small meal appetizer:* Enjoy a spinach salad with tomatoes, chickpeas, green beans, and tuna and a whole-grain baguette. *Carbohydrates: 70 g; Protein: 37 g; Calories: 489*
- *Small meal main course:* Replenish with whole-grain pasta with diced tomatoes. *Carbohydrates: 67 g; Protein: 2 g; Calories: 292*
- *Dessert:* After allowing ample time for the day's snacks and meals to digest, finish your refueling program with one cup of frozen yogurt and berries. *Carbohydrates: 61 g; Protein: 8 g; Calories: 280*

Fluid and Hydration Before, During, and After Exercise

When it comes to fluid balance during exercise, it seems like the proverbial double-edged sword: Drinking too little can lead to **dehydration**—a scary condition exercisers have been cautioned against in every text, handout, and presentation on fluid replacement. But drinking too much plain water—out of fear of not drinking enough—could lead to **hyponatremia** (i.e., low sodium in the blood), a condition less well known and understood, but equally frightening. Here is the good news: the body is very good at handling and normalizing large variations in fluid intake. For this reason, severe hyponatremia and dehydration are rare and generally affect very specific high-risk populations during specific types of activities. Both conditions are highly preventable. To prevent dehydration and hyponatremia, the goal is to drink just the right amount of fluid and/or **electrolytes** before, during, and after exercise to maintain a state of **euhydration,** which is a state of "normal" body water content—the perfect balance between "too much" and "not enough" fluid intake.

Hydration Prior to Exercise

Most people begin exercise euhydrated with little need for a rigorous prehydration regimen. However, if fewer than eight to 12 hours have elapsed since the last intense training session or fluid intake has been inadequate, the athlete may benefit from a prehydration program.

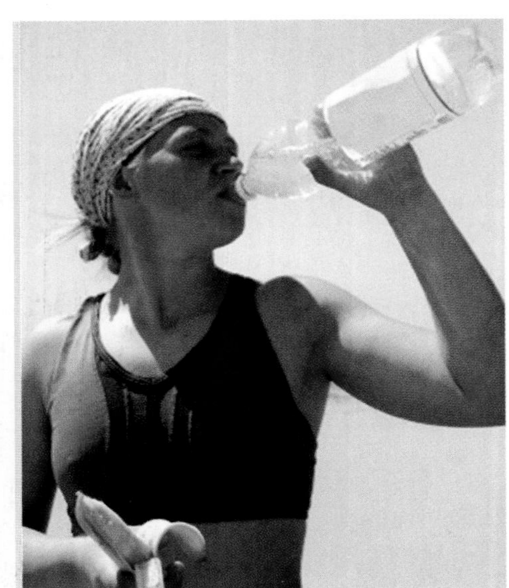

An athlete should begin prehydrating about four hours prior to the exercise session. The athlete should aim to slowly consume about 5 to 7 mL (0.17 to 0.23 oz) of fluid per 1 kg (2.2 lb) of body weight. If after two hours of prehydration no urine is produced or if the urine is dark or highly concentrated, the individual should aim to drink an additional 3 to 5 mL (0.1 to 0.17 oz) of fluid per 1 kg (2.2 lb) of body weight two hours before the event. Drinking fluid that contains 20 to 50 milliequivalents/liter (mEq/L) (460 to 1150 mg/L) of sodium or consuming salt-containing snacks at this time helps stimulate thirst and retain the consumed fluids (Sawka et al., 2007). Some athletes may try to hyperhydrate with glycerol-containing solutions that act to expand the extra- and intra-cellular spaces. While glycerol may be advantageous for certain athletes who meet specific criteria, glycerol is unlikely to be advantageous for athletes who will experience no to mild dehydration during exercise (loss of <2% body weight) and glycerol use may in fact contribute to increased risk of hyponatremia (van Rosendal et al., 2010).

Hydration During Exercise

The goal of fluid intake during exercise is to prevent performance-diminishing or health-altering effects from dehydration or hyponatremia. ACE Fitness Nutrition Specialists can share the following guidelines with clients:

- *Aim for a 1:1 fluid replacement to fluid loss ratio.* Ideally, exercisers should consume the same amount of fluid as they lose in sweat. An easy way to assess post-exercise hydration is to compare pre- and post-exercise body weight. The goal is to avoid weight loss greater than 2%. There is no one-size-fits-all recommendation, though if determining individual needs is not feasible, athletes should aim to drink 0.4 to 0.8 L/h (8 to 16 oz/h), with the higher rate for faster, heavier athletes in a hot and humid environment and the lower rate for slower, lighter athletes in a cool environment (Sawka et al., 2007). Because people sweat at varying rates and exercise at different intensities, this range may not be appropriate for everyone. However, when individual assessment is not possible, this recommendation works for most people.
- *Drink fluids with sodium during prolonged exercise sessions.* If an exercise session lasts longer than two hours or an athlete is participating in an event that stimulates heavy sweat (and consequently, sodium) losses, then the athlete should consider consuming a sports drink that contains elevated levels of sodium. In one study, researchers did not find a benefit from sports drinks that contain only the 18 mmol/L (or 100 milligrams per 8 oz) of sodium typical of most sports drinks and thus concluded that higher levels would be needed to prevent hyponatremia during prolonged exercise (Almond et al., 2005). Table 4-4 presents the sodium content of some popular drinks. The IOM recommends that people exercising for prolonged periods in hot environments consume sports drinks that contain 20 to 30 mEq/L (0.5 to 0.7 g/L) of sodium to stimulate thirst and replace sweat losses and 2 to 5 mEq/L (0.8 to 2.0 g/L) of potassium to replace sweat losses (Rodriguez, Di Marco, & Langley, 2009). Alternatively, exercisers can consume extra sodium with meals and snacks prior to a lengthy exercise session or a day of extensive physical activity. Additional sodium or supplementation with salt tablets seems to be unnecessary based on the limited research on this topic (Hew-Butler et al., 2006; Speedy et al., 2002).

- *Drink carbohydrate-containing sports drinks to reduce fatigue.* Athletes exercising for longer than one hour should also consume carbohydrate with fluids. With prolonged exercise, muscle glycogen stores become depleted and blood glucose becomes a primary fuel source. To maintain performance levels and prevent fatigue, athletes should choose drinks and snacks that provide about 30 to 60 grams of rapidly absorbed carbohydrate for every hour of training. As long as the carbohydrate concentration is about 6 to 8%, it will have little effect on gastric emptying (Rodriguez, Di Marco, & Langley, 2009).

Sports drinks play an important role in replenishing fluids, glucose, and sodium lost during moderate-to-vigorous exercise lasting more than one hour. Although sports drinks may not completely protect against hyponatremia, they serve an important purpose in endurance exercise. Table 4-4 provides nutritional information for some of the most popular sports drinks.

Table 4-4
Evaluating Sports Drinks

Drink	Serving Size (oz)	Calories (kcal)	Sodium (mg)	Carbohydrate (g)	Carbohydrate Concentration (%)
Gatorade	8	50	110	14	6
Gatorade Endurance Formula	8	50	200	14	6
Powerade	8	70	55	19	8
Ultima	8	12.5	37	3	1
Power Bar Endurance	8	70	160	17	7
Propel	8	10	10	3	1
Zico coconut water	8	34	91	7.4	3

EXPAND YOUR KNOWLEDGE

***Myth:* Drinking Fluids Before and During Exercise Causes Gastrointestinal Distress.**

Rationale: Since blood flow is diverted away from the gastrointestinal system during exercise, fluids consumed before or during exercise will just sit around sloshing in the stomach during the workout.

The science: It is true that gastric emptying, or the speed with which the stomach empties its contents into the **small intestine,** slows down during exercise. This is largely because exercise-induced sympathetic stimulation diverts blood flow from the gastrointestinal (GI) system to the heart, lungs, and working muscles. As a result, athletes sometimes experience stomach cramps along with a variety of other uncomfortable GI issues such as reflux, heartburn, bloating, gas, nausea, vomiting, the urge to defecate, and diarrhea. It turns out, though, that good hydration with the right fluids can help increase gastric emptying and lead to reduced GI problems with exercise. Gastric emptying is maximized when the amount of fluid in the stomach is high. On the other hand, high-intensity exercise (>70% $\dot{V}O_2$max), dehydration, hyperthermia, and consumption of high-energy (>7% carbohydrate), **hypertonic** drinks (like juices and some soft drinks) slow gastric emptying.

ACE Fitness Nutrition Specialists can recommend the following practical tips to prepare the gut for competition (Brouns & Beckers, 1993):

- Get acclimatized to heat.
- Stay hydrated.
- Practice drinking during training to improve competition-day comfort.
- Avoid eating too much before and during exercise.
- Avoid high-energy, hypertonic food and drinks before (within 30 to 60 minutes) and after exercise. Limit protein and fat intake before exercise.
- Ingest a high-energy, high-carbohydrate diet.
- Avoid high-fiber foods before exercise.
- Limit **nonsteroidal anti-inflammatory drugs (NSAIDs)** such as ibuprofen and naproxen, alcohol, caffeine, antibiotics, and nutritional supplements before and during exercise, as they can cause gastrointestinal discomfort. The client should experiment during training to identify his or her triggers.
- Urinate and defecate prior to exercise.
- Consult a physician if GI problems persist, especially abdominal pain, diarrhea, or bloody stool.

Post-exercise Hydration

Following exercise, the athlete should aim to correct any fluid imbalances that occurred during the exercise session. This includes consuming water to restore hydration, carbohydrates to replenish glycogen stores, and electrolytes to speed rehydration. If the athlete will have at least 12 hours to recover before the next strenuous workout, rehydration with the usual meals and snacks and water should be adequate. The sodium in the foods will help retain the fluid and stimulate thirst. If rehydration needs to occur quickly, the athletes should drink about 1.5 L of fluid for each kilogram (or 0.70 L of fluid for each pound) of body weight lost (Sawka et al., 2007). This will be enough to restore lost fluid and also compensate for increased urine output that occurs with rapid consumption of large amounts of fluid. A severely dehydrated athlete (>7% body weight loss) with symptoms (nausea, vomiting, or diarrhea) may need intravenous fluid replacement. Those at greatest risk of hyponatremia should be careful not to consume too much water following exercise and instead should focus on replenishing sodium.

NUTRITION APPLICATIONS IN THE LIFECYCLE

A well-balanced eating plan often extends beyond a one-size-fits-all dietary recommendation. At certain times, some individuals need slightly modified dietary recommendations to best meet their lifestyle, nutritional, and cultural needs. While the *Dietary Guidelines* are intended for all Americans ages two and older, some stages of the human lifecycle require special nutritional considerations [U.S. Department of Agriculture (USDA), 2015].

Nutrition in Childhood and Adolescence

The *Dietary Guidelines* recommend that, similar to adults, children eat a diet rich in fruits, vegetables, whole grains, low-fat and nonfat dairy products, beans, fish, and lean meat (USDA, 2010). Specifically, the *Dietary Guidelines* (www.dietaryguidelines.gov) and 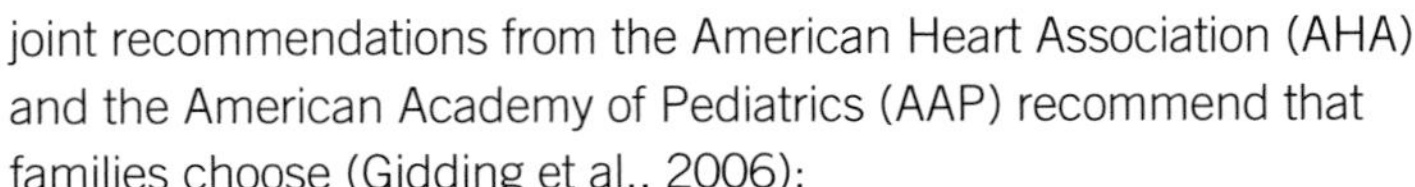 joint recommendations from the American Heart Association (AHA) and the American Academy of Pediatrics (AAP) recommend that families choose (Gidding et al., 2006):

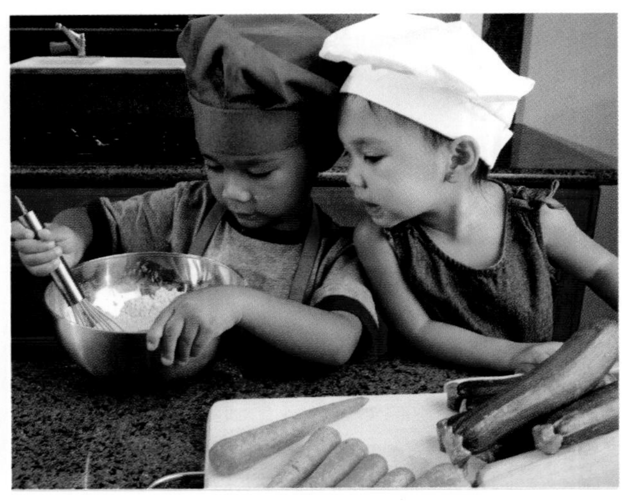

- Mostly whole grains as opposed to refined sugars. Brown bread, brown rice, and brown pasta provide more nutrients than the more heavily processed "white" versions. Cereal should be high in fiber (contain 5 g/serving, or >20% of recommended daily value) and low in sugar [generally considered to be less than 3 grams, although "low sugar" is not defined by the U.S. Food and Drug Administration (FDA) and is not an allowable food claim].
- Ample nutrient-dense dark green and orange vegetables, such as broccoli and carrots, rather than disproportionate amounts of starchy vegetables, such as white potatoes and corn, which contain fewer vitamins and minerals. A general rule of thumb is, the more colorful the vegetable, the more nutrients it contains.
- A variety of fruits, preferably from the whole food sources, as opposed to fruit juices. While the *Dietary Guidelines* still consider 100% juice a serving of fruit, the sugar in juice usually outweighs the benefit from the fruit. (Even though the sugar in 100% juice is **fructose**—a natural fruit sugar—it takes about three apples to make an 8-ounce glass of juice. That is more apple than a child would typically eat in a day and the juice does not contain the healthy fiber contained in the skin.) Children should limit 100% juice to no more than four ounces per day.

- Oils in moderation, with an emphasis on **monounsaturated fats** or **polyunsaturated fats** instead of **trans fats** or **saturated fats.** While fats are calorie dense, some fats are heart-healthy, particularly polyunsaturated fats such as the **omega-3 fatty acids** contained in salmon, tuna, walnuts, and a variety of fortified products (such as milk and eggs) and other foods.
- Low- or nonfat milk products in contrast to regular whole-milk products. Starting at the age of two (and the age of one for kids already **overweight**), all children should consume 2%, 1%, or, preferably, skim or nonfat milk. The higher-fat milk contains a lot more calories and saturated fat, and no additional nutritional value, in terms of nutrients such as protein and calcium.
- Lean meat and bean products instead of higher-fat meats, such as regular (75 to 80% lean) ground beef or chicken with the skin. Lean meats include the white meat from chicken (breast and wings) cooked without the skin and the leanest red meats (typically round or loin).

A summary of the *Dietary Guidelines* for children is presented in Table 4-5.

Table 4-5

Nutrition Needs for Children and Adolescents

	1–3 Years	4–8 Years	9–13 Years	14–18 Years
Calories				
Female	900–1,000	1,200	1,400–1,600	1,800
Male	900–1,200	1,200–1,400	1,600–2,000	2,000–2,400
Milk/dairy	2 cups	2.5 cups	3 cups	3 cups
Lean meat/ beans/nuts/eggs				
Female	2oz	3 oz	5oz	5 oz
Male	3oz	4 oz	6oz	6 oz
Fruits				
Female	1 cup	1.5 cups	1.5 cups	1.5 cups
Male	1 cup	1.5 cups	1.5 cups	2 cups
Vegetables				
Female	1 cup	1.5 cups	2 cups	2.5 cups
Male	1.5 cups	1.5 cups	2.5 cups	3 cups
Grains				
Female	3 oz	4 oz	5 oz	6 oz
Male	3 oz	5 oz	6 oz	7 oz

Estimated calorie needs are based on a sedentary lifestyle. Increased physical activity will require additional calories: by 0–200 kcal/d if moderately physically active; and by 200–400 kcal/d if very physically active.

Appendix 2 and Appendix 3 of U.S. Department of Agriculture (2015). *2015-2020 Dietary Guidelines for Americans* (8th ed.) www.health.gov/dietaryguidelines

A wide gap exists between nutrition recommendations for children and what children actually eat. Currently, children and adolescents eat breakfast less often, away from home more often, a greater proportion of calories from snacks, more fried and nutrient-poor foods, greater portion sizes, fewer fruits and vegetables, excess sodium, more sweetened beverages, and fewer dairy products compared to children from previous generations (Dwyer et al., 2010; French, Story, & Jeffrey, 2001). As a result, children and especially adolescents consume smaller amounts of many nutrients such as calcium and potassium than the recommended values (French, Story, & Jeffrey, 2001).

Children and their parents benefit from tips on how to make healthy choices to support athletic performance. However, more so than the information, families benefit from strategies that support them in teaching their children how to eat healthfully.

EXPAND YOUR KNOWLEDGE

Strategies to Help Teach Families How to Implement the *Dietary Guidelines*

Most parents know *what* their children should eat, but the challenge frequently arises in understanding *how* to make that happen. The following strategies are adapted from recommendations provided by the AHA and the AAP (Gidding et al., 2006).

- Practice what is referred to as the "division of responsibility." Parents choose what foods are available in the home and when the food can be eaten. Children choose, from the food that is offered, *what* they will eat and *how much.* With this approach, the parent has control over nutrient quality and snack and meal times, while the child feels a sense of control in choosing what to eat from the food offered and also is able to use internal feelings of hunger and fullness in deciding how much to eat.
- Arrange for family meals. While family schedules can often be very busy and sometimes chaotic, committing to scheduling family meals as frequently as possible provides many benefits in determining the nutritional value of a child's food intake and provides an opportunity to strengthen the family bond.
- Teach children about food and healthful nutrition by engaging them in choosing food at the grocery store, preparing meals, and possibly gardening, even if it is only a few herbs on a window sill.
- Be a source of quality nutrition information and actively counteract nutrition misinformation in the media and through other sources. Teach children and adolescents how to critically evaluate advertisements and avoid purchases based exclusively on marketing or packaging tactics.
- Discuss nutrition preferences and goals with other adults who provide food to the children, such as other family members, babysitters, carpool participants, after-school program leaders, and coaches.
- Serve as a role models and lead by example.
- Promote and participate in regular daily physical activity.

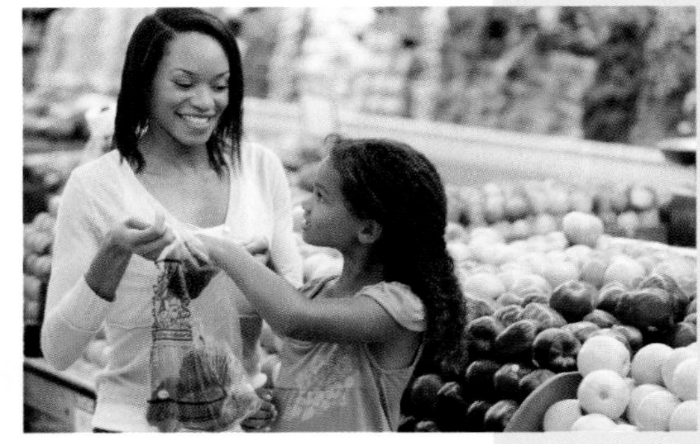

AAP and AHA also recommend that the family and cultural background of the child be considered when making nutrition recommendations (Gidding et al., 2006). Media messages, cultural beliefs that a chubby child is a healthy child, immediate access to inexpensive fast food, and motivation to change are all important determinants of a child's nutrition status.

Adolescents face unique nutritional challenges due to rapid bone growth and other maturational changes associated with the onset of puberty. While caloric and some micronutrient needs increase to support growth, adolescence is also a time of decreasing physical activity for many teens and increased independence when making food choices. Ready access to juice and sports drinks in schools, the prevalence of fast food restaurants, and peer and media pressure to eat fat- and sugar-laden foods make it easy for many teens to eat more calories than they expend, which puts them at greater risk for obesity. While the *Dietary Guidelines* and the MyPlate Food Guidance System provide scientifically sound nutrition guidelines for teens, any nutrition advice offered must be tailored to a teen's readiness to change if it is to be successful (Gidding et al., 2006).

Readers who are interested in serving youth clients should refer to the ACE Youth Fitness Specialty Certification for exercise guidelines and general recommendations for successfully and safely working with this population. Visit ACEfitness.org for more information.

Nutrition for Older Adults

One in eight Americans is an older adult, defined by the Older Americans Act as a person older than 60 years. The main goal for older adults based on *Healthy People 2020* is to "improve health, function, and quality of life" (www.healthypeople.gov). Two major ways to help achieve that objective include physical activity and attention to healthful nutrition.

An ideal eating pattern for older adults closely resembles an ideal eating pattern for the general adult population, with a few notable exceptions and considerations that are depicted in the MyPlate for Older Adults icon developed by Tuft University's Jean Mayer USDA Human Nutrition Research Center on Aging (Figure 4-4).

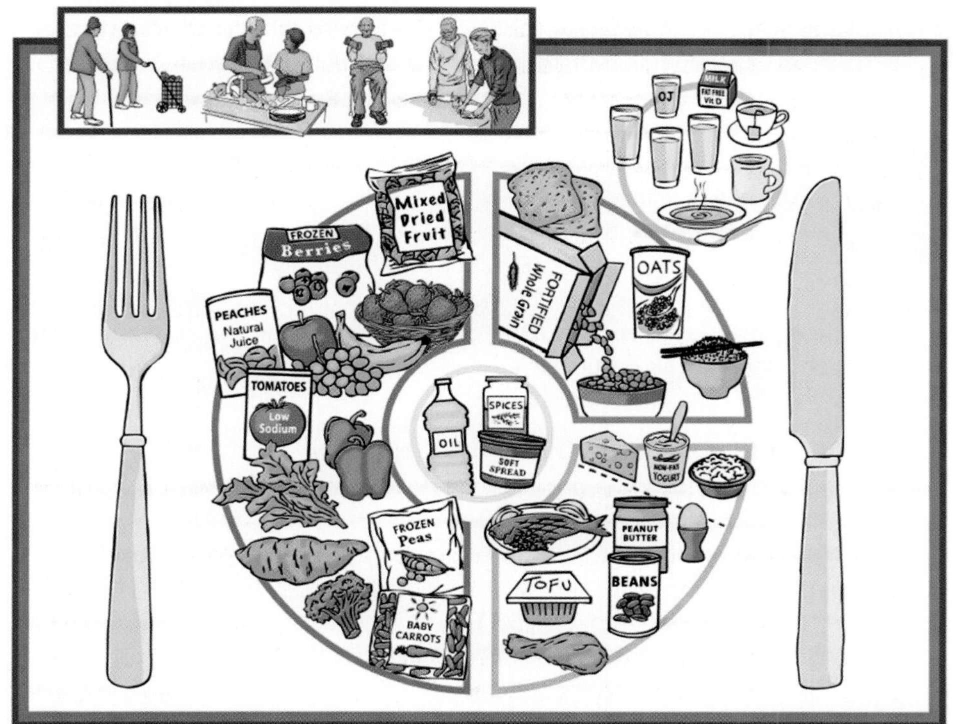

Figure 4-4
MyPlate for Older Adults

Reprinted with permission from Tufts University (2011). *MyPlate for Older Adults.* www.nutrition.tufts.edu/research/myplate-older-adults

As depicted in the icon, on the whole, older adults need to pay particular attention to fluid intake, affordable and easy-to-prepare food, and physical activity. The **Dietary Reference Intakes (DRIs)** provide nutrient recommendations for older adults in categories from 51 to 70 years and >70 years, though actual needs may vary considerably among individuals.

A study that assessed the nutritional intake of older adults and various physical and mental health outcomes found that older adults who ate a diet high in vegetables, fruits, whole grains, poultry, fish, and low-fat dairy products had superior nutritional status, quality of life, and longevity (Anderson, Harris, & Tylavsky, 2011). Unfortunately, many potential barriers may impede an older adult's ability to achieve dietary goals. These barriers include use of multiple medications, each with varying nutritional interactions and restrictions and diet-altering side effects; economic hardships; changes in mental functioning; physiological changes in smell, taste, chewing, swallowing, digestion, and absorption; and social isolation. An ACE Fitness Nutrition Specialist who helps an older adult develop a physical-activity program or improve nutritional intake must take these factors into consideration when providing information and making recommendations. These challenges are most pronounced in individuals older than 85 years.

Though caloric needs decrease with age, many nutrient needs stay the same or increase. Thus, in order to consume appropriate amounts of nutrients without exceeding caloric needs, older adults need to increase the **nutrient density** of their diets, eating more lower-calorie nutrient-packed foods like fruits and vegetables and eating fewer **empty calories**—foods that contain very little nutrition and a large number of calories, such as many desserts and snacks. The majority of older adults struggle to do this and suffer from inadequate nutrient intake, especially calcium, zinc, iron, B vitamins, zinc, and vitamins A, D, E, and K (Bachman et al., 2008; Lichtenstein et al., 2008). Older adults are at particularly high risk of vitamin B12 insufficiency or deficiency (Allen et al., 2009).

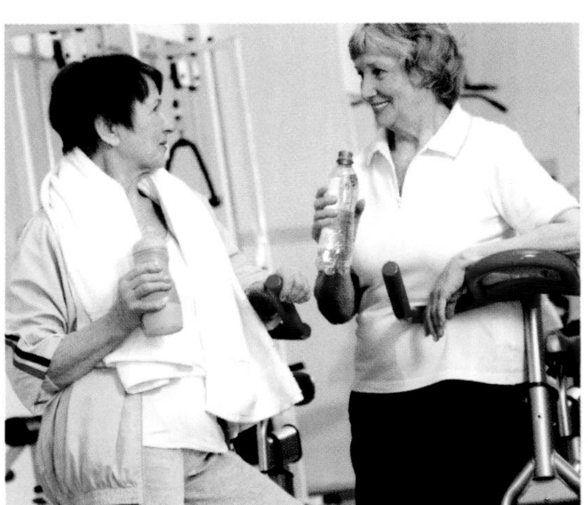

The risk of dehydration is pronounced in older adults, especially those older than 85 years or living in institutionalized settings. Many factors compromise hydration status in older adults. The sensation of thirst decreases with age. The kidneys become less effective at concentrating urine, leading to unnecessary water loss in urine. Medication side effects and interactions interfere with appropriate hydration. Consequently, unless prompted, many older adults may not achieve the adequate intake of fluids, an amount intended to replace normal daily losses and prevent dehydration. Provision of sufficient fluids is especially critical for exercising older adults who have additional exercise-related fluid losses.

Finally, despite decreased appetite and food intake, many older adults struggle with overweight and obesity. This occurs because the age-related decrease in physical activity and metabolic rate is often more pronounced than reduced caloric intake.

Pregnancy and Lactation

Good nutrition habits during pregnancy optimize maternal health and reduce the risk for some birth defects, suboptimal fetal growth and development, and chronic health problems in the developing child. The key components of a health-promoting lifestyle during pregnancy include:

- *Appropriate weight gain:* The IOM (2009) recommends that women gain differing amounts of weight according to their **body mass index (BMI)** (Table 4-6).
- *Appropriate physical activity:* Pregnant women should aim to incorporate 30 minutes or more of moderate-intensity physical activity appropriate for pregnancy on most, if not all, days of the week (ADA, 2008).
- *Consumption of a variety of foods and calories in accordance with the* Dietary Guidelines for Americans: MyPlate offers specialized guidance for optimal nutrition for pregnant and lactating women (www.ChooseMyPlate.gov). Women do not have increased caloric needs until the second trimester, at which time needs increase by 340 calories per day. Women need an additional 450 calories above baseline in the third trimester.
- *Appropriate and timely vitamin and mineral supplementation:* Pregnant women need 600 µg of **folic acid** daily from fortified foods or supplements in addition to food forms of folate from a varied diet (ADA, 2008). Folic acid reduces the risk of neural tube defects if taken prior to conception through the sixth week of pregnancy and may reduce birth defects if taken later in pregnancy. Many pregnant women suffer from **iron-deficiency anemia** and may benefit from iron supplementation.
- *Avoidance of alcohol, tobacco, and other harmful substances:* Pregnant women are advised to avoid alcohol, tobacco, and other harmful substances due to their real and potential negative effects on the developing fetus.

Table 4-6
Appropriate Weight Gain During Pregnancy

Body mass index (kg/m²)	Recommended Weight Gain
<18.5	28–40 lb (12.7–18.2 kg)
18.5–24.9	25–35 lb (11.4–15.9 kg)
25.0–29.9	15–25 lb (6.8–11.4 kg)
>30	11–20 lb (5.0–9.1 kg)

Source: Institute of Medicine (2009). *Weight Gain During Pregnancy.* Washington, D.C.: National Academy Press.

- *Limit caffeine intake:* Pregnant women and women who could become pregnant should avoid caffeine intakes above 300 mg/day due to increased risk of delayed conception, miscarriage, and low birth weight (ADA, 2008).
- *Safe food handling:* Pregnant women and their fetuses are at higher risk of developing foodborne illness and should take extra precautions to prevent consumption of contaminated foods by avoiding:
  - ✓ Soft cheeses not made with pasteurized milk
  - ✓ Deli meats, unless they have been reheated to steaming hot
  - ✓ Raw or unpasteurized milk or milk products, raw eggs, raw or undercooked meat, unpasteurized juice, raw sprouts, and raw or undercooked fish, such as sushi and sashimi
  - ✓ Cat litter boxes
  - ✓ Handling pets when preparing foods
  - ✓ Shark, swordfish, king mackerel, or tilefish. Pregnant women can safely consume 12 ounces or less of fish or shellfish per week, provided that it is low in mercury, such as shrimp, canned light tuna, salmon, pollock, and catfish. Consumption of albacore tuna should be limited to 6 ounces or less per week.

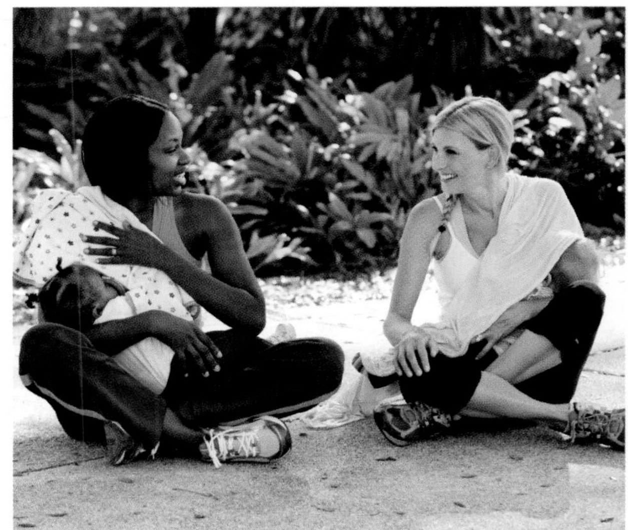

Prior to the child's birth, most women will make the decision as to whether they plan to breastfeed. Breastfeeding provides optimal nutrition and health protection for the first six months of life. Exclusive breastfeeding for the first six months of life is also associated with decreased risk of the following: infection, including ear infections, upper respiratory infections, and lower respiratory infections such as pneumonia and bronchiolitis; gastroenteritis; asthma; necrotizing enterocolitis (NEC); eczema; chronic disease including obesity, **type 2 diabetes, type 1 diabetes,** inflammatory bowel disease, and celiac disease; sudden infant death syndrome (SIDS); and cancer, especially leukemia (AAP, 2012). From six to 12 months, breastfeeding combined with the introduction of complementary foods is optimal. Women who breastfeed require approximately 500 additional calories per day for weight maintenance. Thus, breastfeeding generally quickens postpartum weight loss. The ACE Fitness Nutrition Specialist can help women return to their pre-pregnancy weight by reinforcing the positive nutrition changes made during pregnancy, such as increased fruit, vegetable, and whole-grain consumption. Also, the ACE Fitness Nutrition Specialist should facilitate entry or re-entry into a regular physical-activity program. When in doubt about the nutritional needs for a pregnant or lactating client, the fitness professional should refer her to an RD specializing in this area and/or a certified lactation consultant.

NUTRITION AND SPECIAL CONSIDERATIONS

Many clients may require special consideration due to adherence to a particular eating plan such as a vegetarian or gluten-free diet or due to a health condition or illness. In these cases, the ACE Fitness Nutrition Specialist can be an important source of information and also a link to other health professionals, when appropriate.

Vegetarian Diets

A growing number of Americans are vegetarians, meaning that they may not eat meat, fish, poultry, or products containing these foods. Vegetarian diets come in several forms, all of which are healthful, nutritionally adequate, and effective in disease prevention if carefully planned. A **lacto-ovo vegetarian** does not eat meat, fish, or poultry, but does consume milk and eggs. A **lacto-vegetarian** does not eat eggs, meat, fish, or poultry, but does consume milk. A **vegan** does not consume any animal products, including dairy products such as milk and cheese, and some may not even consume products like gelatin because it is made from animal cartilage.

Vegetarian diets provide several health advantages. They are usually low in saturated fat, cholesterol, and animal protein and high in fiber, folate, vitamins C and E, **carotenoids,** and some **phytochemicals.** Compared to omnivores, vegetarians have lower rates of obesity, death from cardiovascular disease, **hypertension,** type 2 diabetes, and prostate and colon cancer. However, if poorly planned, vegetarian diets may include insufficient amounts of protein, iron, vitamin B12, vitamin D, calcium, and other nutrients (ADA, 2009).

Quality protein intake is crucial for vegetarians. A main determinant of protein quality is whether a food contains all of the essential amino acids. Most meat-based products are higher-quality proteins because they have varying amounts of the essential amino acids, while plant proteins other than soy are incomplete proteins because they do not contain all eight to 10 essential amino acids (see page 17). However, complementary plant products such as rice and beans together provide all of the essential amino acids. Research suggests that most vegetarians consume adequate amounts of complementary plant proteins throughout the day to meet their protein needs (see Figure 4-2). Thus, the complementary proteins do not need to be consumed in the same meal (ADA, 2009).

Too few well-conducted research studies exist to determine whether or not a vegetarian diet affects athletic performance (Venderley & Campbell, 2006). However, if vegetarian athletes do not consume enough calories to fuel exercise, protein for maintenance and repair, and vitamins and minerals for physiological processes, performance may suffer. Some suggestions to increase caloric intake include the following:

- Eat more frequent meals and snacks
- Include meat alternatives
- Add dried fruit, seeds, nuts, and other healthful calorie-dense foods

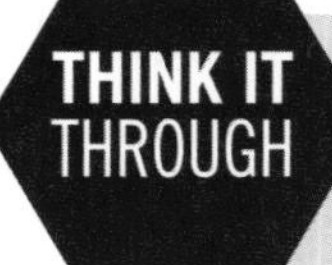

Vegetarianism is becoming more of a common practice in today's society. Thus, fitness professionals will most likely encounter clients who choose to eat a vegetarian diet. What will you do to educate and coach clients who choose to practice one of the many vegetarian eating plans about how to maintain adequate nutritional status while meeting their performance and weight-management goals?

Gluten-free Diet

Over the past several years, a growing number of people have experimented with gluten-free diets to help alleviate symptoms like abdominal pain, cramping, and generalized fatigue. While historically (and, until recently, scientifically) a gluten-free diet only has been considered necessary for people with celiac disease (a condition defined by an allergy to gluten-containing products), many people who do not have celiac disease attest to the benefits of a gluten-free diet. A growing body of scientific evidence is beginning to support the notion of non-celiac wheat sensitivity (Caroccio et al., 2012).

Gluten is a protein compound made of two proteins called gliadin and glutenin. Gluten is found joined with starch in the grains wheat, rye, and barley. People with celiac disease mount a severe immune reaction when the gastrointestinal system is exposed to gliadin.

Ultimately, the small intestine loses its capacity to effectively absorb nutrients, leading to vitamin deficiencies, anemia, weight loss, abdominal pain, diarrhea, and, in some cases, neurologic dysfunction. Anyone who suffers from the symptoms of celiac disease should be evaluated by a physician, who will order laboratory testing and possibly arrange for a biopsy of the small intestine to confirm the diagnosis. The only definitive treatment for the disease is strict avoidance of gluten-containing foods, and patients with this condition should seek the guidance of an RD who can provide a therapeutic diet.

Gluten sensitivity is much more common, and less understood, than celiac disease. This occurs when the body has a pronounced response to gluten-containing foods, leading to feelings of tiredness, abdominal pain, and other GI symptoms like diarrhea or constipation. Many people report experiencing these symptoms after eating gluten-containing foods (or more commonly, they report these symptoms going away after avoiding gluten), but it is not clear what causes these symptoms or the body's actual response to the gluten. It is very important for anyone who believes they might have a gluten sensitivity to see a physician and RD prior to adopting a gluten-free diet. The physician can test for celiac disease (the tests are not accurate if done after a person has eliminated gluten from the diet) and the RD can help develop a therapeutic eating plan to manage the symptoms. Typically, people with gluten sensitivity will test negative for celiac disease but still feel that gluten-containing foods make their symptoms worse.

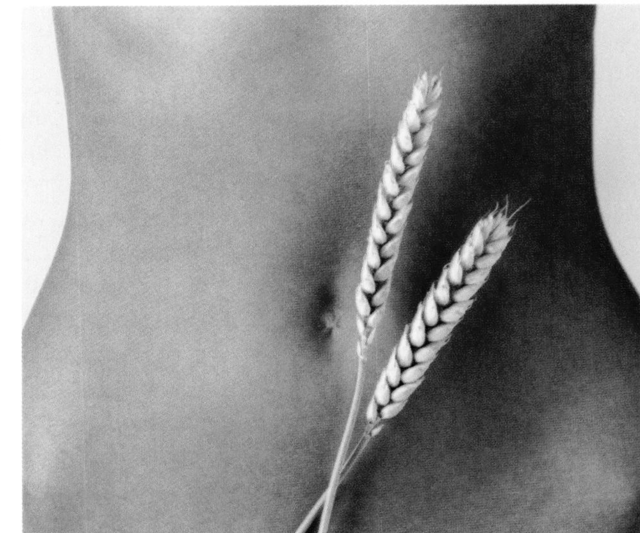

The *Dietary Guidelines* recommend that most adults get anywhere from six to eight servings of grains per day. Grains are an excellent source of B-vitamins and fiber. Most standard grains such as bread, cereal, and pasta contain wheat, rye, or barley and thus include gluten. Many foods contain gluten and, without appropriate dietary planning, complete elimination of gluten-containing grains can lead to nutritional deficiencies including B vitamins, calcium, vitamin D, iron, zinc, magnesium, and fiber. In fact, a Swedish research study of people with celiac disease who had been gluten-free for 10 years found that half of the patients had vitamin deficiencies, including low levels of vitamin B-6 or folate, or both (Hallert et al., 2002). A survey of people on a gluten-free diet in the United States found that more than half had inadequate fiber, iron, and calcium intake (Thompson et al., 2005). Though it is true that a multivitamin may be able to provide "insurance" and protect from overt nutritional deficiencies, it is preferable to get the body's needed nutrients from food sources when possible. While adhering to a gluten-free diet is a challenge, thanks to the 2004 Food Allergen Labeling and Consumer Protection Act, food labels must state if they contain any of the top eight food allergens, which includes wheat. While it is possible to buy gluten-free bread, pasta, cereal, and various other products, these tend to cost substantially more than their gluten-containing counterparts. However, many fresh fruits and vegetables and healthy unprocessed foods are affordable and naturally gluten-free. Other naturally gluten-free foods include rice, corn, soy, potato, tapioca, beans, quinoa, millet, buckwheat, flax, nut flours, uncontaminated (with wheat) oats, milk, butter, cheese, meat, fish, poultry, eggs, beans, and seeds.

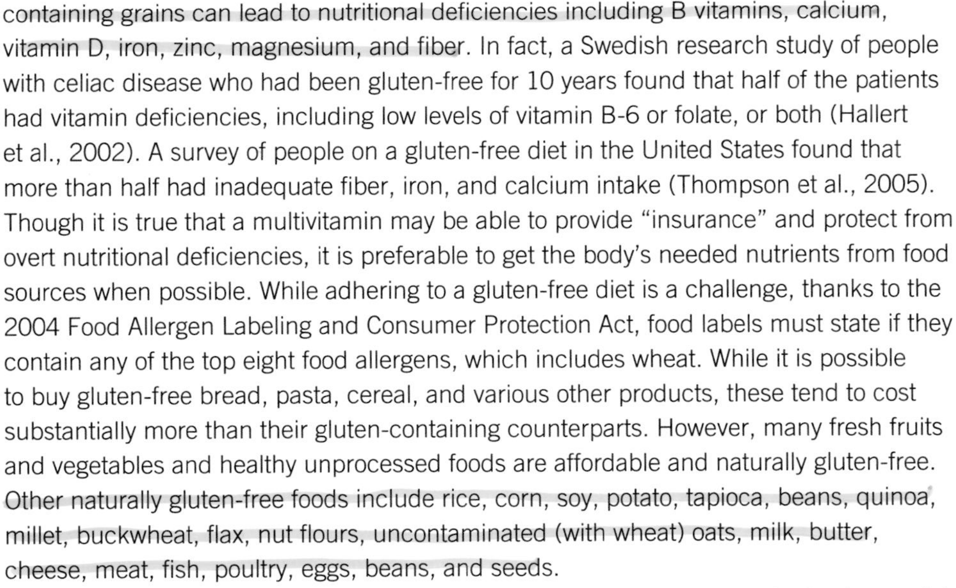

Importantly, adopting a gluten-free diet is not recommended as a method to lose weight or to "become healthier." The diet is restrictive and if poorly planned could lead to serious vitamin deficiencies and contribute to disordered eating behaviors. And, unlike saturated and trans fat, for example, gluten itself is not inherently unhealthy.

Eating Disorders

Most fitness professionals will at some point face the challenge of helping someone overcome the powerful grips of an eating disorder such as **anorexia nervosa, bulimia nervosa, binge eating disorder,** or other disordered eating. Fitness professionals and coaches who work with young people and others at risk for eating disorders play a critically important role in helping prevent the onset of an obsession with weight, body image, and exercise. The National Eating Disorders Association (www.nationaleatingdisorders.org) offers the following tips for coaches and fitness professionals to help prevent eating disorders:

- Take warning signs seriously (see page 109). If an ACE Fitness Nutrition Specialist believes that someone may have an eating disorder, he or she should share those concerns in an open, direct, and sensitive manner, keeping in mind the following "don'ts" when confronting someone with a suspected eating or exercise disorder: Don't oversimplify, diagnose, become the person's therapist, provide exercise advice without first helping the individual get professional help, or get into a battle of wills if the person denies having a problem.
- De-emphasize weight. Avoid weighing individuals who may have an eating disorder. Also eliminate comments about weight.
- Do not assume that reducing body fat or weight will improve performance.
- Help other allied health professionals recognize the signs of eating disorders and be prepared to address them.
- Provide accurate information about weight, weight loss, **body composition,** nutrition, and sports performance. Have a broad network of referrals (such as physicians, mental health specialists, and registered dietitians) that may also be able to help educate individuals when appropriate.
- Emphasize the health risks of low weight, especially for female athletes with menstrual irregularities (in which case, referral to a physician, preferably one who specializes in eating disorders, is warranted).
- Avoid making any derogatory comments about weight or body composition to or about anyone.
- Do not curtail athletic performance and gym privileges to an athlete or exerciser who is found to have eating problems unless medically necessary. Consider the individual's physical and emotional health and self-image when deciding how to modify exercise participation level.
- Strive to promote a positive self-image and self-esteem in exercisers and athletes.
- Carefully assess one's own assumptions and beliefs as they relate to self-image, body composition, exercise, and dieting.

EXPAND YOUR KNOWLEDGE

What can or should I do to help an individual I believe may have an eating disorder?

If you suspect that someone has an eating disorder, consider using the "CONFRONT" approach advocated by the National Association of Anorexia Nervosa and Associated Disorders (ANAD) (www.anad.org):

C—Concern. Share that the reason you are approaching the individual is because you care about his or her mental, physical, and nutritional needs.

O—Organize. Prepare for the confrontation. Think about who will be involved, the best environment for the conversation to take place, why you are concerned, how you plan to talk to the person, and the most appropriate time.

N—Needs. What will the individual need after the confrontation? Have referrals to professional help and/or support groups available should the individual be ready to seek help.

F—Face the confrontation. Be empathetic but direct. Be persistent if the individual denies having a problem.

R—Respond by listening carefully.

O—Offer help and suggestions. Be available to talk and provide other assistance when needed.

N—Negotiate another time to talk and a timeframe in which to seek professional help, preferably from a physician or registered dietitian who specializes in eating disorders as well as an experienced psychologist.

T—Time. Remember that the individual will not be "fixed" overnight. Recovery takes time and patience.

A fitness professional can play an important role in helping to identify individuals who may be suffering from an eating disorder and referring them to the appropriate trained professional. As such, it is important to keep in mind that it is outside the scope of practice of an ACE Fitness Nutrition Specialist to attempt to counsel and treat individuals with a suspected eating disorder.

In addition to being a source of help and **empathy,** ACE Fitness Nutrition Specialists can play an important role in developing structured exercise programs for people recovering from eating and exercise disorders who have already sought help from a qualified medical professional. An important first step is to develop a partnership with the individual's treating physician. Seek medical clearance and general recommendations from the physician regarding the maximal duration and intensity of exercise. Note that individuals with a BMI of less than 20 kg/m² may not receive clearance to exercise until they gain a specified amount of weight. When working with the individual, emphasize the positive psychological and health benefits of appropriate exercise and minimize focus on physical appearance and weight. Fitness professionals should always strive to develop a balanced and well-rounded program that includes cardiovascular training, resistance training, and flexibility exercises. The goal is to help the individual learn how to exercise in moderation.

EXPAND YOUR KNOWLEDGE

Signs and Symptoms of Eating Disorders

Anorexia nervosa: Extreme thinness; excessive exercise; fine, soft hair that covers the body; easily broken bones; obsessive behavior; cognitive impairment; depression; low self-esteem; extreme perfectionism; self-consciousness; self-absorption; and ritualistic behavior

Bulimia nervosa: "Chubby cheeks" from swollen parotid glands, eroded dental enamel, scars on back of hands from repeated self-induced vomiting, irregular menstruation, loss of normal bowel function, acid reflux, depressed mood, anxiety, alcohol and drug use, low self-esteem, irritability, impulsive spending, shoplifting, sexual impulsivity, and concentration and memory impairments

Binge eating disorder: No definitive physical cues, repeated overconsumption of large amounts of food in a short period of time, mental health disorders such as anxiety and depression, eating when full or not hungry, eating until uncomfortably full, feeling ashamed or guilty about eating habits, feeling isolated, and losing and gaining weight repeatedly (i.e., yo-yo dieting)

Obesity

Obesity is described as a BMI of ≥30 kg/m², a measurement based on height and weight. While not a perfect measure of body fatness, BMI accurately categorizes most people. Obesity results from an imbalance of caloric intake and caloric expenditure. It makes sense that obesity treatments target either decreased caloric intake (or in some cases, decreased absorption of calories consumed) or increased caloric expenditure either via increased exercise or by revving up the body's metabolism. In all, there are four potential treatment options: dietary changes, lifestyle changes including exercise and behavioral modification, medications, and surgery.

While pills are never a "quick fix" for an unhealthy lifestyle, in some cases medications may be beneficial for people who are not successful with improved eating and exercise habits. Research suggests that overweight or obese people who eat healthfully, exercise regularly, and take a weight-loss medication may lose more weight than those who use the drug alone or lifestyle treatment alone at one year (Wadden et al., 2005). The two most well-studied weight-loss medications are sibutramine and orlistat. Sibutramine (Meridia®) works by decreasing appetite. In 2010, Meridia was withdrawn from the U.S. market due to clinical trial data in which the drug increased the risk of cardiovascular events, including heart attack and **stroke.** Orlistat (Xenical® and Alli®) blocks fat absorption. While orlistat used to be available by prescription only, Alli can be purchased over the counter. Weight loss is modest—about 6 pounds (2.7 kg)—and the cost reaches about $170 per month for the prescription version (Li et al., 2005). In general, an effective weight-loss medication will lead to a 4-lb (1.8-kg) loss within four weeks.

In 2012, Lorcaserin became the first new FDA–approved weight-loss drug in more than 13 years, followed soon after by Qnexa. Lorcaserin (Lorquess) binds to cell receptors that help control appetite. Two clinical drug trials found that lorcaserin's weight-loss-promoting effects are modest—about 5.8% of body weight in one year (participants in the placebo group lost 2.5%). That said, a sizeable number of people taking the drug experienced these weight improvements—47% compared to just 23% in the placebo group (Hiatt, Thomas, & Goldfine, 2012). Qnexa is the combination of two older medications—phenteramine, an appetite suppressant, and topiramate, which is classically used to control seizures and headache (topiramate's physiologic role in weight loss is unclear). The combination appears to contribute to a 10% weight loss when combined with improved nutrition and exercise, and 62% of treated individuals lost 5% of body weight by one year, compared to 20% in the placebo group (Hiatt, Thomas, & Goldfine, 2012). In clinical trials, the drug also decreased blood pressure and diabetes risk, but it may increase heart rate and risk of birth defects when taken by pregnant women. Each of the FDA-approved weight-loss drugs carries significant potential side effects, which a client should discuss with a physician prior to beginning treatment.

When dietary, lifestyle, and pharmacological approaches do not work, some people may benefit from weight-loss surgery, such as gastric banding and gastric bypass procedures. Ideal candidates are severely obese (BMI >40 kg/m^2) or have a BMI >35 kg/m^2 with other high-risk conditions, such as diabetes, sleep apnea, or life-threatening cardiopulmonary problems; have an "acceptable" operative risk determined by age, degree of obesity, and other pre-existing medical conditions; have been previously unsuccessful at weight loss with a program integrating diet, exercise, behavior modification, and psychological support; and are carefully selected by a multidisciplinary team that has medical, surgical, psychiatric, and nutritional expertise (Consensus Development Conference Panel, 1991). Weight-loss surgery is generally not recommended for the overweight or mildly obese person trying to lose 20 or 30 lb (9.1–13.6 kg). However, in 2011 the FDA approved laparoscopic adjustable gastric banding for select individuals with a BMI ≥30 kg/m^2 and an obesity-related comorbidity. Only those individuals who are committed to permanent lifestyle changes—including regular physical activity and a healthy diet—are considered good candidates for surgery (Consensus Development Conference Panel, 1991).

EXPAND YOUR KNOWLEDGE

Alli

In June 2007, Alli became the first over-the-counter diet pill approved by the FDA. It remains the only FDA-approved weight-loss medication available over-the-counter (Steffen et al., 2010). It is a half-strength version of the prescription weight-loss drug Xenical (orlistat), approved for nonprescription use in the United States by overweight patients ages 18 and older who are also on a reduced-calorie, low-fat diet. For best results, Alli should be taken before every meal that contains fat. It works by decreasing the amount of fat absorbed by the gastrointestinal tract during the digestive process. When taken at the recommended dosage, Alli reduces dietary fat absorption by approximately 25% (Johnson et al., 2007; Zhi et al., 1994). Research has shown that when individuals use Alli in combination with diet and exercise, they lose up to 50% more weight on average compared to dieting and exercising alone. As with any drug, Alli has several documented side effects, including excessive flatulence, abdominal pain, and oily, difficult-to-control bowel movements. Those individuals hailing Alli as the next "magic bullet" for weight loss should bear in mind that most weight-loss experts contend that without the contributory effects of diet and exercise, Alli's beneficial weight-loss effects will be very limited.

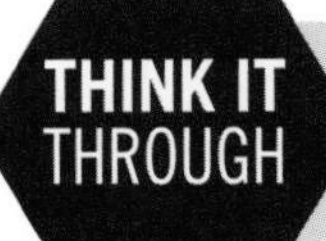

How would you respond to overweight or obese clients who ask you for recommendations on the best over-the-counter weight-loss drug to take?

Childhood Obesity

It is no secret that the United States faces an epidemic of childhood obesity. Obesity prevalence among children increased from 5% in the 1960s to 17% in the 2000s (Ogden et al., 2012). Black girls (24%), Mexican-American boys (24%), and children from lower-income communities with little access to healthful foods and physical-activity opportunities suffer the highest rates (Ogden et al., 2012). While genes and environment both contribute to obesity risk, the increasing prevalence of childhood obesity has occurred too rapidly to be explained by a genetic shift; rather, changes in physical activity and nutrition are responsible (Barlow et al., 2007).

As with adults, behavior-based weight loss and subsequent weight maintenance prove to be extremely challenging for children. In fact, obesity in childhood, especially among older children and those with the highest BMIs, is likely to persist into adulthood (Brisbois, Farmer, & McCargar, 2012; Whitaker et al., 1997). Social marginalization, type 2 diabetes, cardiovascular disease, and myriad other morbidities are real threats for overweight children during childhood and into adulthood (Halfon et al., 2013; Lobstein, Baur, & Uauy, 2004). Alarmed by these sobering statistics, stakeholders—including schools, communities, healthcare providers, and nutrition and activity experts—have responded with the development of numerous policies, programs, and interventions aimed to prevent and treat childhood obesity. The multifaceted strategies may be beginning to pay off, with many cities starting to show in 2012 stabilization and even small decreases in the rates of obesity (Robert Wood Johnson Foundation, 2012).

Heart Disease

Coronary heart disease (CHD), a leading killer of both men and women in the United States, develops from **atherosclerosis,** or an accumulation of fat and cholesterol in the lining of the arteries that supply oxygen and nutrients to the heart muscle. Over time, blood flow is reduced and oxygenation to the heart can become limited, leading to **angina** (chest pain) and **myocardial infarction** (heart attack). Though atherosclerosis usually is not deadly until middle age and beyond, it begins to develop in childhood (McMahan et al., 2006; Haust, 1990). High blood cholesterol levels—in particular, **low-density lipoprotein (LDL)**—and cholesterol's susceptibility to oxidation are main culprits in the development of atherosclerosis.

Fitness professionals can play an important role in helping people minimize their cardiovascular disease risk by educating them about risk factors and encouraging them to talk with their physicians about their own personal risk. It is important to emphasize the importance of keeping close tabs on risk factors, not only for older adults who may have already developed one or more risk factors and now must vigorously work to reverse them, or at least prevent their progression, but also for younger individuals who appear to be perfectly healthy.

EXPAND YOUR KNOWLEDGE

Questions Clients Should Ask Their Doctors

- What is my risk for heart disease?
- What is my blood pressure? What does it mean for me, and what do I need to do about it?
- What are my cholesterol numbers? (These include total cholesterol, LDL "bad" cholesterol, HDL "good" cholesterol, and triglycerides.) What do they mean for me, and what do I need to do about them?
- What are my BMI and waist measurement? Do they indicate that I need to lose weight for my health?
- What is my blood sugar level? Does it mean I am at risk for diabetes?
- What other screening tests for heart disease do I need? How often should I return for checkups for my heart health?
- For smokers: What can you do to help me quit smoking?
- How much physical activity do I need to help protect my heart? What kinds of activities are helpful?
- What is a heart healthy eating plan for me? Should I see a registered dietitian to learn more about healthy eating?
- How can I tell if I am having a heart attack?

Regardless of a person's overall risk, everyone should be encouraged to follow these nutrition recommendations to optimize heart health:

- Eat a diet rich in fruits and vegetables, whole grains, and high-fiber foods.
- Consume at least 3 ounces of fish (in particular oily fish like salmon, trout, and tuna) twice per week.
- Limit saturated fat to <10% of total caloric intake (preferably <7%), cholesterol to <300 mg/day, alcohol to no more than one drink per day, and sodium intake to <2.3 g/day (1 tsp of salt).
- Keep trans fat intake as low as possible.

Studies have shown that following these basic dietary recommendations leads to beneficial changes in reported dietary intake as well as measurable decreases in blood pressure, total cholesterol, and LDL cholesterol (Brunner et al., 2007). Still, implementation is overwhelming and extremely difficult for many people. In fact, only 3% of Americans eat healthfully, engage in regular physical activity, maintain a healthy weight, and do not smoke (Sandmaier, 2007).

Hypertension

Hypertension is defined as having a **systolic blood pressure (SBP)** of ≥140 mmHg, a **diastolic blood pressure (DBP)** of ≥90 mmHg, and/or being on antihypertensive medication. According to these criteria, about 30% of adults (75 million people) in the United States have hypertension [Centers for Disease Control and Prevention (CDC), 2011; National Heart, Lung, and Blood Institute (NHLBI), 2009]. Millions more are **prehypertensive,** with a blood pressure greater than 120/80 mmHg (CDC, 2011). Hypertension is the leading cause of stroke in the United States; therefore, blood pressure should be carefully controlled. While prescription medications are highly effective in reducing blood pressure, nutrition and physical activity are also important in the treatment and prevention of hypertension. In fact, multiple studies have shown that the **Dietary Approaches to Stop Hypertension (DASH) eating plan** combined with decreased salt intake can substantially reduce blood pressure levels and potentially make blood-pressure medications unnecessary (Champagne, 2006).

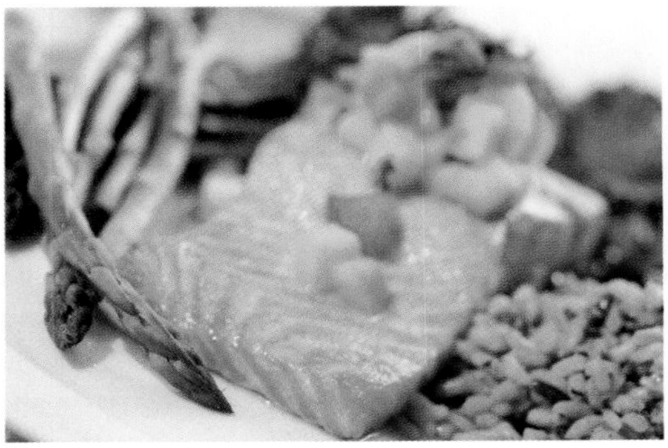

The DASH eating plan, while developed to reduce blood pressure, is an overall healthy eating plan that can be adopted by anyone regardless of whether he or she has elevated blood pressure. In fact, some studies suggest that the DASH eating plan may also reduce CHD risk by lowering total cholesterol and LDL cholesterol in addition to lowering blood pressure (Champagne, 2006). The DASH eating plan is low in saturated fat, cholesterol, and total fat. The staples are fruits, vegetables, and low-fat dairy products. Fish, poultry, nuts, and other unsaturated fats as well as whole grains are also encouraged. Red meat, sweets, and sugar-containing beverages are very limited. The DASH eating plan recommends that men drink 2 or fewer and women drink 1 or fewer alcohol beverages per day. One drink is equivalent to 12 ounces beer, 5 ounces wine, or 1.5 ounces hard liquor. The DASH eating plan is described in detail in Chapter 2.

Diabetes

An estimated 21 million people in the United States have diabetes, with more than 6 million undiagnosed cases, while prevalence is approximately 7.0% of the population (CDC, 2011). Diabetes mellitus is a condition that results from abnormal regulation of blood glucose. Type 1 diabetes results from the inability of the pancreas to secrete **insulin,** the **hormone** that allows the cells to take up glucose from the bloodstream. Type 2 diabetes results from the cells' decreased ability to respond to insulin. In most cases, the nutrition recommendations for individuals with diabetes closely resemble the *Dietary Guidelines.* Approximately 90 to 95% of cases of diabetes are type 2 (CDC, 2011). However, it is especially important for people with diabetes to balance nutrition intake with exercise and insulin or other medications in order to maintain a regular blood sugar level throughout the day. All individuals with diabetes who have not already had a comprehensive nutrition consultation prior to beginning an exercise program should be referred to an RD for nutrition education and an individualized therapeutic diet. Nutrition management from an RD is a Medicare-covered service for individuals with diabetes.

Osteoporosis

Osteoporosis is defined as a weakening of the bones, which can lead to bone fracture of the hip, spine, and other skeletal sites. It is estimated that more than 50% of all women and 20% of all men over the age of 50 will suffer an osteoporotic fracture at some time in their lives (U.S. Department of Health & Human Services, 2004). The disease most often affects elderly women, although it can occur in men and younger women. Nutrition therapy for the prevention and treatment of osteoporosis includes adequate calcium intake, which is modestly correlated with **bone mineral density,** and adequate vitamin D intake. Vitamin D deficiency is associated with higher bone turnover, reduced calcium absorption, and decreased bone mass. Adequate vitamin K (found primarily in green leafy vegetables and some vegetable oils) intake might also help decrease fracture risk (Cockayne et al., 2006). Smoking and a sedentary lifestyle also increase the risk of osteoporosis, while engaging in weight-bearing physical activity decreases the risk (Mahan, Escott-Stump, & Raymond, 2011).

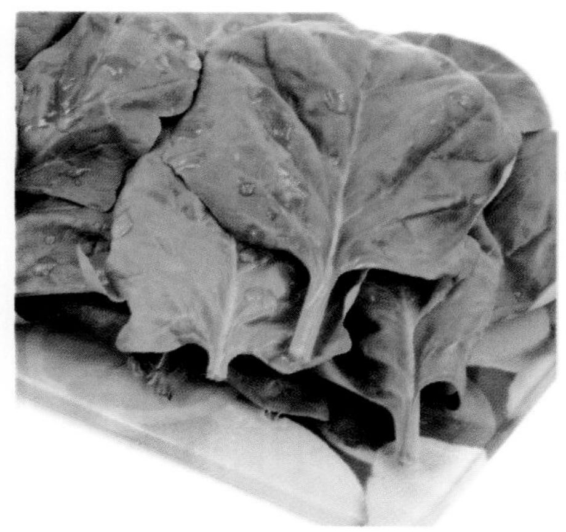

Iron-deficiency Anemia

Up to 20% of women age 18 to 44 have iron-deficiency anemia (ADA, 2004). Iron is an important component of **hemoglobin,** the protein complex responsible for delivering oxygen to muscles and the body's other cells. With iron deficiency, less oxygen is available for cells to use to make energy. As a result, iron deficiency decreases energy levels and endurance capacity. It also can induce preterm labor and result in low birth weight. Infants, adolescent girls, pregnant women, endurance athletes, and elderly women are at highest risk of iron-deficiency anemia (ADA, 2004). To prevent iron-deficiency anemia, advise clients to consume recommended amounts of iron-rich foods (refer to the DRIs included on page 36 for recommended amounts by gender and age); consume a source of vitamin C at each meal to increase iron absorption; include a serving of meat, fish, or poultry at each meal; and avoid consuming iron and coffee or tea within a few hours of each other since coffee and tea contain tannins that interfere with iron absorption (Mahan, Escott-Stump, & Raymond, 2011).

Cultural Considerations

Flavor, price, tradition, and emotional and social meaning of food are critical factors to consider when providing dietary recommendations. It is important to recommend healthful food choices that are compatible with the client's typical eating patterns, cultural beliefs about food, and overall lifestyle. In most situations, retaining pieces of the individual's customary eating habits is advisable. After all, adopting a more Westernized diet often leads to increased intake of calories, refined carbohydrates, fat, processed foods, and sodium, and reduced consumption of complex carbohydrates, fruits, and vegetables. Together, these changes lead to dramatic increases in obesity. However, some traditional eating patterns, such as the typical diet in the Southeastern United States, are less healthy than the standard American fare. In those cases, it may be advisable to help individuals adopt more mainstream eating habits, or better yet, make healthy substitutions for high-fat and low-nutrient-density foods in their traditional diets (Kumanyika, 2006).

SUMMARY

The ACE Fitness Nutrition Specialist plays an important in providing credible nutrition information to clients with special nutritional needs and linking them to other qualified experts, when appropriate. By sharing the guidelines and recommendations presented in this chapter, fitness professionals can provide a valuable service to a wide variety of clientele, from elite athletes seeking a competitive edge to fitness facility members looking for help with weight management, while staying within their scope of practice.

REFERENCES

Allen, L. et al. (2009). How common is vitamin B12 deficiency? *American Journal of Clinical Nutrition*, 89, 2, 712s–716s.

Almond, C.S.D. et al. (2005). Hyponatremia among runners in the Boston Marathon. *New England Journal of Medicine,* 352, 15, 1550–1556.

American Academy of Pediatrics, Section on Breastfeeding (2012). Breastfeeding and the use of human milk. *Pediatrics,* 129, 3, e827–e841.

American Dietetic Association (2009). Position of the American Dietetic Association and Dietitians of Canada: Vegetarian diets. *Journal of the American Dietetic Association,* 109, 1266–1282.

American Dietetic Association (2008). Position of the American Dietetic Association: Nutrition and lifestyle for a healthy pregnancy outcome. *Journal of the American Dietetic Association,* 108, 3, 556–561.

American Dietetic Association (2004). Position of the American Dietetic Association and Dietitians of Canada: Nutrition and women's health. *Journal of the American Dietetic Association,* 104, 6, 984–1001.

Anderson, A.L., Harris, T.B., & Tylavsky, F.A. (2011). Dietary patterns and survival of older adults. *Journal of the American Dietetic Association*, 111, 1, 84–91.

Bachman, J.L. et al. (2008). Sources of food group intakes among the U.S. population, 2001–2002. *Journal of the American Dietetic Association*, 108, 5, 804–814.

Barlow S.E. et al. (2007). Expert committee recommendations regarding the prevention, assessment, and treatment of child and adolescent overweight and obesity: Summary report. *Pediatrics,* 120, S4, S164–S193.

Brisbois, T.D., Farmer, A.P., & McCargar, L.J. (2012). Early markers of adult obesity: A review. *Obesity Reviews*, 13, 347–367.

Brouns, F. & Beckers, E. (1993). Is the gut an athletic organ? Digestion, absorption and exercise. *Sports Medicine,* 15, 242–257.

Brunner E.J. et al. (2007). Dietary advice for reducing cardiovascular risk. *Cochrane Database of Systematic Reviews*, 4: CD002128.

Centers for Disease Control and Prevention (2011). *Health, 2011 With Chartbook on Trends in the Health of Americans.* Retrieved November 20, 2011: www.cdc.gov/nchs/data/hus/hus10.pdf#066

Champagne, C.M. (2006). Dietary interventions on blood pressure: The Dietary Approaches to Stop Hypertension (DASH) trials. *Nutrition Reviews,* 64, 2, (II), S53–S56.

Cockayne S. et al. (2006). Vitamin K and the prevention of fractures. *Archives of Internal Medicine,* 166, 1256–1261.

Caroccio, A. et al. (2012). Non-celiac wheat sensitivity diagnosed by double-blind placebo-controlled challenge: Exploring a new clinical entity. *American Journal of Gastroenterology*, 107, 12, 1898–1906.

Consensus Development Conference Panel (1991). Gastrointestinal surgery for severe obesity. *Annals of Internal Medicine,* 115, 956–961.

Dansinger, M.L. et al. (2005). Comparison of the Atkins, Ornish, Weight Watchers, and Zone diets for weight loss and heart disease risk reduction: A randomized trial. *Journal of the American Medical Association,* 293, 1, 43–53.

Dwyer, J.T. et al. (2010). Feeding infants and toddlers study 2008: Progress, continuing concerns, and implications. *Journal of the American Dietetic Association,* 110, S60–67.

Foster, G.D. et al. (2003). A randomized trial of a low-carbohydrate diet for obesity. *New England Journal of Medicine,* 348, 21, 2082–2090.

French, S.A., Story, M., & Jeffrey, R.W. (2001). Environmental influences on eating and physical activity. *Annual Reviews of Public Health,* 22, 309–335.

Gardner, C.D. et al. (2007). Comparison of the Atkins, Zone, Ornish, and LEARN diets for change in weight and related risk factors among overweight premenopausal women: The A TO Z Weight Loss Study: A randomized trial. *Journal of the American Medical Association,* 297, 9, 969–977.

Gidding, S.S. et al. (2006). Dietary recommendations for children and adolescents: A guide for practitioners. *Pediatrics,* 117, 544–559.

Halfon, N. et al. (2013). Associations between obesity and comorbid mental health, developmental, and physical health conditions in a nationally representative sample of U.S. children aged 10 to 17. *Academy of Pediatrics,* 13, 1, 6–13.

Hallert, C. et al. (2002). Evidence of poor vitamin status in celiac patients on a gluten-free diet for 10 years. *Alimentary Pharmacology & Therapeutics,* 16, 1333–1339.

Haust, M.D. (1990). The genesis of atherosclerosis in pediatric age-group. *Pediatric Pathology,* 10, 1–2, 253–271.

Hew-Butler, T.D. et al. (2006). Sodium supplementation is not required to maintain serum sodium concentrations during an Ironman triathlon. *British Journal of Sports Medicine,* 40, 3, 255–259.

Hiatt, W.R., Thomas, A., & Goldfine, A.B. (2012). What cost weight loss? *Circulation*, 125, 9, 1171–1177.

Institute of Medicine (2009). *Weight Gain During Pregnancy.* Washington, D.C.: National Academy Press.

Institute of Medicine (2005). *Dietary Reference Intakes for Energy, Carbohydrate, Fiber, Fat, Fatty Acids, Cholesterol, Protein, and Amino Acids.* Washington, D.C.: National Academy Press.

Johnson S. et al. (2007). A predictive model for gastrointestinal side effects due to dietary fat with orlistat [abstract 010-27]. In: *2007 IFT Annual Meeting Technical Program Book of Abstracts.* Chicago, Ill.: Institute of Food Technologists.

Kreider, R.B. et al. (2010). ISSN exercise & sport nutrition review: Research & recommendations. *Journal of the International Society of Sports Nutrition,* 7, 7.

Kumanyika, S. (2006). Nutrition and chronic disease prevention: Priorities for U.S. minority groups. *Nutrition Reviews,* 64, 2, (II), S9–S14.

Lappe, F.M. (1992). *Diet for a Small Planet.* New York: Ballantine Books.

Li, Z. et al. (2005). Meta-analysis: Pharmacologic treatment of obesity. *Annals of Internal Medicine,* 5, 142, 532–546.

Lichtenstein, A.H. et al. (2008). Modified MyPyramid for older adults. *Journal of Nutrition,* 138, 1, 5–11.

Lobstein, T., Baur, L., & Uauy, R. (2004). Obesity in children and young people: A crisis in public health. *Obesity Reviews,* 5, Suppl. 1, 4–85.

Mahan, L.K., Escott-Stump, S., & Raymond, J.L. (2011). *Krause's Food Nutrition and Diet Therapy* (13th ed.). Philadelphia: W.B. Saunders Company.

McMahan, C.A. et al. (2006). Pathological determinants of atherosclerosis in youth risk scores are associated with early and advanced atherosclerosis. *Pediatrics,* 118, 4, 1447–1455.

Moore, D.R. et al. (2009). Ingested protein dose response of muscle and albumin protein synthesis after resistance exercise in young men. *American Journal of Clinical Nutrition,* 89, 1, 161–168.

National Heart, Lung, and Blood Institute (2009). *Morbidity and Mortality: 2009 Chart Book on Cardiovascular, Lung, and Blood Diseases.* Rockville, Md.: US Department of Health and Human Services, National Institutes of Health. www.nhlbi.nih.gov/resources/docs/2009_ChartBook.pdf

Ogden, C.L. et al. (2012). Prevalence of overweight and trends in body mass index among U.S. children and adolescents, 1999–2010. *Journal of the American Medical Association*, 307, 5, 483–490.

O'Reilly, J., Wong, S.H., & Chen, Y. (2010). Glycaemic index, glycaemic load and exercise performance. *Sports Medicine*, 40, 27–39.

Robert Wood Johnson Foundation (2012). *Health Policy Snapshot: Childhood Obesity.* www.rwjf.org/healthpolicy

Rodriguez, N.R., Di Marco, N.M., & Langley, S. (2009). American College of Sports Medicine position stand: Nutrition and athletic performance. *Medicine & Science in Sports & Exercise,* 41, 709–731.

Rosenbloom, C. & Coleman, E. (Eds.) (2012). *Sports Nutrition: A Practice Manual for Professionals* (5th ed.). Washington, D.C.: Academy of Nutrition and Dietetics.

Sandmaier, M. (2007). *The Healthy Heart Handbook for Women.* Bethesda, Md.: U.S. Department of Health and Human Services: National Institutes of Health, National Heart, Lung, and Blood Institute. Retrieved November 21, 2011: nhlbi.nih.gov/health/public/heart/other/hhw/hdbk_wmn.pdf

Sawka, M.N. et al. (2007). American College of Sports Medicine position stand: Exercise and fluid replacement. *Medicine & Science in Sports & Exercise,* 39, 2, 377–390.

Speedy, D.B. et al. (2002). Oral salt supplementation during ultradistance exercise. *Clinical Journal of Sport Medicine,* 12, 5, 279–284.

St. Jeor, S.T. et al. (2001). Dietary protein and weight reduction: A statement for healthcare professionals from the nutrition committee of the Council on Nutrition, Physical Activity, and Metabolism of the American Heart Association. *Circulation,* 104, 1869–1874.

Steffen, K.J. et al. (2010). A prevalence study and description of Alli use by patients with eating disorders. *International Journal of Eating Disorders,* 43, 472–479.

Stevenson, E.J. et al. (2009). Dietary glycemic index influences lipid oxidation but not muscle or liver glycogen oxidation during exercise. *American Journal of Physiology, Endocrinology, and Metabolism,* 296, E1140–1147.

Thomas, D.E., Elliott, E., & Baur, L. (2007). Low glycemic index or low glycemic load diets for overweight and obesity. *Cochrane Database of Systematic Reviews,* 18, 3, CD005105.

Thomas, D.E. & Elliott, E.J. (2009). Low glycemic index, or low glycaemic load, diets for diabetes mellitus. *Cochrane Database of Systematic Reviews*, 21, 1, CD006296.

Thompson, T. et al. (2005). Gluten-free diet survey: Are Americans with celiac disease consuming recommended amounts of fiber, iron, calcium and grain foods? *Journal of Human Nutrition and Dietetics*, 18, 163–169.

Trenell, M.I. et al. (2008). Effect of high and low glycaemic index recovery diets on intramuscular lipid oxidation during aerobic exercise. *British Journal of Nutrition,* 99, 326–332.

U.S. Department of Agriculture (2015). *2015-2020 Dietary Guidelines for Americans* (8th ed.) www.health.gov/dietaryguidelines

U.S. Department of Health & Human Services (2004). *Bone Health and Osteoporosis: A Report of the Surgeon General.* Rockville, Md.: U.S. Department of Health & Human Services, Office of the Surgeon General.

van Rosendal S.P. et al. (2010). Guidelines for glycerol use in hyperhydration and rehydration associated with exercise. *Sports Medicine,* 40, 2, 113–129.

Venderley, A.M. & Campbell, W.W. (2006). Vegetarian diets: Nutritional considerations for athletes. *Sports Medicine*, 36, 4, 293–305.

Wadden, T.A. et al. (2005). Randomized trial of lifestyle modification and pharmacotherapy for obesity. *New England Journal of Medicine*, 353, 2111–2120.

Whitaker, R.C. et al. (1997). Predicting obesity in young adulthood from childhood and parental obesity. *New England Journal of Medicine,* 337, 869–873.

Zhi, J. et al. (1994). Retrospective population-based analysis of the dose-response (fecal fat excretion) relationship of orlistat in normal and obese volunteers. *Clinical Pharmacology and Therapeutics,* 56, 82–85.

SUGGESTED READING

Clark, N. (2008). *Nancy Clark's Sports Nutrition Guidebook* (4th ed.). Champaign, Ill.: Human Kinetics.

National Heart Lung and Blood Institute. *The DASH Eating Plan.* www.nhlbi.nih.gov/health/health-topics/topics/dash/

Rodriguez, N.R., Di Marco, N.M., & Langley, S. (2009). American College of Sports Medicine position stand: Nutrition and athletic performance. *Medicine & Science in Sports & Exercise,* 41, 709–731.

U.S. Department of Agriculture (2015). *2015-2020 Dietary Guidelines for Americans* (8th ed.) www.health.gov/dietaryguidelines

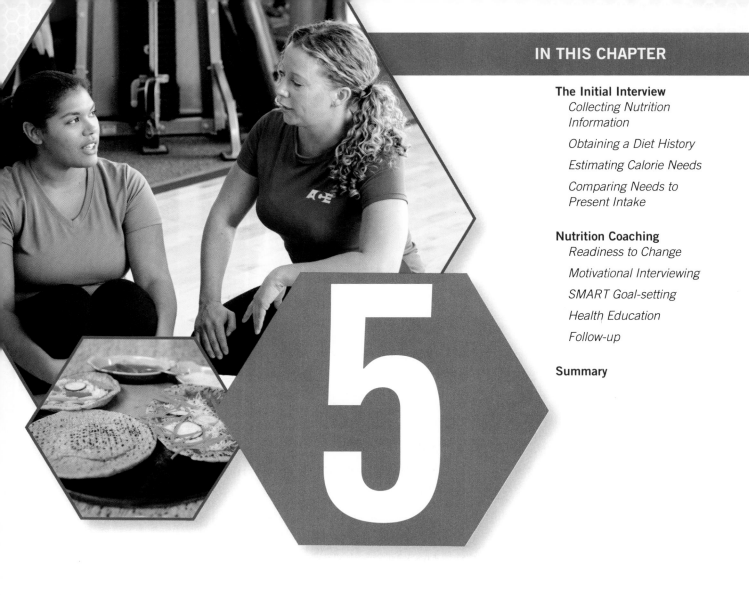

5

IN THIS CHAPTER

LEARNING OBJECTIVES

AFTER READING THIS CHAPTER, YOU WILL BE ABLE TO:

- LIST THE ESSENTIAL COMPONENTS OF THE INITIAL INTERVIEW
- DESCRIBE THE IMPORTANCE OF HEALTH SCREENING
- LIST SEVERAL SITUATIONS IN WHICH A CLIENT SHOULD BE REFERRED TO ANOTHER HEALTH PROFESSIONAL
- DESCRIBE THE COMMON TOOLS USED TO COLLECT NUTRITION INFORMATION
- DESCRIBE HOW UNDERSTANDING A CLIENT'S READINESS TO CHANGE MAY IMPACT NUTRITION RECOMMENDATIONS
- IMPLEMENT MOTIVATIONAL INTERVIEWING IN NUTRITION COACHING SESSIONS
- EXPLAIN HOW TO DEVELOP SMART GOALS
- SUMMARIZE ADULT LEARNING THEORY AND HOW IT MAY BE APPLIED IN TEACHING CLIENTS ABOUT BODY COMPOSITION AND NUTRITION COACHING

NUTRITION COACHING

> *"I get tired of people who say, 'It's simple, just eat less and move more…' We don't do dieters any favors by telling them that it's easy and simple."*
>
> —Tara Parker Pope, *The New York Times* blogger on her struggles with weight (Nolan, 2012)

With about 108 million Americans (54% of adults) on a diet at any given time, 65 billion dollars spent each year on weight-loss products (MarketData Enterprises, 2012), and the devastating health consequences resulting from excess weight and **obesity,** efforts to control weight and body size permeate the everyday lives of most Americans. While not everyone who seeks the services of an ACE Fitness Nutrition Specialist will be seeking help with weight loss, the mantra will be similar—changes in exercise and nutrition are essential to achieve a named goal, whether it be weight loss, muscle gain, optimal athletic performance, improved health status, or management of disease.

To best help a client achieve behavioral goals, an ACE Fitness Nutrition Specialist must employ a repertoire of tools and skills to not only provide effective nutrition coaching, but also to assess a person's readiness to change, anticipate and overcome barriers, help make it easier to adopt desired changes, and take steps to continually increase a client's commitment to change.

THE INITIAL INTERVIEW

The initial interview provides the ACE Fitness Nutrition Specialist an opportunity to build **rapport** with clients. To be effective in helping a client achieve nutrition and **body composition** goals, it is essential to have a trusting relationship with the client. The ACE Fitness Nutrition Specialist can begin to build rapport with a client from the start of the initial interview with a warm welcome and use of **active listening** techniques, including reflecting, summarizing, and the use of **empathic statements.**

After the initial introductions and greetings, the client may be asked to complete a lifestyle and health-history questionnaire as part of the initial **health screening.** Health screening is the systematic assessment of the client's health history and risk factors to identify clients who require evaluation by other health professionals. Alternatively, the client may have received and completed the questionnaire prior to the initial meeting. In either case, the initial interview should include discussion of the questionnaire to identify health risks. A sample health, nutrition, and fitness questionnaire is presented in Figure 5-1.

Figure 5-1
Health, nutrition, and fitness questionnaire

CONFIDENTIAL

HEALTH, NUTRITION, AND FITNESS QUESTIONNAIRE

Date ________________

Name ____________________________________ Age ________ Gender ______

Email ______________________________ Phone number ____________________

HEALTH GOALS

1. Please describe your major health, nutrition, and/or fitness goals:______________________________

____

2. What are the two to three biggest barriers to achieving these goals?______________________________

____

3. What are the two to three greatest strengths that will help you to achieve these goals?____________________

____

4. Please check the box that best describes how ready you are to make changes to your lifestyle to achieve these goals.
   - ❑ Do not believe I need to change
   - ❑ Would like to change, but don't think that I can
   - ❑ Will make changes soon
   - ❑ Recently started to make changes (past 6 months)
   - ❑ Would like to intensify changes
   - ❑ Made changes, but relapsed

5. On a scale of 1–10, how important is this change to you? _______

6. On a scale of 1–10, how confident are you that you will achieve this change? _______

MEDICAL INFORMATION

7. How would you describe your health? ❑ Excellent ❑ Good ❑ Fair ❑ Poor

8. Are you taking any prescription or over-the-counter medications or dietary herbs or supplements? ❑ Yes ❑ No

   If yes, please list the medications and state the reason for taking: ______________________________

   ____

9. When was the last time you visited your physician? ____________________

10. Do I have permission to communicate with your physician? ❑ Yes ❑ No

    If yes, please state your physician's name and contact phone number. See HIPAA release form.

    ____

11. Do you have or has your doctor or another licensed healthcare professional told you that you have any of the following conditions?

❑ Allergies (specify: ________)
❑ Amenorrhea or absence of menstrual period >3 months
❑ Anemia
❑ Anxiety
❑ Arthritis
❑ Asthma
❑ Cancer
❑ Cardiovascular disease
❑ Celiac disease
❑ Chronic sinus condition
❑ Cigarette smoker
❑ Crohn's disease
❑ Depression
❑ Diabetes
❑ Disordered eating
❑ Intestinal problems
❑ Gastroesophageal reflux disease (GERD)
❑ High blood pressure/ hypertension
❑ High cholesterol
❑ Hyper/hypo-thyroidism
❑ Hypoglycemia
❑ Insomnia
❑ Intestinal problems
❑ Irritable bowel syndrome
❑ Osteoporosis
❑ Polycystic ovary disease
❑ Currently pregnant or <3 months postpartum
❑ Skin problems Describe:____________ ____________
❑ Surgeries Describe:____________ ____________
❑ Past injuries Describe:____________ ____________
❑ Describe any other health conditions you have, or for which you take medication: ____________ ____________ ____________

12. Has anyone in your immediate family been diagnosed with any of the following? If yes, please describe.

	Relationship (e.g., father)	Age of diagnosis
❑ Heart disease	____________	______
❑ High cholesterol	____________	______
❑ High blood pressure	____________	______
❑ Cancer	____________	______
❑ Diabetes	____________	______
❑ Osteoporosis	____________	______

NUTRITION HISTORY

13. Have you ever followed a modified diet to manage a health condition? ❑ Yes ❑ No
If yes, please describe: ____________

14. Do you follow a specialized diet (low-carb, gluten-free, vegan, etc). ❑ Yes ❑ No
If yes, please describe the diet and reasons for following: ____________
____
Was the diet prescribed by a physician? ❑ Yes ❑ No

15. Who purchases and prepares your food? ____________

PHYSICAL-ACTIVITY HISTORY

16. Are you currently physically active? ❑ Yes ❑ No
If yes, please describe: _____ minutes of cardiovascular activity, ________ times per week
_____ minutes of strength or resistance training, ________ times per week
_____ minutes of flexibility training, ________ times per week

17. Please list your favorite physical activities:____________
____

WEIGHT HISTORY

18. What would you like to do regarding your weight? ❑ Lose ❑ Maintain ❑ Gain
19. What was your lowest weight in the past five years ? ________ Your highest? ________
20. What is your current weight? ________ What is your height? ________

OTHER

Is there any other information that you think I should know? Please use this space.____________
____

Thank you for your time and for sharing this information. It will be used to help develop a plan that will best meet your needs and help you to safely achieve your goals.

In addition to reviewing health history, the questionnaire presented in Figure 5-1 also asks questions about nutrition, physical activity, and behavior to better understand the client's motivation for seeking help. A "yes" answer to any of the medical or family history questions should warrant further evaluation by a physician. Other common situations in which a referral is indicated—and to whom these individuals should be referred—are highlighted in Table 5-1.

Table 5-1
Making Referrals

Concern	Refer To....
Requests comprehensive individualized sports nutrition program for optimal athletic performance	Registered dietitian who is a board-Certified Specialist in Sports Dietetics (CSSD)
Demonstrates signs or symptoms of eating disorder	Primary care physician, mental health specialist, registered dietitian with focus in eating disorders
Any significant underlying medical condition such as cardiovascular problems, hypertension, kidney disease, diabetes, arthritis, gastrointestinal problems	Primary care physician
Takes multiple medications or supplements or is considering starting new supplement	Primary care physician, registered dietitian
Pregnant or lactating	Primary care physician, registered dietitian
Recent injury and would like nutrition plan to enhance healing and recovery	Primary care physician, registered dietitian
Obese child, adolescent, or adult	Primary care physician

Prior to initiating referrals to other allied health professionals, it is essential to ask a client to sign a **Health Insurance Portability and Accountability Act (HIPAA)** release form, which provides authorization to share certain health information with other healthcare providers. A sample form is presented in Figure 5-2. If this form is not available, or if a client declines to sign it, the allied health professional can verbally

Figure 5-2
Authorization to share health information

I, ______________________________ (client's name) authorize ______________
______________________ (allied health professional's name) to share the following information:

- ❑ nutrition intake
- ❑ nutrition concerns
- ❑ body composition assessment results
- ❑ nutrition and body composition goals
- ❑ eating behaviors
- ❑ medication and supplement use
- ❑ any information deemed necessary to improve health or athletic performance

With the following individual or organization:
(Insert name, address, and phone number of individual or organization with whom the information will be shared)

____
____
____

This consent will be revoked on: ______________________. If no date is listed, it will be revoked one year from the date of signature.

Signature: ______________________________ Date: ______________

recommend to the client to see his or her primary care physician and arrange for follow-up once the client has documented clearance from the health provider.

Collecting Nutrition Information

Nutrition assessment as it historically has been defined (the evaluation of an individual's nutritional status and unique nutritional needs) is the domain of the **registered dietitian (RD).** However, certain nutrition assessment tools can be utilized by ACE Fitness Nutrition Specialists to help clients better understand their nutritional behaviors without providing an individualized assessment of nutritional status or crossing outside the boundaries of professional **scope of practice** and potentially causing harm to the client or exposing the allied health professional to unanticipated legal liability. ACE Fitness Nutrition Specialists who are very interested in providing *detailed* and *individualized* nutrition assessments and recommendations may consider pursuing a credential as an RD.

The Path to Becoming a Registered Dietitian and Certified Specialist in Sports Dietetics

How to Become a Registered Dietitian

The following information represents the required qualifications to become a registered dietitian as defined by the Commission on Dietetic Registration (www.cdrnet.org).

To take the certifying examination to become a registered dietitian, applicants must meet the following academic and supervised practice requirements:

- Academic requirements
  - ✓ Minimum of a bachelor's degree
- Completion of a Didactic Program in Dietetics Accredited by the Accreditation Council for Education in Nutrition and Dietetics (ACEND) of the Academy of Nutrition and Dietetics. A listing of accredited programs is available at www.eatright.org/becomeanRDorDTR.
  - ✓ Supervised practice requirements
  - ✓ Completion of an ACEND-accredited dietetic internship program, which consists of a minimum of 1,200 hours of supervised practice, *or*
  - ✓ Completion of an accredited coordinated program through integration of didactic instruction with a minimum of 1,200 hours of supervised practice

How to Become a Board-certified Specialist in Sports Dietetics

The following are the required qualifications to become a Board-certified Specialist in Sports Dietetics from the Commission on Dietetic Registration (www.cdrnet.org):

- Current registered dietitian (RD) status
- Maintenance of the RD status for a minimum of two years
- Documentation of 1,500 hours of sports nutrition–related experience as an RD
- Pass a written multiple-choice exam

While rules vary by state, it is generally accepted that it is within the scope of practice of the allied health professional to use government tools and guidelines, published position papers, and research studies and published texts to provide clients with nutrition information. The tools outlined in this chapter fall within these domains.

Obtaining a Diet History

Obtaining a diet history not only provides the ACE Fitness Nutrition Specialist with baseline nutritional information about the client's typical eating habits, but also provides clients with insight into their own behaviors that they may not have considered previously. Several commonly used tools to obtain a diet history include **food diaries/food records, 24-hour recalls,** and **food-frequency questionnaires.** These tools are best used in combination with an exercise and training log when working with active clients.

Food Diary/Food Record

Keeping a food diary involves having clients describe a "typical" eating day, including all foods and beverages. Clients should be urged to be specific and estimate amounts as best they can. Be sure to discuss weekends versus weekdays. Space is provided in the food diary for the client to note how hungry he or she is when the food is consumed. Additional space could be added to include information on mood, location, and time of day for more detailed intake information.

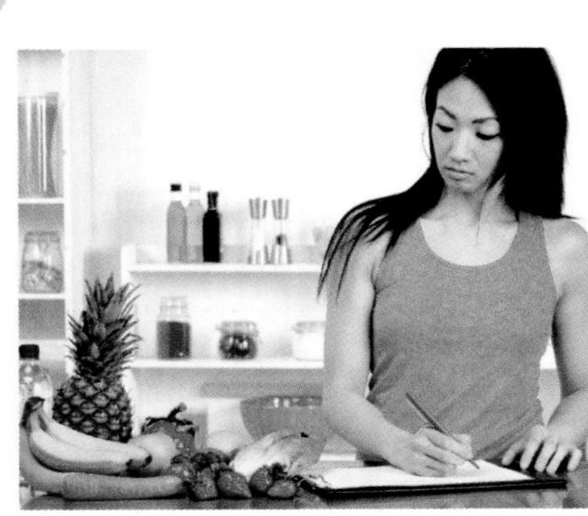

One thing to consider is that people generally underestimate or under-report their caloric intake and tend to eat more salads, vegetables, and lower-calorie foods when using a food diary than their weight might suggest. Experience with probing the client, asking nonjudgmental questions, and offering a supportive environment is likely to reveal a more truthful picture of a client's eating pattern.

Proper instruction on how to keep food records will often yield better results than just handing a client a sheet of paper and instructing him or her to "write down what you eat." ACE Fitness Nutrition Specialists should adhere to the following guidelines to help clients more accurately report their food intakes (Figure 5-3):

- Have clients keep a record for three consecutive days, including one weekend day (i.e., Thursday-Friday-Saturday or Sunday-Monday-Tuesday). Advise them to choose three days that would be typical of their usual intake (to obtain the most accurate picture of each client's diet).
- Have clients record everything they eat or drink during those days, including water, any added salt, candies, gum, condiments, **vitamin/mineral** supplements, sports drinks, coffee, tea, medications, and alcoholic beverages.
- Clients should use a separate sheet of paper for each day and create columns with the following titles: Meal/Snack Time, Food/Beverage & Amount, Food Group Servings, Hunger Level, Mood/Thoughts, Location, and Challenges.
- In the first column, clients record whether the foods and/or beverages were part of a meal (and which one) or consumed as part of a snack, as well as the time when all foods and beverages were consumed. It is also important to record everything immediately after each meal or snack so that they do not forget what was eaten.
- In the second column, clients should give as much specific information as possible:
  - ✓ Method of cooking (e.g., baked, broiled, fried, boiled, or toasted)
  - ✓ Brand names of commercial products
  - ✓ Descriptive words on the packaging such as low-fat or low-sodium
  - ✓ Specific foods and drinks
    - Bread (whole wheat, white, rye; number of slices per loaf)
    - Milk (whole, low-fat, skim, protein-enriched)
    - Margarine (stick, tub, diet)
    - Vegetables (canned, fresh, frozen)
    - Meats (fat trimmed, weighed with bone, skinned)
    - Drinks (light, low-calorie, diet, low-fat), including additions such as cream and sugar
    - Snacks (pretzels, chips, dry roasted or raw nuts)
    - Size of fruits or vegetables (small, medium, large, extra large)
    - Ingredients/condiments used in salads, sandwiches, or on food items (e.g., mayonnaise, ketchup, mustard, gravy, sauce, grated cheese, salad dressing, lettuce, and tomato)

Clients should also list the amount of food or beverage consumed, measured by a scale (for weight in ounces or grams), a ruler (for height, length, and width), or via a household measure (for volume: cups, tablespoons, or teaspoons). If possible, clients should weigh and measure foods after preparation and indicate when it was done. They can use package-label information on commercially made products.

Meal/Snack Time		Food/Beverage & Amount	Food Group Servings	Hunger Level	Mood/ Thoughts	Location	Challenges
BREAKFAST							
SNACK							
LUNCH							
SNACK							
DINNER							

Figure 5-3
Sample food diary/record

Clients should also record any significant feelings or emotions they were experiencing before and after eating, their hunger level, where the food was eaten, and any obstacles that were faced when making decisions and choices.

There are also a number of websites and phone applications now available that enable users to track their daily food intake in a convenient fashion via the phone, tablet device, or computer. These websites and "apps" provide a database of foods to choose from, as well as detailed **nutrient** information for all foods entered. Users can then track their daily calorie, protein, **fat,** and **carbohydrate** intake along with **micronutrients.** Many of these resources also provide an exercise diary that allows individuals to view their calorie expenditure and/or workout history.

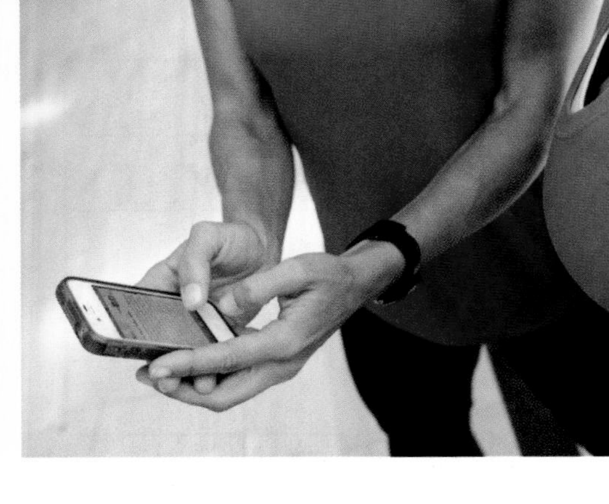

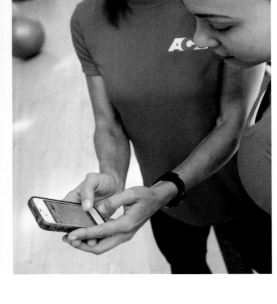

Description and Procedure

Sources: Bountziouka et al., 2010; Nataranjan et al., 2010; Svendsen et al., 2006

- The client records intake throughout the day, including water and beverages. The client also records daily physical activity. The client is solely responsible for the foods and beverages consumed throughout the day, as well as for recording them.
- By reviewing food intake along with the calories and fat consumed, the fitness professional can easily pinpoint any trouble spots with food (e.g., late-night eating or meal skipping).
- The client must be very specific. Instead of writing "ham sandwich," he or she should write down how much ham was actually on the sandwich. Was it 3 ounces (105 calories) or 8 ounces (280 calories)? It is important to include what types of condiments were used as well.

Necessary Components

- The client only needs to record his or her food intake in a food diary booklet, in a notebook, or on pieces of paper. Fitness professionals should teach clients that it is best to record food intake immediately after consumption, instead of writing it down at the end of the day when it is easy to forget foods consumed.

Pros

- Easy to administer
- Economical
- Increased awareness of habits and foods consumed

Cons

- Dependent on the literacy of the client
- Respondent burden
- Recall bias: Records may not reflect "typical" intakes because interest in "pleasing" the ACE Fitness Nutrition Specialist may alter consumption or tracking
- Lack of knowledge on estimating **portion** sizes, calories, and fat content of foods consumed

24-hour Recall

The same tools used for the food diary can be used when administering the 24-hour recall (see Figure 5-3). Obviously, a major limitation of the 24-hour recall is that "yesterday" may not truly reflect the scope of a person's typical eating patterns. In addition, this tool relies heavily on memory.

Description and Procedure

Sources: Takachi et al., 2011; Schatzkin et al., 2003

- Obtain information on food and fluid intake for the previous day or previous 24 hours.
- The 24-hour recall is based on the assumption that the intake described is typical of daily intake.
- A five-pass method can be used that includes the following:
  - ✓ A "quick list" pass in which the respondent is asked to list everything consumed in the previous day
  - ✓ A "forgotten foods" pass in which a standard list of foods and beverages that are often forgotten is read to prompt recall
  - ✓ A "time and occasion" pass in which the time and name for each eating occasion is collected
  - ✓ A "detailed" pass in which the detailed descriptions and portion sizes are collected and the time interval between meals is reviewed to check for additional foods
  - ✓ The "final" pass: one last opportunity to recall the foods consumed

Necessary Components

- Time that the food or beverage was consumed
- The food or beverage item
- **Serving** size of the food or beverage item
- How the food was prepared
- Where the client consumed the food or beverage item
- Any relevant notes regarding the meal or food item

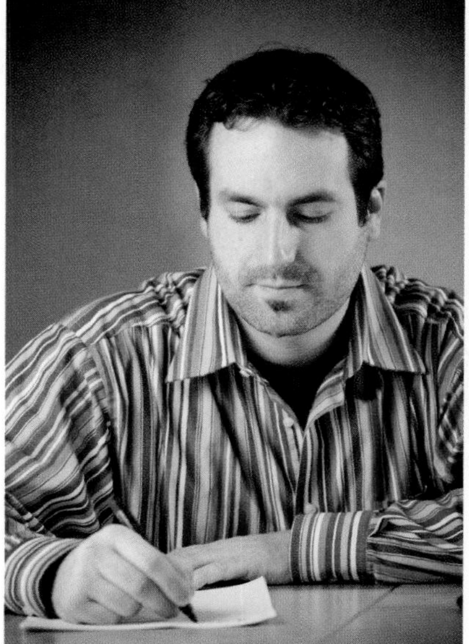

Pros

- Easy to administer
- Not dependent on the literacy of the respondent
- Precision and, when multiple days are assessed, reliability
- Low administration costs

Cons

- The need to obtain multiple recalls to reliably estimate usual intake
- Participant burden
- Difficulty of the estimation of portion sizes
- Recall bias: Records may not reflect "typical" intakes because interest in "pleasing" the ACE Fitness Nutrition Specialist may alter consumption or tracking

Food-frequency Questionnaire

A complete food-frequency questionnaire (FFQ) is a multipage list of hundreds of different foods or food types and the client is asked to indicate how often each of the foods is consumed on a daily, weekly, or monthly basis. This method is frequently used in population-based research studies such as the National Health and Nutrition Examination Survey (NHANES) to characterize typical intake. While it provides useful information into typical eating patterns, it can be overwhelming for an ACE Fitness Nutrition Specialist to use effectively in practice due to the large amount of information obtained. With that said, an ACE Fitness Nutrition Specialist may encounter the FFQ and should have familiarity with its procedure, advantages, and disadvantages. Figure 5-4 presents a portion of a sample food-frequency questionnaire.

Description and Procedure

Sources: Takachi et al., 2011; Bountziouka et al., 2010; Svendsen et al., 2006; Schatzkin et al., 2003; Willett, 2001

- The FFQ identifies foods that the client most commonly eats.

Figure 5-4
Sample food-frequency questionnaire

Food	Every Day (Always)	3 or 4 Times/Week (Often)	Every 2 or 3 Weeks (Sometimes)	Don't Eat (Never)
Dairy Products				
Milk, whole				
Milk, reduced fat				
Milk, nonfat				
Cottage cheese				
Cream cheese				
Other cheeses				
Yogurt				
Ice cream				
Sherbet				
Puddings				
Margarine				
Butter				
Other				
Meats				
Beef, hamburger				
Poultry				
Pork, ham				
Bacon, sausage				
Cold cuts, hot dogs				
Other				
Fish and Other Protein Sources				
Canned tuna				
Breaded fish				
Fresh or frozen fish				
Eggs				
Peanut butter				
Grain Products				
Bread, white				
Bread, whole wheat				
Rolls, muffins				
Pancakes, waffles				
Bagels				
Pasta, spaghetti				
Pasta, macaroni and cheese				
Rice				
Crackers				
Other				

Figure 5-4
Continued

Food	Every Day (Always)	3 or 4 Times/Week (Often)	Every 2 or 3 Weeks (Sometimes)	Don't Eat (Never)
Cereals				
Sugar-coated				
High-fiber (bran)				
Natural (granola)				
Plain (e.g., Cheerios®)				
Fortified				
Other				
Fruits				
Oranges, orange juice				
Tomatoes, tomato juice				
Grapefruit, grapefruit juice				
Strawberries				
Cranberry juice				
Apples, apple juice				
Grapes, grape juice				
Fruit drink				
Peaches				
Bananas				
Other				
Vegetables				
Peppers				
Potatoes				
Lettuce				
Broccoli				
Spinach				
Carrots				
Corn				
Squash				
Peas				
Green beans				
Beets				
Other				
Snacks and Sweets				
Chips (potato, corn)				
Pretzels				
Popcorn				
French fries				
Cookies				
Pastries				
Candy				
Sugar, honey, jelly				
Soda, regular				
Soda, diet				
Cocoa				
Other				

- The client indicates, on average, how much and how often he or she consumes different foods.
- Analysis of the FFQ data provides information about the daily intake of many nutrients.

Necessary Components

- Vary among FFQs, but typically include a large list of foods with their corresponding frequency of consumption

Pros

- Relatively low administrative costs
- Ability to assess usual and longer-term intake

Cons

- Inaccuracy of absolute nutrient values
- Fluctuation of nutrient values depending on instrument length and structure
- Lack of detail regarding specific foods
- General imprecision
- Recall bias: Records may not reflect "typical" intakes because interest in "pleasing" the ACE Fitness Nutrition Specialist may alter consumption or tracking
- Seasonal variability
- Cultural/diet variability (e.g., vegetarians or individuals on therapeutic diets)

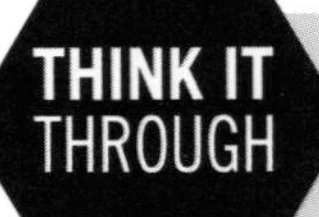

In what scenarios would each of the following nutrition interview techniques be most helpful: food record, 24-hour recall, and food frequency questionnaire?

SuperTracker

While ACE Fitness Nutrition Specialists may choose to use their own tools and forms to collect dietary information, the federal government provides resources that not only collect the essential information but also provide an assessment of the food intake based on how well it conforms to the *Dietary Guidelines for Americans* [U.S. Department of Agriculture (USDA), 2015]. For example, the online SuperTracker provides tools to estimate calorie needs and to track, analyze, and evaluate nutrition and physical activity (www.supertracker.usda.gov) (Figure 5-5).

By using a government-endorsed tool such as the SuperTracker, an ACE Fitness Nutrition Specialist provides a client with a valuable service but stays within the scope of practice of an allied health professional who is not a licensed or registered dietitian. Those fitness professionals who choose to use their own forms or nutrient analysis databases or programs should avoid *diagnosing* vitamin or nutrient deficiencies, *prescribing* supplements or other nutritional regimens, *advising* clients of a specific nutrition plan, or providing a *nutritional analysis* in response to data collected. Rather, the allied health professional can use the forms as tools to help a client recognize areas of potential improvement or concerns based on the *Dietary Guidelines* (USDA, 2015) or position statements, such as the position of the American College of Sports Medicine and the American Dietetic Association Position Statement on Nutrition and Athletic Performance (Rodriguez, Di Marco, & Langley, 2009).

Estimating Calorie Needs

The SuperTracker also provides a useful tool to approximate caloric needs for individuals. The SuperTracker accounts for broad ranges of physical-activity level (<30 minutes per day, 30–60 minutes per day, >60 minutes per day). This estimation

10 tips
Nutrition Education Series

use SuperTracker your way

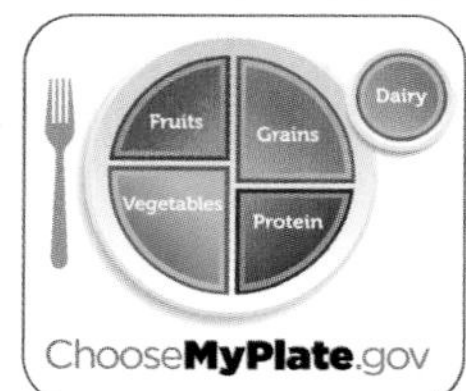

10 tips to get started

SuperTracker is an online tool where you can get a personalized nutrition and activity plan. Track what you eat and your activities to see how they stack up, and get tips and support to help you make healthy choices.

1 create a profile
Enter information about yourself on the **Create Profile** page to get a personal calorie limit and food plan; register to save your data and access it any time.

2 compare foods
Check out **Food-A-Pedia** to look up nutrition info for over 8,000 foods and compare foods side by side.

3 get your plan
View **My Plan** to see your daily food group targets—what and how much to eat within your calorie allowance.

4 track your foods and activities
Use **Food Tracker** and **Physical Activity Tracker** to search from a database of over 8,000 foods and nearly 800 physical activities to see how your daily choices stack up against your plan; save favorites and copy for easy entry.

5 build a combo
Try **My Combo** to link and save foods that you typically eat together, so you can add them to meals with one click.

6 run a report
Go to **My Reports** to measure progress; choose from six reports that range from a simple meal summary to an indepth analysis of food group and nutrient intakes over time.

7 set a goal
Explore **My Top 5 Goals** to choose up to five personal goals that you want to achieve. Sign up for **My Coach Center** to get tips and support as you work toward your goals.

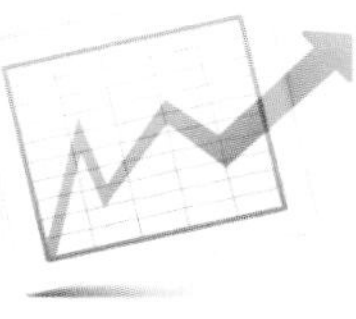

8 track your weight
Visit **My Weight Manager** to enter your weight and track progress over time; compare your weight history to trends in your calorie intake and physical activity.

9 record a journal entry
Use **My Journal** to record daily events; identify triggers that may be associated with changes in your health behaviors and weight.

10 refer a friend!
Tell your friends and family about **SuperTracker**; help them get started today.

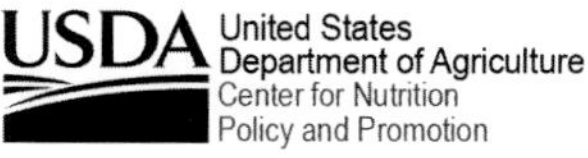

Go to www.ChooseMyPlate.gov for more information.

DG TipSheet No. 17
December 2011
USDA is an equal opportunity provider and employer.

Figure 5-5
Use SuperTracker your way

will work for most people. However, individuals who would like the most accurate estimation of caloric needs may benefit from use of the Mifflin-St. Jeor equation, which is generally considered to be the most accurate estimation of **resting metabolic rate (RMR)** for overweight or obese individuals (Frankenfield, Roth-Yousey, & Compher, 2005). Other RMR equations are available (Table 5-2).

Table 5-2
Resting Metabolic Rate (RMR) Prediction Equations (kcal/day)

Mifflin-St. Jeor Equations
(Frankenfield, Roth-Yousey, & Compher, 2005; Frankenfield et al., 2003; Mifflin et al., 1990)

Men: RMR = (9.99 x weight) + (6.25 x height) – (4.92 x age) + 5
Women: RMR = (9.99 x weight)+ (6.25 x height) – (4.92 x age) – 161

Multiply the RMR value derived from the prediction equation by the appropriate activity correction factor:
1.200 = sedentary (little or no exercise)
1.375 = lightly active (light exercise/sports one to three days per week)
1.550 = moderately active (moderate exercise/sports three to five days per week)
1.725 = very active (hard exercise/sports six to seven days per week)
1.900 = extra active (very hard exercise/sports and a physical job)

Note: This equation is more accurate for obese than non-obese individuals.

Schofield Equation
(Tverskaya et al., 1998; Schofield, 1985; Harris & Benedict, 1919)

Age	Males	Females
15–18	BMR = 17.6 x weight + 656	BMR = 13.3 x weight + 690
18–30	BMR = 15.0 x weight + 690	BMR = 14.8 x weight + 485
30–60	BMR = 11.4 x weight + 870	BMR = 8.1 x weight + 842
>60	BMR = 11.7 x weight + 585	BMR = 9.0 x weight + 656

Note: This equation slightly underestimates for women and slightly overestimates for men.

Owen Equation
(Owen et al., 1987; 1986)

Males: RMR = (10.2 x weight) + 879	Females: RMR = (7.18 x weight) + 795

Cunningham Equation
(Cunningham, 1991)

All subjects: REE (kcal/day) = (21.6 x FFM) + 370

Note: This is considered one of the better prediction equations for athletes because it takes into account fat-free mass.

Wang Equation
(Bauer, Reeves, & Capra, 2004)

All subjects: REE (kcal/day) = (21.5 x FFM) + 407

Note: This equation is potentially better for athletes because it takes into account fat-free mass.

Note: All methods of determining RMR are estimates only; Equations use weight in kilograms (kg) and height in centimeters (cm); REE = Resting energy expenditure; FFM = Fat-free mass; RMR = Resting metabolic rate; BMR = Basal metabolic rate; Note that RMR and BMR are sometimes used interchangeably.

DO THE MATH

Use the Mifflin-St. Jeor equation to calculate the calorie needs of Audrey, a 30-year-old female who is 5'7" (1.7 m), weighs 145 pounds (66 kg), and engages in 40 to 60 minutes of moderate-intensity physical activity most days of the week.

For women: RMR = 9.99 x wt (kg) + 6.25 x ht (cm) – 4.92 x age (yrs) – 161

For Audrey: RMR = 9.99 x 66 kg + 6.25 x 170 cm – 4.92 x 30 – 161
= 659 + 1,063 – 148 – 161
= 1,413

The RMR is then multiplied by an activity factor of 1.550 (see Table 5-2) to yield the number of calories Audrey needs to consume for weight maintenance:
1,413 x 1.550 = **2,190 calories**

Comparing Needs to Present Intake

Once a client has determined the appropriate total number of calories to consume per day to maintain weight, together with an ACE Fitness Nutrition Specialist the client should determine performance and weight-management goals. This can come from increased energy expenditure through physical activity, decreased caloric intake through dietary changes, or both. Very active athletes may have opposite concerns, in which they need to make a focused effort to consume an adequate number of calories to fuel particularly prolonged or intense activity.

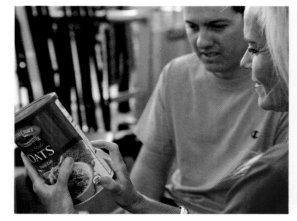

The client's nutritional goals form the basis for comparing needs to present intake. If the client would like to follow a generally healthy eating plan that conforms to the **Dietary Reference Intakes (DRIs)** and other general nutritional standards such as the MyPlate recommendations, an analysis available from www.supertracker.usda.gov provides an excellent tool to help evaluate how a person's typical eating plan compares to the *Dietary Guidelines.* If the client would like to use a different eating plan as the standard, he or she should compare the dietary recommendations from that eating plan with the assessment of actual intake. The "ideal" eating plan should overall be healthy and an eating approach that the client will be able to follow. ACE Fitness Nutrition Specialists should exercise caution when helping an athlete to conform to a non-government-endorsed eating plan, as this may cross into the scope of an RD. Note that the *Dietary Guidelines* do endorse the **Dietary Approaches to Stop Hypertension (DASH) eating plan** and **Mediterranean diet** (see page 67).

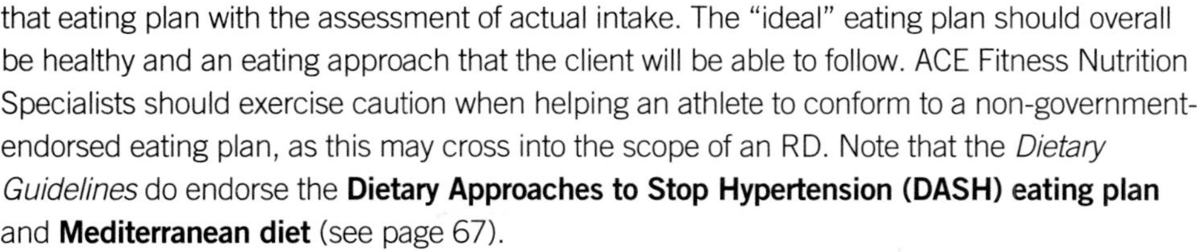

NUTRITION COACHING

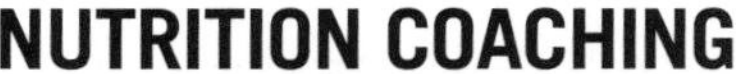

Nutrition assessment tools help to form the basis upon which an athlete develops goals and accompanying actionable strategies to achieve those goals. Nutrition coaching consists of assessing the athlete's readiness to change, goal-setting including the development of an action plan, and ongoing health education and follow-up.

Readiness to Change

Whether a client's goals are related to weight loss, muscle gain, optimal athletic performance, improved health status, or management of disease, most people recognize that improvements in exercise and nutrition are essential to achieve success. The challenge is that making changes to long-standing, ingrained behaviors requires more than knowledge. It demands significant changes in the way a person lives, from how he or she responds to cues of hunger and fullness to the mental self-talk that either supports or impedes a person's efforts to start or complete a workout. An exercise or nutrition program will not be successful without a behavioral assessment and plan to ensure that the client follows the recommended changes to activity and diet. This can only happen if the client is psychologically ready to make changes. One way to assess whether or not a client is ready for change is to administer a readiness-to-change questionnaire (Figure 5-6).

THINK IT THROUGH

How will you handle clients who hire you to help them make important behavioral changes for health improvement, yet are not quite ready for the kind of effort it takes to make those changes? What kind of policies will you put in place to evaluate clients' readiness to change?

Figure 5-6
Readiness-to-change questionnaire

	YES	NO
Are you looking to change a specific behavior?	❑	❑
Are you willing to make this behavioral change a top priority?	❑	❑
Have you tried to change this behavior before?	❑	❑
Do you believe there are inherent risks/dangers associated with not making this behavioral change?	❑	❑
Are you committed to making this change, even though it may prove challenging?	❑	❑
Do you have support for making this change from friends, family, and loved ones?	❑	❑
Besides health reasons, do you have other reasons for wanting to change this behavior?	❑	❑
Are you prepared to be patient with yourself if you encounter obstacles, barriers, and/or setbacks?	❑	❑

Stages of Change

The **transtheoretical model of behavioral change (TTM),** which is also called the **stages-of-change model,** initially was developed in an effort to increase the effectiveness of smoking-cessation programs (Prochaska, 1979). Over the years, this model has gained acceptance as an effective model of behavioral change across many disciplines, including weight management. The model consists of several constructs, of which the stages of change are the best known.

The stages of change construct acknowledges that behavioral change is a process that develops over time. The stages are based on a client's readiness to change and the anticipated or actual changes that are already in place. A client may progress through the stages linearly, waver between stages, or progress then **relapse.**

The **precontemplation** stage occurs when a person does not believe there is a problem and does not anticipate making any changes in the foreseeable future. This is a person who would benefit from educational information about the value of health-behavior changes, but who would not be receptive to a fitness training or nutrition coaching program. Indications that a person is in the precontemplation stage include comments such as, "My doctor made me see you," "I don't understand why I am here," "I am not interested in making any changes," or "I don't think that changes in my nutrition will affect my sports performance." People in this stage may have unsuccessfully attempted changes in the past, do not believe they can successfully make changes, or do not believe that changes are necessary.

The **contemplation** stage occurs when a person believes that change is necessary and plans to take action within the next six months. A person in this stage believes that the benefits of change outweigh the drawbacks, but is acutely aware of the downsides of change and is not ready yet to commit to an intervention. This weighing of the pros and cons is commonly referred to as **decisional balance** (Table 5-3). A person may remain in this stage for months to years. A prospective client in the contemplation stage may not be willing to commit to a program that is scheduled to begin soon, but may be receptive to information about a program planned for the future. An athlete in this stage may state "I want to improve my game, but I don't think I can spend any more time on this sport than I already do."

Table 5-3
Sample Decisional Balance Worksheet

Behavior	Disadvantages	Advantages
Snacking on highly processed, sugary foods throughout the day	Continued weight gain Blood-sugar spikes, which lead to pronounced fatigue about 30 minutes after snacking Feelings of guilt about giving in to sugar cravings	Taste Temporary energy boost from blood-sugar spike Convenient snack (no preparation required) Low cost
Replace unhealthy snacks with fresh, whole foods (fruits, vegetables, nuts, or whole grains)	Takes time for taste buds to readjust to enjoy whole-food flavors Increased preparation time (must buy snacks ahead of time and bring them from home instead of purchasing them from the vending machine)	Achieve weight-loss goal and improve health profile Level blood sugar throughout the day (more energy and less fatigue) Feelings of success and achievement for eating healthy Setting a good example for kids and providing them with healthier snacks as well

The **preparation** stage occurs when a person intends to take action in the immediate future, typically within the next month. This person already may have made significant changes within the past year and may have plans to initiate change, such as joining a health club, discussing weight with a physician, training for a physical event such as a 5K, or seeking out the services of a fitness trainer or nutrition coach. A person in this stage is an ideal client who will benefit most from a well-designed program.

The **action** stage describes individuals who have made and maintained substantial lifestyle changes within the past six months. These individuals have overcome significant obstacles and barriers to change. An example may be a novice runner who recently began running three mornings per week with a friend with the goal to "get in shape." A client in the action stage is at highest risk for beginning a program but struggling to make a permanent change, as many fitness and nutrition programs are short-lived, with **adherence** progressively decreasing over the first several months after initiation.

The **maintenance** stage describes individuals who have committed to a significant behavioral change for longer than six months. At this stage, relapses occur less frequently, though they still occur at a rate greater than 7% until change has been maintained for five years (U.S. Department of Health and Human Services, 1990). Individuals in maintenance have high **self-efficacy** that they can maintain the positive change and rely less frequently on **processes of change** than individuals in the earlier stages of change.

Processes of Change

The processes of change refer to the tools that people both knowingly and unknowingly use to progress through the stages of change. An awareness of these processes is useful for ACE Fitness Nutrition Specialists aiming to help ready someone to make a change and also to adhere to behavioral changes. While many processes exist, the following 10 have received the most support in studies of the model (Prochaska, Redding, & Evers, 2002).

- *Consciousness raising* involves increasing awareness of the benefits of change and the potential harms of inaction. For example, fitness professionals should explain that physical activity decreases stress and a sedentary lifestyle increases the risk of disease and early death. This is most useful for people in the precontemplation and contemplation stages of change.
- *Dramatic relief* describes implementation of emotionally moving testimony, documentary, or role playing to increase motivation to make change. Examples include sharing the story of a person in a similar situation as the client who achieved an impressive feat after committing to a lifestyle change, or having an overweight or obese client watch the HBO/National Institute of Health's documentary "The Weight of the Nation" (available to view for free at http://theweightofthenation.hbo.com).
- *Self-reevaluation* prompts the person to envision him- or herself both with and without the unhealthy behavior. For example, an ACE Fitness Nutrition Specialist may use this technique to help a college athlete who makes unhealthy food choices in the dorm cafeteria to envision herself overeating high-fat and high-salt meals, how she feels afterwards, and how it affects her performance. She may then envision herself choosing healthier options and the resulting benefits.
- *Environmental reevaluation* prompts clients to consider how their behaviors affect the people around them. For example, a fitness professional using this method may ask an athlete how he feels his behavior affects his teammates or his family members.
- *Helping relationships* or **social support** greatly enhance success with behavioral change. An ACE Fitness Nutrition Specialist can help improve social support for a client through rapport-building, follow-up calls and emails, and buddy systems.
- *Contingency management* offers rewards for making planned behavioral changes. Contingency contracts, positive reinforcements, and group recognition are all powerful motivators for most people. Importantly, food rewards typically do more harm than good for children and for people trying to manage their weight.
- *Social liberation* relies on the power of peer influence and changing societal norms and policies to induce behavioral change. Several research studies support the notion that people are more likely to make healthful (or unhealthful) behavioral changes when they associate with peers who practice those behaviors (Bond et al., 2012; Cunningham et al., 2012; Howland, Hunger, & Mann, 2012; Christakis & Fowler, 2007). In addition, emerging evidence suggests that large-scale policy changes and changes to the built environment improve nutrition habits and support physical activity (Sallis et al., 2012; Tester, 2009; Gordon-Larsen et al., 2006).
- *Self-liberation*, also known as willpower, employs making a commitment to change and acting on that commitment. A public assertion of this commitment (such as a declaration to family members or a Facebook post or Tweet) can help enhance adherence. However, an undue reliance on willpower to achieve lasting change can be counterproductive.
- *Counterconditioning*, or behavioral substitution, refers to substitution of healthier behaviors for less healthy ones. For example, a person who always drinks a regular soda when he gets home from work might replace it with a glass of lemon water or unsweetened iced tea.

- *Stimulus control* can be used by an ACE Fitness Nutrition Specialist to help clients reduce cues for undesirable behavior and increase cues for desirable behavior. For example, a fitness professional can advise an athlete who is striving to lose weight to keep junk food out of the pantry and stock up on fruits and vegetables, limit time with friends and colleagues with destructive eating habits and attitudes, make an effort to spend more time with active and healthy individuals, and eat small well-planned meals throughout the day to avoid a starvation binge or pit stop at the closest vending machine or fast food restaurant.

Willpower

Legendary football coach Vince Lombardi once said: "The difference between a successful person and others is not a lack of strength, not a lack of knowledge, but rather a lack of will." Lombardi suggests that mental fortitude and self-restraint are essential for success. While willpower is a desirable attribute that is important for successful weight loss for many people, endless efforts to exert willpower often lead to feelings of deprivation, bingeing, and diet failure. In fact, restrained eating (or attempting to cognitively control intake by imposing strict rules on the kinds of food and number of calories allowed) and the subsequent perceived deprivation has been associated with weight gain rather than the desired weight loss.

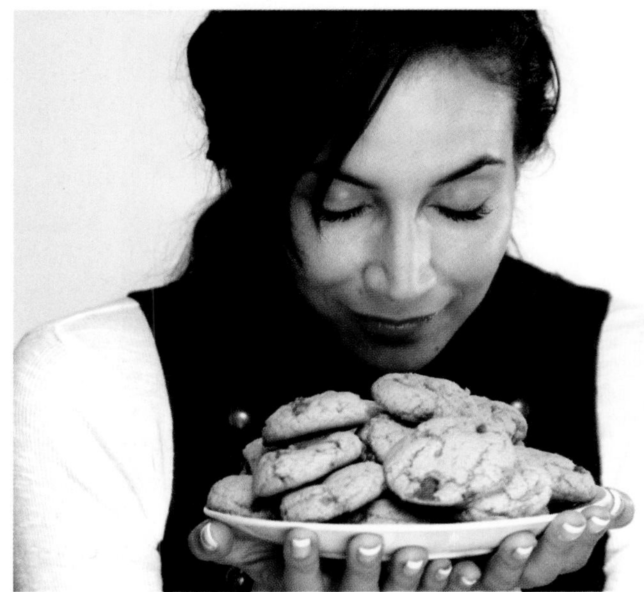

For restrained eaters, and others who rely heavily on willpower to make healthy nutrition and exercise choices, behavioral changes can help put an end to the cognitive war and allow eating and exercise to be healthful and enjoyable guilt-free daily activities. People trying to lose weight can diminish the importance of willpower in achieving success by ditching the diet mentality and instead committing to permanent lifestyle changes including balanced and healthy nutrition choices (to control caloric intake), regular physical activity (to maximize caloric expenditure), and behavioral modification (to facilitate adherence to nutrition and activity goals). Refer to the *ACE Health Coach Manual* for more detail on how to assess a client's stage of change and then use that information to individualize the client's program.

Motivational Interviewing

Motivational interviewing is a technique that prompts the client to develop a plan of action. Through open-ended questions and other active listening techniques such as reflective listening and summarizing, the interviewer gains insights into the client's readiness to change, motivations, and barriers, as well as possible approaches the client may implement to achieve his or her goals (Miller & Rollnick, 2002). This is in contrast to the traditional counseling technique in which a counselor provides advice and the client is expected to listen and follow the counselor's advice. Motivational interviewing has proven to be effective in helping to improve nutrition and physical-activity behaviors and promote weight loss (Armstrong et al., 2011).

The process of motivational interviewing can be simplified to five basic steps:

- *Ask open-ended questions:* Open-ended questions allow for deeper conversation and for the client to share his or her stories. Clients do most of the talking while the fitness professional listens and responds with reflective or summary statements.

Sample questions might include the following:
- ✓ "What will be the biggest challenges in making this change?"
- ✓ "Why is this time different?"

- *Elicit "change talk":* This technique asks clients to identify reasons for wanting to change. This helps clients and fitness professionals address discrepancies between what the client states that he or she would like to do and what he or she actually does. For example, a client states that he would like to lose weight but then continues to eat a high-calorie diet. Sample questions might include the following:
  - ✓ "What changes would you like to make?"
  - ✓ "What will happen if you don't make any changes?"
  - ✓ "How will your life be different as a result of the changes you make today?"

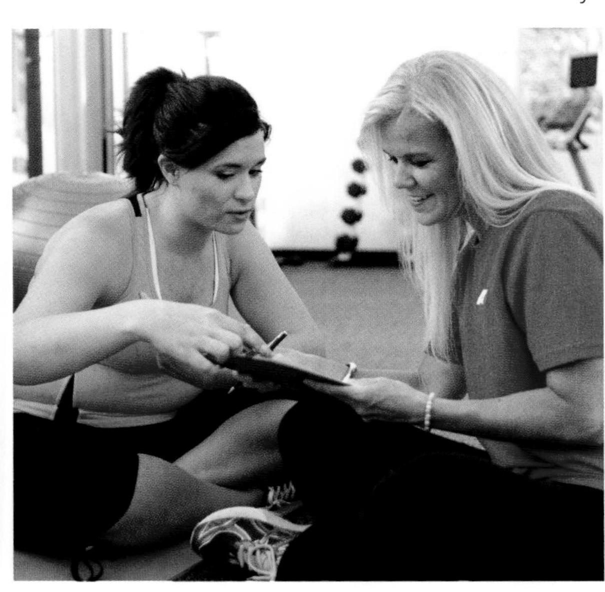

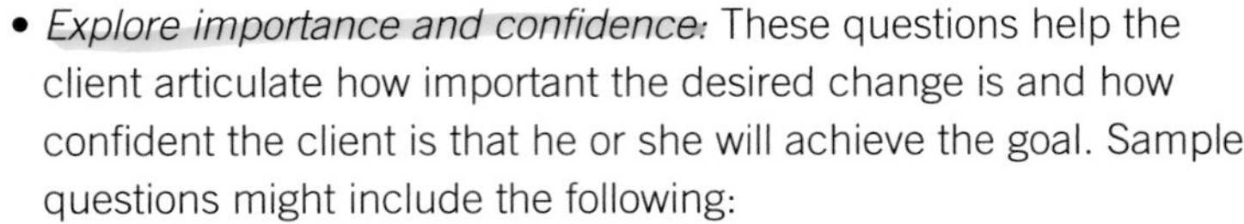

- *Explore importance and confidence:* These questions help the client articulate how important the desired change is and how confident the client is that he or she will achieve the goal. Sample questions might include the following:
  - ✓ "On a scale of 1 to 10, how confident are you that you can make this change and how important do you feel this change is to your quality of life?"
  - ✓ "Why did you choose that number, instead of one more or one less?"
- *Practice reflective listening and summarizing:* Reflective listening involves carefully listening to the client and then stating back to the client what was heard. For example, a fitness professional might say, "It sounds like what you're saying is that you are highly motivated to change, but think that it is going to be very difficult." This technique helps the client identify the need for change, anticipated challenges, and how to overcome them. Summarizing statements are longer reflections, which may link different pieces of the conversation or provide a recap of a notable portion of the discussion.
- *Affirm:* Affirming statements voice support and confidence in the client's commitment to behavioral change. An example might be as follows:
  - ✓ "I think that your idea to take the stairs instead of the elevator will provide you with great health benefits and help you achieve your weight-loss goal. I have a lot of confidence that you are going to be successful."

For more information on how to effectively use motivational interviewing with clients, refer to the *ACE Health Coach Manual.*

SMART Goal-setting

Athletes can begin to tackle their most challenging health struggles with goal-setting. When it comes to nutrition and physical-activity goals, **SMART goals** (i.e., specific, measurable, attainable, relevant, and time-bound) help set the stage for success by transforming vague visions into a specific plan for a healthier lifestyle.

- *Specific:* "What do you hope to achieve?"
- *Measurable:* "How will you know if you got there?"
- *Attainable:* "Is this a goal you believe you can realistically achieve with a reasonable amount of effort?"
- *Relevant:* "When you achieve this goal, how will you feel?" Clients should choose a goal that is really meaningful to them so that they feel a sense of pride and accomplishment when they achieve the goal.
- *Time-bound:* "When do you want to achieve this goal?" Encourage clients to set a specific date by which the goal will be realized.

Short-term **process-centered goals** can also be very effective to help a client celebrate smaller successes more frequently. Process-centered goals are the steps that lead to achieving an **outcome-centered goal.** For example, if a client had a goal to lose 5 pounds (2.3 kg) (an outcome-centered goal), smaller process-centered goals (e.g., walking for 45 minutes, five days per week) would help get him or her closer to the weight-loss goal.

At the completion of the motivational interviewing and SMART goal-setting process, the ACE Fitness Nutrition Specialist may consider asking the client to sign a behavioral contract. In the contract, the client explicitly states his or her goal, identifies his or her confidence level that the goal will be achieved on a 0 to 10 scale, and identifies a reward for success. A sample behavioral contract is shown in Figure 5-7.

Figure 5-7
Behavioral contract

Using Behavioral Contracting to Promote Lifestyle Change

Behavioral contracting is an effective behavior-modification strategy. With behavioral contracting, the client establishes a system of non-food rewards for maintaining goal lifestyle changes. Behavioral contracting is most effective when the rewards are outlined by, and meaningful to, the client. If the rewards are not meaningful, the client may not find them to be worth working toward. Behavioral contracting works differently for each individual and fitness professionals have to be careful not to push certain rewards on clients. Additionally, behavioral contracting is most effective when it is used consistently. Once certain goals are met, contracts need to be reconstructed throughout the duration of program participation.

Below are the elements of a typical behavioral contract.

I Will: (Do what) ______________________________

(When) ______________________________

(How often) ______________________________

(How much) ______________________________

How confident am I that I will do this? ______________________________

If I successfully make this positive lifestyle change by ________, I will reward myself with

____

____

______________________________.

If I fail to successfully make this positive lifestyle change, I will forfeit this reward.

I, ______________________________, have reviewed this contract
(Client)

and I agree to discuss the experience involved in accomplishing or not accomplishing this health-

behavior improvement with ______________________________ on ______________.
(Fitness Professional) (Date)

Signed (Client): ______________________________

Signed (ACE Fitness Nutrition Specialist): ______________________________

Health Education

An essential function of an ACE Fitness Nutrition Specialist is to provide health education to clients. For adult learners, the most effective health education does not come from lectures, Powerpoint presentations, or study guides—the standard teaching fare in elementary, high school, and college classrooms. Adult learners are more likely to retain and act upon information when it is presented in a way that is highly relevant, based on prior experiences, practical, and perceived to be important (Knowles, Swanson, & Holton, 2011). For example, while a child might memorize or learn something esoteric because the information is necessary to pass a test written by an authority figure, adult learners retain new information that is deemed by them (rather than by an authority figure) to be important and useful for their daily lives. A fitness professional who understands the essentials of adult learning will experience increased success in helping clients learn, retain, and apply new information to their everyday lives.

EXPAND YOUR KNOWLEDGE

Tools for Nutrition Coaching

Many tools are readily accessible to help provide effective health and nutrition education to clients, while staying within the scope of practice of an ACE Fitness Nutrition Specialist.

- *Dietary Guidelines for Americans:* Every five years, the United States Department of Agriculture releases *Dietary Guidelines,* the federal government's best recommendations for how to eat a healthy diet. These *Guidelines* offer a great deal of information that can be parlayed into weekly email tips, social media posts, client handouts, or any of a number of ways to provide clients with information in an easy-to-digest and memorable format (refer to Chapter 2).
- *Food diary:* The food diary is more than a tool for a client to record intake. It also provides a client direct insight into eating behaviors. The mere act of maintaining a food log influences the dietary choices a person makes, making it a very effective strategy for inducing behavioral change even in the absence of direct advice to the client (see Figure 5-3).
- *Recipes:* Clients may struggle to consistently prepare healthy meals or develop new ways to meet their nutritional needs. Sharing recipes from reputable sources that are healthy and appropriate for the client offers a practical approach to making it easier for the client to achieve his or her nutrition or body composition goals (refer to the Appendix).
- *Cooking demonstrations:* Hands-on cooking demonstrations turn vague pieces of nutritional information into easy-to-remember and useful strategies to achieve goals. For example, telling a client to "eat carbohydrates and protein" after exercise for optimal recovery is forgettable. Providing several examples of healthy snacks that meet the recommended intakes is not only memorable, but also much more likely to influence future dietary choices.
- *Position statements and research studies:* Fitness professionals rely heavily on position statements and research studies that highlight what works and what does not in achieving nutrition or body-composition goals. Many individuals, particularly athletes, generally are very interested in the newest nutrition advances and findings. Sharing brief recaps of these studies helps individuals to stay informed, helps to counter the large amount of circulating nutrition misinformation, and increases the credibility of the ACE Fitness Nutrition Specialist.

Follow-up

The context in which an ACE Fitness Nutrition Specialist helps a client improve food choices or body composition varies considerably. As such, the most appropriate method to follow up with a client's nutrition and body-composition goals, challenges, and successes also will vary. In any case, the fitness professional should regularly follow up or check in with the client to assess progress toward goals and provide continual information and reassurance to help the client be successful. This could be in the form of individual consultation and follow-up visits, ongoing workshops, electronic or online communication, or other modes of communication.

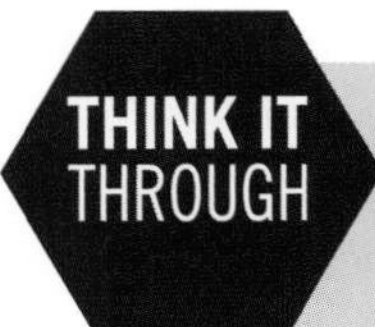

It is common for clients to feel overwhelmed by all of the information they learn in the beginning of a weight-loss or lifestyle-modification program. How would you help clients set up their environments for success without giving them too much information to handle all at once?

SUMMARY

An exercise or nutrition program is only successful if the recommended changes to activity and diet are followed. To best help a client achieve behavioral goals, an ACE Fitness Nutrition Specialist must employ a repertoire of tools and skills to not only provide effective nutrition evaluation, coaching, and education, but also to assess a person's readiness to change, anticipate and overcome barriers, help make it easier to adopt desired changes, and take steps to continually increase a client's commitment to change. ACE Fitness Nutrition Specialists who take a systematic and evidence-based approach to nutrition coaching are likely to have satisfied clients with the highest likelihood of safely achieving their nutrition, fitness, and health goals.

REFERENCES

Armstrong, M.J. et al. (2011). Motivational interviewing to improve weight loss in overweight and/or obese patients: A systematic rview and meta-analysis of randomized controlled trials. *Obesity Reviews,* 12, 709–712.

Bauer, J., Reeves, M.M., & Capra, S. (2004). The agreement between measured and predicted resting energy expenditure in patients with pancreatic cancer: A pilot study. *Journal of the Pancreas,* 5, 1, 32–40.

Bond, R.M. et al. (2012). A 61-million-person experiment in social influence and political mobilization. *Nature,* 489, 7415, 295–298.

Bountziouka, V. et al. (2010). Statistical methods used for the evaluation of reliability and validity of nutrition assessment tools used in medical research. *Journal of Current Pharmaceutical Design,* 34, 3770–3775.

Christakis, N.A. & Fowler, J.H. (2007). The spread of obesity in a large social network over 32 years. *New England Journal of Medicine,* 357, 4, 370–379.

Cunningham, J.D. (1991). Body composition as a determinate of energy expenditure: A synthetic review and a proposed general prediction equation. *American Journal of Clinical Nutrition,* 54, 963–969.

Cunningham, S.A. et al. (2012). Is there evidence that friends influence body weight? A systematic review of empirical research. *Social Science Medicine,* 75, 7, 1175–1183.

Frankenfield, D., Roth-Yousey, L., & Compher, C. (2005). Comparison of predictive equations for resting metabolic rate in healthy nonobese and obese adults: A systematic review. *Journal of the American Dietetic Association,* 105, 5, 775–789.

Frankenfeld, D. et al. (2003). Validation of several established equations for resting metabolic rate in obese and nonobese people. *Journal of the American Dietetic Association,* 103, 9, 1152–1159.

Gordon-Larsen, P. et al. (2006). Inequality in the built environment underlies key health disparities in physical activity and obesity. *Pediatrics,* 117, 2, 417–424.

Harris, J. & Benedict, F. (1919). A biometric study of basal metabolism in man. *Key Facts in Clinical Nutrition.* Washington, D.C.: Carnegie Institute of Washington.

Howland, M., Hunger, J.M., & Mann, T. (2012). Friends don't let friends eat cookies: Effects of restrictive eating norms on consumption among friends. *Appetite,* 59, 2, 505–509.

Knowles, M.S., Swanson, R.A., & Holton, E.F. (2011). *The Adult Learner: The Definitive Classic in Adult Education and Human Resource* (7th ed.). Burlington, Mass.: Elsevier.

MarketData Enterprises, Inc. (2012). *Press Release: Number of American Dieters Soars to 108 Million.* Retrieved January 31, 2013: www.marketdataenterprises.com

Mifflin, M.D. et al. (1990). A new predictive equation for resting energy expenditure in healthy individuals. *American Journal of Clinical Nutrition,* 51, 241–247.

Miller, W.R. & Rollnick, S. (2002). *Motivational Interviewing: Preparing People for Change Behavior* (2nd ed.). New York: Guilford Press.

Nataranjan, L. et al. (2010). Measurement error of dietary self-report in intervention trials. *American Journal of Epidemiology,* 172, 819–827.

Nolan, R. (2012). *Behind the Cover Story: Tara Parker-Pope on Weight Loss. The New York Times.* Retrieved October 28, 2012: www.6thfloor.blogs.nytimes.com/2012/01/03/behind-the-cover-story-tara-parker-pope-on-obesity/.

Owen, C.E. et al. (1987). A reappraisal of caloric requirements of men. *American Journal of Clinical Nutrition,* 46, 75–85.

Owen, C.E. et al. (1986). A reappraisal of caloric requirements in healthy women. *American Journal of Clinical Nutrition,* 44, 1–19.

Prochaska, J.O. (1979). *Systems of Psychotherapy: A Transtheoretical Analysis.* Pacific Grove, Calif.: Brooks-Cole.

Prochaska, J.O., Redding, C.A., & Evers, K.E. (2002). The transtheoretical model and stages of change. In: Glanz, K., Rimer, B.K., & Lewis, F.M. (Eds.). *Health Behavior and Health Education* (3rd ed.). San Francisco: Jossey-Bass.

Rodriguez, N.R., Di Marco, N.M., & Langley, S. (2009). American College of Sports Medicine position stand: Nutrition and athletic performance. *Medicine & Science in Sports & Exercise,* 41, 709–731.

Sallis, J.F. et al. (2012). Role of built environments in physical activity, obesity, and cardiovascular disease. *Circulation,* 125, 5, 729–737.

Schatzkin, A. et al. (2003). A comparison of a food-frequency questionnaire with a 24-hour recall for use in an epidemiological cohort study: Results from the biomarker-based Observing Protein and Energy Nutrition (OPEN) study. *International Journal of Epidemiology,* 32, 1054–1062.

Schofield, R. (1985). Equations for estimating basal metabolic rate (BMR). *Human Nutrition: Clinical Nutrition,* 39C, 5–41.

Svendsen, M. et al. (2006). Accuracy of food

intake reporting in obese subjects with metabolic risk factors. *British Journal of Nutrition,* 95, 640–649.

Takachi, R. et al. (2011). Validity of a self-administered Food Frequency Questionnaire for middle-aged urban cancer screenees: Comparison with 4-day weighed dietary records. *Journal of Epidemiology,* 1–12.

Tester, J.M. (2009). The built environment: Designing communities to promote physical activity in children. *Pediatrics,* 123, 6, 1591–1598.

Tverskaya, R. et al. (1998). Comparison of several equations and derivation of a new equation for calculating basal metabolic rate in obese children. *Journal of the American College of Nutrition,* 17, 4, 333–336.

U.S. Department of Agriculture (2015). *2015-2020 Dietary Guidelines for Americans* (8th ed.) www.health.gov/dietaryguidelines

U.S. Department of Health and Human Services (1990). *The Health Benefits of Smoking Cessation: A Report of the Surgeon General.* U.S. Department of Health and Human Services Publication no. CDC 90-8416. Washington, D.C.: U.S. Government Printing Office.

Willett, W. (2001). Commentary: Dietary diaries versus food frequency questionnaires—A case of undigestible data. *International Journal of Epidemiology,* 30, 317–319.

SUGGESTED READING

American Council on Exercise (2013). *ACE Health Coach Manual.* San Diego, Calif.: American Council on Exercise.

Maxwell, J.C. (2010). *Everyone Communicates, Few Connect.* Nashville, Tenn.: Thomas Nelson.

Rodriguez, N.R., Di Marco, N.M., & Langley, S. (2009). American College of Sports Medicine position stand: Nutrition and athletic performance. *Medicine & Science in Sports & Exercise,* 41, 709–731.

U.S. Department of Agriculture (2015). *2015-2020 Dietary Guidelines for Americans* (8th ed.) www.health.gov/dietaryguidelines

6

IN THIS CHAPTER

LEARNING OBJECTIVES

AFTER READING THIS CHAPTER, YOU WILL BE ABLE TO:

- DESCRIBE SEVERAL PRACTICAL TIPS TO HELP A CLIENT LEARN HOW TO COOK
- APPLY SEVERAL BASIC COOKING ESSENTIALS
- HOST A GROCERY STORE TOUR AND EXPLAIN TIPS AND STRATEGIES FOR SELECTING FOODS AT THE VARIOUS SECTIONS OF THE GROCERY STORE, INCLUDING COMPARING AND ANALYZING NUTRITION LABELS
- OFFER SEVERAL TIPS TO HELP MAKE EATING MEALS AT HOME EASIER
- LIST SEVERAL WAYS TO REDUCE PORTIONS AND CALORIES WHEN EATING OUT
- SELECT THE HEALTHIEST CHOICES FROM A RESTAURANT MENU BASED ON ENTRÉE DESCRIPTIONS

ESSENTIALS OF MEAL SELECTION AND PREPARATION

Many clients understand what they need to eat for optimal health, but they do not know how to choose and prepare healthful meals. An ACE Fitness Nutrition Specialist who understands the essentials of meal preparation can be an invaluable source of information and guidance in helping a client translate nutrition knowledge into action.

Despite the popularity of the Food Network cable channel and televised cooking programs, many people struggle to consistently prepare healthy meals. With schedules to balance, jobs to work, and homework to do, mealtimes are often considered a chore. It is no surprise, then, that many families declare success when an assortment of food makes it to the dinner table, even if the meal is neither healthy nor tasty. Though a large percentage of people would like to eat healthier, most people perceive that they do not have enough time, money, or know-how to cook "gourmet" meals.

COOKING HEALTHY MEALS: FROM ASPIRATION TO REALITY

A haphazard approach to meal preparation may be part of the reason for the disconnect between what Americans know is a healthy meal and what they actually eat. The primary predictor of whether a person likes a food is whether it tastes good. Many people believe that healthy food not only does not taste as good as food heavy in **solid fats and added sugars**, but also that it costs more. But it does not necessarily have to be that way. As a client makes the commitment to prepare healthier meals, it is essential that it does not add a significant amount of time in the kitchen or an increased strain on the operating budget. To achieve this objective, clients should learn how to (1) build a healthy meal; (2) prepare quick, easy, healthful, and delicious meals; (3) save time and money and optimize health by planning meals in advance; and (4) make informed purchasing decisions.

Learn to Build a Healthy Meal

A healthy meal contains a balance of food groups to help provide for nutrient needs. Creating a healthy meal is the act of turning nutrition knowledge into action. One effective approach to building a healthy meal is to prepare combinations of foods that resemble the MyPlate recommendations—½ vegetables and fruits, ¼ whole grains, ¼ lean protein, and a serving of a calcium-rich food. When clients take this simple approach to meal planning, they ensure a balance of nutrients and set the stage for meeting the nutrition standards set forth by the *Dietary Guidelines for Americans* (U.S. Department of Agriculture, 2015). For more information on the essential steps to building a healthy meal, refer to Figure 6-1.

10 tips
Nutrition Education Series

build a healthy meal

10 tips for healthy meals

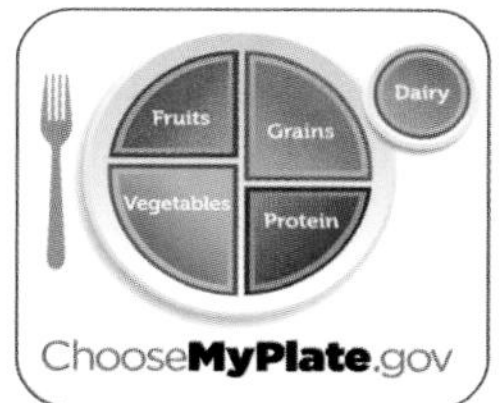

A healthy meal starts with more vegetables and fruits and smaller portions of protein and grains. Think about how you can adjust the portions on your plate to get more of what you need without too many calories. And don't forget dairy—make it the beverage with your meal or add fat-free or low-fat dairy products to your plate.

1 make half your plate veggies and fruits

Vegetables and fruits are full of nutrients and may help to promote good health. Choose red, orange, and dark-green vegetables such as tomatoes, sweet potatoes, and broccoli.

2 add lean protein

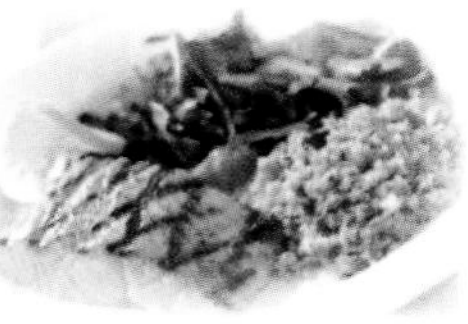

Choose protein foods, such as lean beef and pork, or chicken, turkey, beans, or tofu. Twice a week, make seafood the protein on your plate.

3 include whole grains

Aim to make at least half your grains whole grains. Look for the words "100% whole grain" or "100% whole wheat" on the food label. Whole grains provide more nutrients, like fiber, than refined grains.

4 don't forget the dairy

Pair your meal with a cup of fat-free or low-fat milk. They provide the same amount of calcium and other essential nutrients as whole milk, but less fat and calories. Don't drink milk? Try soymilk (soy beverage) as your beverage or include fat-free or low-fat yogurt in your meal.

5 avoid extra fat

Using heavy gravies or sauces will add fat and calories to otherwise healthy choices. For example, steamed broccoli is great, but avoid topping it with cheese sauce. Try other options, like a sprinkling of low-fat parmesan cheese or a squeeze of lemon.

6 take your time

Savor your food. Eat slowly, enjoy the taste and textures, and pay attention to how you feel. Be mindful. Eating very quickly may cause you to eat too much.

7 use a smaller plate

Use a smaller plate at meals to help with portion control. That way you can finish your entire plate and feel satisfied without overeating.

8 take control of your food

Eat at home more often so you know exactly what you are eating. If you eat out, check and compare the nutrition information. Choose healthier options such as baked instead of fried.

9 try new foods

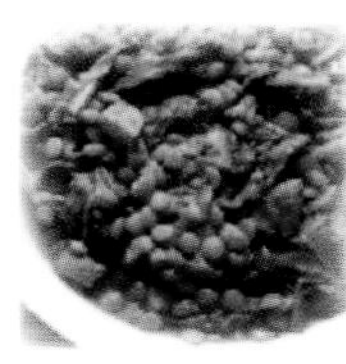

Keep it interesting by picking out new foods you've never tried before, like mango, lentils, or kale. You may find a new favorite! Trade fun and tasty recipes with friends or find them online.

10 satisfy your sweet tooth in a healthy way

Indulge in a naturally sweet dessert dish—fruit! Serve a fresh fruit cocktail or a fruit parfait made with yogurt. For a hot dessert, bake apples and top with cinnamon.

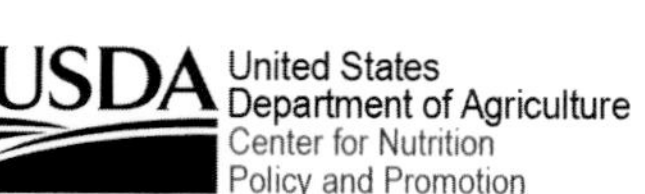

Go to www.ChooseMyPlate.gov for more information.

DG TipSheet No. 7
June 2011
USDA is an equal opportunity provider and employer.

Figure 6-1
Build a healthy meal

Apply Basic Cooking Essentials

Inspiring individuals to eat healthy home-cooked meals extends far beyond sharing governmental nutrition recommendations such as the MyPlate guidelines (www.ChooseMyPlate.gov). In order for people to feel inspired to prepare their own food, they also need to feel like they have the knowledge and skills to make healthy food taste good. Stated simply, they need to learn how to cook. The ACE Fitness Nutrition Specialist can help clients to use their nutrition knowledge to make healthy and tasty meals by teaching them some basic cooking fundamentals.

- *Keep it simple:* The first rule of thumb for a novice cook is to keep it simple. If a client describes "lack of time" or "I hate to cook" as major reasons for struggling to eat healthy, then that client may benefit from an introduction to some very quick and simple recipes that taste good, promote health, are easy to prepare, and are difficult to "mess up." The "intro" recipes should contain only a few ingredients and be easy to follow. Remind the client to read the entire recipe before starting.
- *Consider substitutions:* Once clients feel comfortable with the recipes and have gained experience in the kitchen, they can get more creative by substituting ingredients and experimenting with spices and herbs. For example, instead of ground beef for taco night, a client might try baking mahi-mahi with cumin and lemon for a lighter, healthier, and more adventurous version. Or a client may use thinly sliced eggplant and zucchini as substitutes for pasta in his or her favorite lasagna recipe. Clients may also want to make substitutions to some recipes to reduce **saturated fat,** sugar, and/or sodium. Here are a few tips from the "Eat Healthy, Move More" workshop adjunct to the *Dietary Guidelines*:
  - ✔ Cook using low-fat methods such as baking, broiling, boiling, or microwaving, rather than frying.
  - ✔ Season foods with herbs, spices, lime or lemon juice, and vinegar rather than salt.
  - ✔ Use oils and spray oils instead of solid fats like butter and margarine.
  - ✔ Increase the amount of vegetables and/or fruit in a recipe—remember, you want to fill half of your plate with vegetables or fruits.
  - ✔ Take the skin off chicken and turkey pieces before cooking them.
  - ✔ Reduce the amount of sugar by one-quarter to one-third. For example, if a recipe calls for 1 cup, use 2/3 cup. To enhance the flavor when sugar is reduced, add vanilla, cinnamon, or nutmeg.
- *Enhance flavor and appeal:* The success of a new recipe or meal idea extends beyond the quality of the recipe. Encourage clients to incorporate flavorful ingredients into recipes that also smell delicious. Such ingredients as onions, garlic, and many herbs and spices create a mouth-watering aroma.
- In fact, spices and herbs can transform a bland meal into a truly gourmet experience. Spices are components of aromatic plants, such as bark, roots, buds, flowers, fruits, and seeds that are grown in the tropics and add a sweet, spicy, or hot flavor to foods. Herbs are leaves and stems of plants that grow in temperate climates. Such seeds as caraway and sesame, which come from tropical and temperate regions, and dehydrated vegetables (such as celery and garlic powder) also add flavor to foods. Figure 6-2 includes a detailed description of the most common spices and herbs and when to use them.
- *Remember that timing is everything:* The temperature, texture, and overall taste of a food depend in large part on timing. Clients should be careful to serve hot foods hot and cold foods cold. A delicious steamed vegetable may turn a person off to vegetables if it is overcooked and served soggy.
- *Make it look good:* If a meal looks attractive and appealing, it is much more likely that family members will eagerly give it a try.

Figure 6-2
Herbs and spices

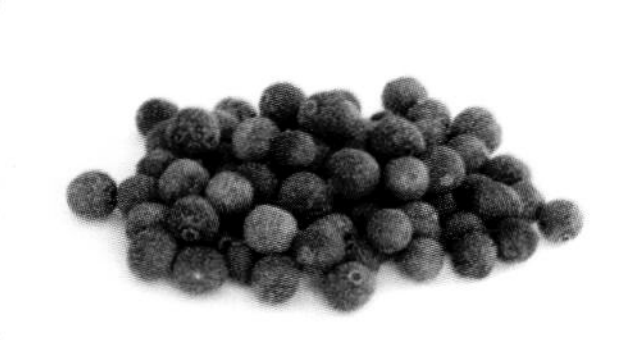

ALLSPICE: Berry of the evergreen "pimento tree." Commonly used in Jamaican cooking. Tastes like mix of cinnamon, nutmeg, and cloves, thus the name "allspice."

Uses: Chicken, beef, fish (key ingredient in "jerk" dishes), fruit desserts, cakes, cookies, and apple cider

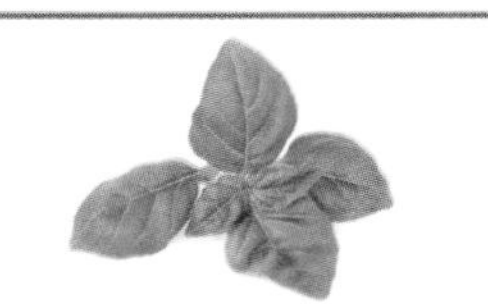

BASIL: Aromatic leaf of the bay laurel. Pungently aromatic, sweet, spicy flavor.

Uses: Essential ingredient in Italian and Thai dishes; main ingredient in pesto

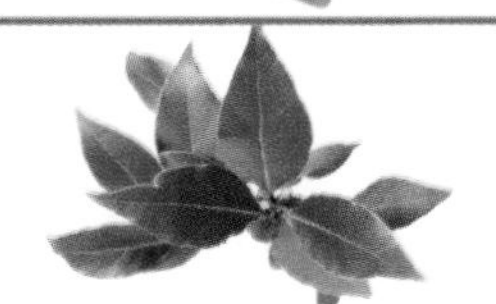

BAY LEAF: Leaf of evergreen laurel. Aromatic, bitter, spicy, pungent flavor.

Uses: Soups, stews, braises, and pâtés; used often in Mediterranean cuisine

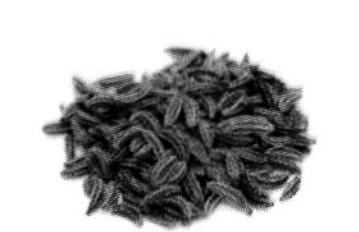

CARAWAY SEED: Seeds from the fruit of perennial herb of ginger family. Grown mostly in India; Very expensive. Sweet and pungent flavor, highly aromatic.

Uses: Rye breads and baked goods; often used in European cuisine

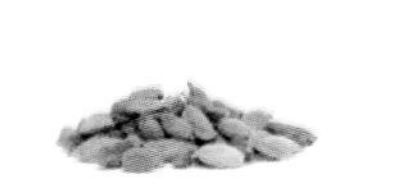

CARDAMOM: Seeds from fruit of perennial herb of ginger family; grown mostly in India; very expensive. Sweet and pungent flavor, highly aromatic.

Uses: Indian curry dishes, lunch meats

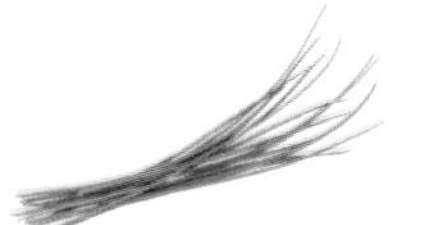

CHIVES: Smallest species of the onion family. Onion flavor.

Uses: Soups, salad dressings, and dips

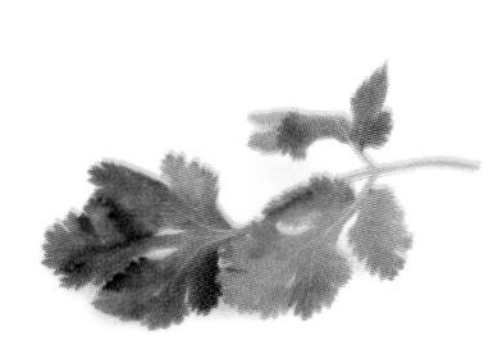

CILANTRO (CORIANDER): Annual flowering herb. Can be cultivated for leaves, seeds, flower, and roots. May have "soapy" versus "herby" taste depending on the genetics of the taster.

Uses: Often used in Latin American, Indian, and Chinese dishes, and in salsa and guacamole, stir fries, and grilled chicken or fish; best when used fresh

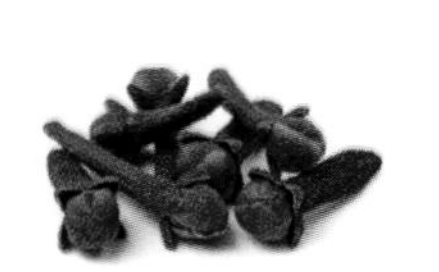

CLOVES: Dried flower buds from evergreen of myrtle family. Warm, spicy, astringent, fruity, slightly bitter flavor.

Uses: Whole gloves on ham or pork roast; ground cloves to season pear or apple desserts, beets, beans, tomatoes, squash, and sweet potatoes

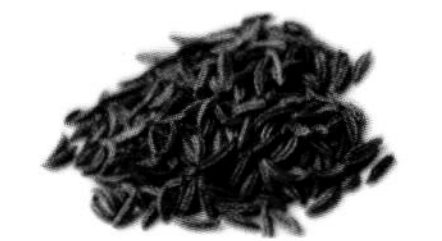

CUMIN SEED: Seeds of flowering plant of parsley family. Earthy and warming flavor.

Uses: Curry powder and chili; used throughout the world (second most common seasoning after black ground pepper)

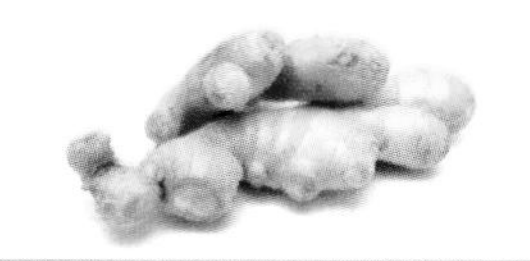

GINGER: Underground stem of perennial tropical plant. Biting flavor, fragrant.

Uses: Asian dishes, marinade for chicken and fish, gingerbread, cookies, and processed meats

MARJORAM: Leaves and flowers of perennial of mint family. Sweet pine and citrus flavor.

Uses: Meats, fish, poultry, vegetables, and soups

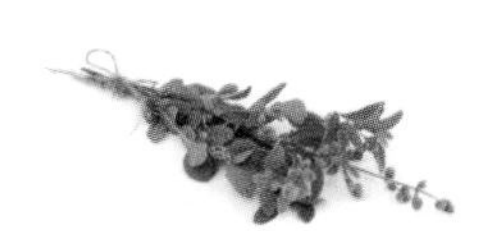

NUTMEG: Seed of fruit of evergreen tree. Sweet, warm, pungent, aromatic, bitter flavor.

Uses: Eggnog, French toast, cooked fruits, sweet potatoes, and spinach

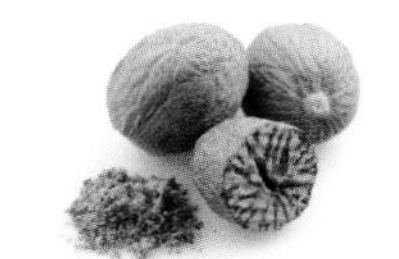

OREGANO: Leaves of perennial of the mint family. Related to majoram, but very different flavor. Strong, pungent, aromatic, bitter flavor.

Uses: Italian dishes, chili, beef stew, pork, and vegetables

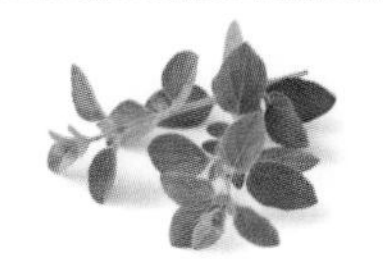

PARSLEY: Leaves of a biennial herbaceous plant; curly and flat leaf varieties. Grassy, bitter flavor.

Uses: Widely used throughout world, including in meat, soup, and vegetables; often used as garnish

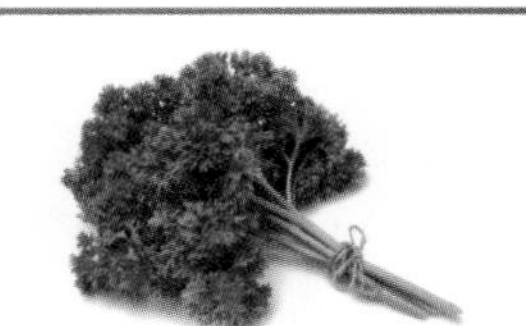

ROSEMARY: Woody perennial herb of evergreen shrub of mint family. Sweet, spicy, peppery flavor.

Uses: Flavoring in stuffing and roast lamb, pork, chicken, and turkey

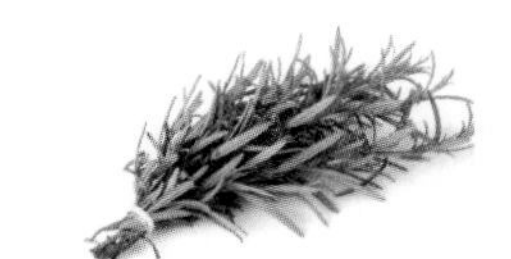

SAFFRON: Spice derived from flower of iris family. Very expensive. Earthy, sweet flavor.

Uses: Baked goods and rice dishes

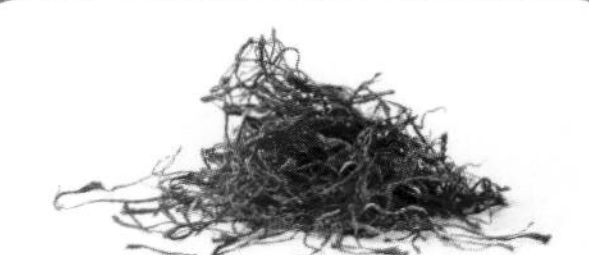

SAGE: Medicinal plant of mint family. Slightly peppery flavor.

Uses: Often used to flavor fatty meals

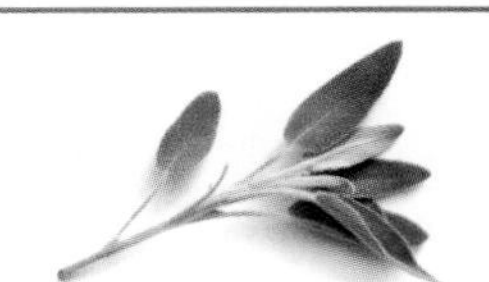

TARRAGON: Flowering tops and leaves of a perennial herb. Often called "dragon herb." Minty "anise-like" (resembles licorice) flavor.

Uses: Chicken, fish, and egg dishes; one of four "fine herbs" of French cooking

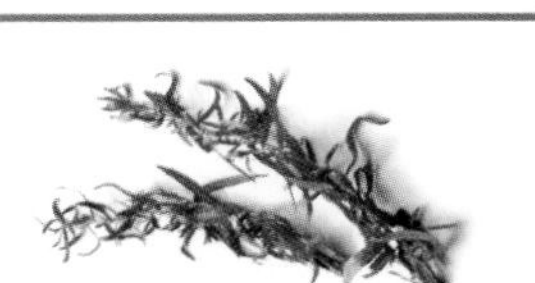

THYME: Leaves and flowering tops of a shrublike perennial of the mint family. Biting, sharp, spicy, herbaceous flavor. Blends well with other herbs.

Uses: Meats, soups, and stews

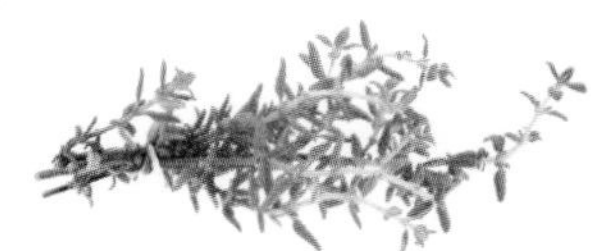

TURMERIC: Stem of plant of tropical perennial herb. Mild, peppery, mustardy, pungent taste.

Uses: Curry powders, mustards, and condiments

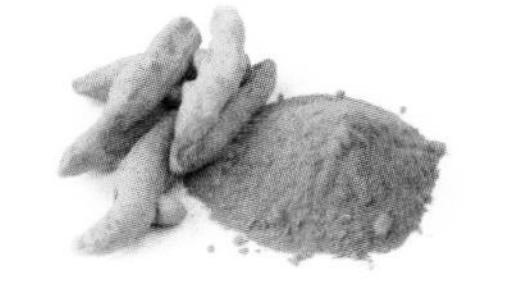

Sources: Bennion, M.B. & Scheule, B.S. (Eds.) (1999). *Introductory Foods* (13th ed.) New York: Prentice Hall; University of Tennessee Extension (2002a). *Eat Smart: Get Your Family to the Table. Cooking Basics.* https://utextension.tennessee.edu/publications/Documents/SP732.pdf

Plan Ahead

While clients may attend a cooking class, collect recipes, and fully intend to cook more frequently, if it is not convenient and cost-effective to prepare healthy meals, many clients will not do it. When clients plan ahead, they will be more likely to prepare healthy home-cooked meals.

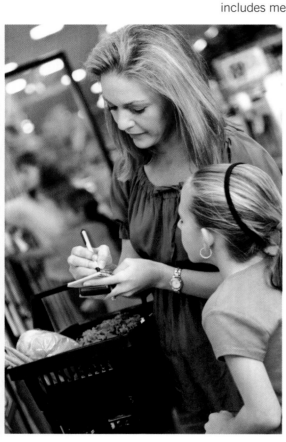

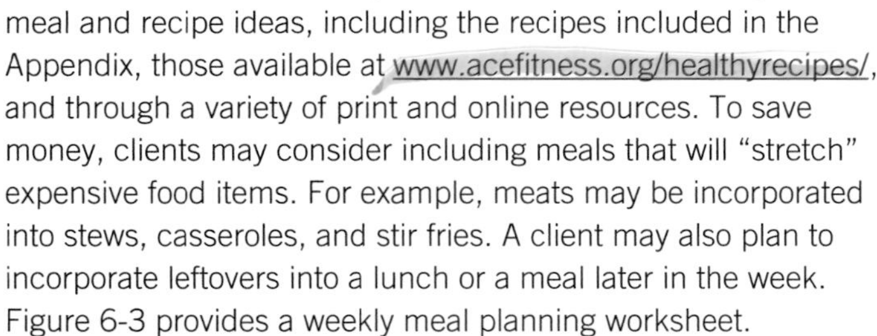

- *Make a weekly meal plan:* Encourage clients to create a weekly meal plan that includes meals and snacks for the week. Many resources are available to get healthy meal and recipe ideas, including the recipes included in the Appendix, those available at www.acefitness.org/healthyrecipes/, and through a variety of print and online resources. To save money, clients may consider including meals that will "stretch" expensive food items. For example, meats may be incorporated into stews, casseroles, and stir fries. A client may also plan to incorporate leftovers into a lunch or a meal later in the week. Figure 6-3 provides a weekly meal planning worksheet.
- *Use a grocery list:* Encourage clients to create a detailed grocery list that includes all of the ingredients needed for the week's meals, as well as a detailed list of other snacks and beverages the family may need for the week. This way, the client will have all of the needed ingredients on hand for the week's meals, making it easier to eat at home rather than going through a fast-food restaurant on the way home from an exhausting day at work. Figure 6-4 offers a sample grocery store list template.
- *Save time:* Clients may consider reviewing the week's recipes and doing as much preparation as possible on the weekend or another day when more time is available. For example, a client may wash and cut vegetables and place them in baggies corresponding to specific recipes. The extras are then ready for snacking on and incorporating into packed lunches. A client may even consider making portions of the week's meals over the weekend and then freezing them for easy reheating. This planning helps to save time and makes it easier to continue to eat healthy even when life becomes hectic.

Clients can also save time by soliciting help from other family members or roommates. A busy client may give other family members tasks in helping prepare a meal, whether that is setting the table, washing and cutting produce, mixing the salad, or cleaning the dishes. Having help not only saves time, but it also gets the other family members involved in cooking, a potent way to help picky kids (and adults) develop a taste for healthy foods.

GROCERY SHOPPING FUNDAMENTALS

Without a plan, an undiscerning client can enter a grocery store and become immediately unfettered. A hungry client may be quick to go over the grocery list and add a variety of additional and unnecessary foods to the shopping cart. Brought kids along? A trip through the diaper aisle could lead to a tantrum over sugar-sweetened cereal or some other colorful, sugar-laden snack. (Grocery stores often place unhealthy, highly processed "kid foods" across from essential baby and child necessities like diapers in an effort to appeal to kids to convince their parents to buy the junk food). A client not only needs to plan meals for the week, but also plan an approach to tackling the grocery store experience.

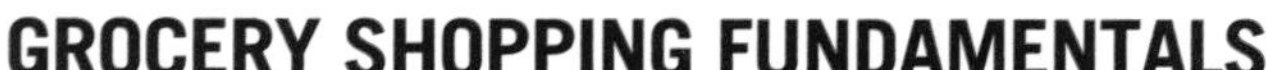

Day	Breakfast	Lunch	Dinner
Sunday			
Monday			
Tuesday			
Wednesday			
Thursday			
Friday			
Saturday			

Figure 6-3
Weekly meal planning worksheet

Figure 6-4
Sample grocery list template

Fruits and Vegetables	Breads, Rice, Cereal, and Pasta	Meat, Poultry, Fish, Eggs, Beans, and Nuts
Milk, Cheese, and Yogurt	**Fats and Oils**	**Other**

General Tips

The following general tips will help clients to have an overall positive experience at the grocery store:

- Buy groceries when not hungry and not rushed.
- Follow the grocery list. Avoid aisles that contain items not on the list.
- Shop the perimeter of the grocery store. This helps to emphasize the healthier options and minimize purchase of highly processed foods that are usually shelved in the center aisles.
- Cut coupons and combine with items on sale to save money.
- Find and compare unit prices listed on shelves to get the best price. Price per unit information is generally included in small print under an item's price label.
- Buy generic and store brands if they are less expensive.
- Purchase items in bulk or as family packs to save money, when appropriate (but do not do this if it means purchasing more food that may go bad sitting on the shelf or counter at home).
- Avoid purchasing unhealthy foods marketed to children.

Figure 6-5 offers several money-saving tips for cost-conscious consumers and those clients who express concern that they cannot afford to eat healthy.

The Grocery Store Tour

The ACE Fitness Nutrition Specialist can provide clients a valuable service by helping them understand how to make wise choices at the grocery store. One way to do this is through a grocery store tour, in which the ACE Fitness Nutrition Specialist provides clients nutrition information and tips section-by-section through the store.

THINK IT THROUGH

Taking a tour through the grocery store can be a valuable experience for both the ACE Fitness Nutrition Specialist and the client. The client learns essential information about how to make the best food choices while shopping and the ACE Fitness Nutrition Specialist gets a better understanding of the current nutrition knowledge of the client. If you decide to offer grocery store tours as part of your training services, how much will you charge? Will you travel to the client's most frequently visited store, or will you require the client to meet at a store close to your location? Will you provide educational handouts and shopping lists for the tour? Spend some time thinking about the approach you will take in leading grocery store tours.

Choose Quality Ingredients

While clients should search for the best deal and the most affordable groceries, it also important to shop for quality to optimize taste and nutritional value. ACE Fitness Nutrition Specialists can share the following tips with clients for choosing quality ingredients:

- *Meat, poultry, and seafood:* Choose the healthiest cuts of meat. The leanest cuts of meat are the round and loin. The most tender cuts of beef include the short loin and sirloin (as well as the very fatty ribs). The round is a medium tender cut. Poultry and fish are generally healthier than red meat and beef. Fish is very high in **protein** and essential nutrients, such as **omega-3 fatty acids.** While the typical American eats nowhere near the recommended frequency of eating fish twice per week, doing so goes a long way toward optimizing health.
- *Produce:* Encourage clients to seek out the most colorful and freshest fruits and vegetables. For the best taste (and smallest impact on the environment), clients should choose produce that is locally grown and in season, whenever possible. Not only do these purchases support the local farmer, but they also help to ensure that the client gets the freshest produce available. With that said, during times of the year when few fruits and vegetables are in season, or for families on a tight budget, frozen or canned fruits and vegetables may be a better choice and they usually retain the same nutritional value. For more information on choosing the highest quality produce, refer to Table 6-1.

10 tips
Nutrition Education Series

eating better on a budget

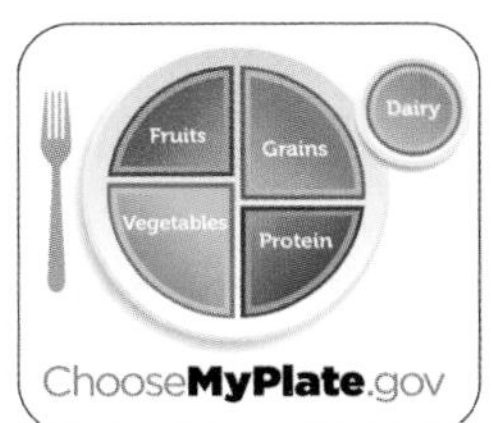

10 tips to help you stretch your food dollars

Get the most for your food budget! There are many ways to save money on the foods that you eat. The three main steps are planning before you shop, purchasing the items at the best price, and preparing meals that stretch your food dollars.

1 plan, plan, plan!

Before you head to the grocery store, plan your meals for the week. Include meals like stews, casseroles, or stir-fries, which "stretch" expensive items into more portions. Check to see what foods you already have and make a list for what you need to buy.

2 get the best price

Check the local newspaper, online, and at the store for sales and coupons. Ask about a loyalty card for extra savings at stores where you shop. Look for specials or sales on meat and seafood—often the most expensive items on your list.

3 compare and contrast

Locate the "Unit Price" on the shelf directly below the product. Use it to compare different brands and different sizes of the same brand to determine which is more economical.

4 buy in bulk

It is almost always cheaper to buy foods in bulk. Smart choices are family packs of chicken, steak, or fish and larger bags of potatoes and frozen vegetables. Before you shop, remember to check if you have enough freezer space.

5 buy in season

Buying fruits and vegetables in season can lower the cost and add to the freshness! If you are not going to use them all right away, buy some that still need time to ripen.

6 convenience costs... go back to the basics

Convenience foods like frozen dinners, pre-cut vegetables, and instant rice, oatmeal, or grits will cost you more than if you were to make them from scratch. Take the time to prepare your own—and save!

7 easy on your wallet

Certain foods are typically low-cost options all year round. Try beans for a less expensive protein food. For vegetables, buy carrots, greens, or potatoes. As for fruits, apples and bananas are good choices.

8 cook once...eat all week!

Prepare a large batch of favorite recipes on your day off (double or triple the recipe). Freeze in individual containers. Use them throughout the week and you won't have to spend money on take-out meals.

9 get your creative juices flowing

Spice up your leftovers—use them in new ways. For example, try leftover chicken in a stir-fry or over a garden salad, or to make chicken chili. Remember, throwing away food is throwing away your money!

10 eating out

Restaurants can be expensive. Save money by getting the early bird special, going out for lunch instead of dinner, or looking for "2 for 1" deals. Stick to water instead of ordering other beverages, which add to the bill.

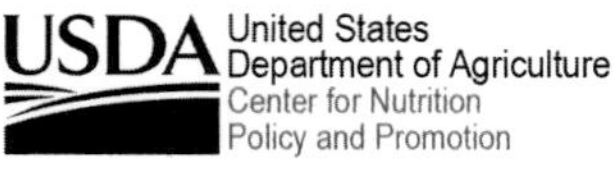

Go to www.ChooseMyPlate.gov for more information.

DG TipSheet No. 16
December 2011
USDA is an equal opportunity provider and employer.

Figure 6-5
Eating better on a budget

Table 6-1

How to Choose Fresh Fruits and Vegetables

Fruit/Vegetable	January	February	March	April	May	June	July	August	September	October	November	December	The best fruit/vegetable is/has...
Apples	■	■	■	■	■				■	■	■	■	Firm with no soft spots
Apricot						■	■						Golden yellow, plump, and firm. Not yellow or green, very hard or soft, or wilted
Artichoke			■	■	■								Plump and compact with green, fresh-looking scales
Asparagus			■	■	■	■							Straight, tender, deep green stalks with tightly closed buds
Avocado	■	■	■	■	■	■	■	■	■	■	■	■	Firm but yields to gentle pressure
Banana	■	■	■	■	■	■	■	■	■	■	■	■	Firm with no bruises
Bell pepper	■	■	■	■	■	■	■	■	■	■	■	■	Firm skin and no wrinkles
Blueberries						■	■	■					Firm, plump, and brightly colored
Broccoli	■	■	■	■	■					■	■	■	Dark green bunches
Brussels sprouts										■	■		Tight outer leaves, bright green color, and firm body
Cantaloupe					■	■	■	■					Slightly golden with light fragrant smell
Carrots	■	■	■	■	■	■	■	■	■	■	■	■	Deep orange and not cracked or wilted
Cauliflower									■	■	■		Bright green leaves enclosing firm and closely packed white curd
Celery	■	■	■	■	■	■	■	■	■	■	■	■	Fresh, crisp branches with light green to green color
Cherries					■	■							Fresh appearing, firm
Coconuts	■	■	■						■	■	■	■	Good weight for size with inside milk still fluid
Cranberries			■	■	■	■	■		■	■	■	■	Firm, plump, and brightly colored
Corn					■	■	■	■					Green, tight, and fresh-looking husk; ears with tightly packed row of plump kernels
Cucumber					■	■	■						Firm with rich green color and no soft spots
Eggplant						■	■	■	■				Firm, heavy, smooth, and uniformly dark purple
Grapefruit	■	■	■	■	■	■				■	■	■	Firm, well rounded, and heavy for size; avoid puffy/rough skinned
Grapes					■	■	■	■	■				Firm, plump, and has well-colored clusters
Honeydew		■	■	■	■	■	■	■	■	■			Creamy yellow rounds and pleasant aroma
Kiwi						■	■	■					Soft
Lettuce	■	■	■	■	■	■	■	■	■	■	■	■	Fresh, crisp leaves without wilting
Mushrooms	■	■	■	■									Firm, moist, and blemish-free
Onion	■	■	■	■	■	■	■	■	■	■	■	■	Dry and solid with no soft spots or sprouts
Orange	■	■	■	■	■						■	■	Firm, heavy for size, and has brightly colored skin
Peach						■	■	■	■				Soft to touch with fragrant smell
Pear	■	■	■	■	■			■	■	■	■	■	Yields gently to pressure at stem end
Peas				■	■	■							Bright green and full
Peppers	■	■	■	■	■	■	■	■	■	■	■	■	Firm with thick flesh and glossy skin
Persimmon	■									■	■	■	Firm, plump, and orange-red
Pineapple		■	■	■	■	■	■	■					Slightly soft; ripe when leaves are easily removed with small tug

Table 6-1 (continued)
How to Choose Fresh Fruits and Vegetables

Fruit/Vegetable	January	February	March	April	May	June	July	August	September	October	November	December	The best fruit/vegetable is/has...
Plum						■	■	■	■				Plump, yield to slight pressure
Pomegranate									■	■	■		Thin-skinned and bright purple-red
Spinach			■	■	■								Large, bright leaves; avoid coarse stems
Strawberries				■	■	■	■						Dry, firm, and bright red in color
Summer squash						■	■	■					Firm with bright and glossy skin
Sweet potato									■	■	■	■	Firm, dark, and smooth
Tomato					■	■	■	■					Plump with smooth skin and no blemishes

Note: Shaded box indicates the prime growing season for the fruit or vegetable

Sources: www.fruitsandveggiesmatter.gov; University of Tennessee Extension (2002b). *A Guide to Buying Fruits and Vegetables.* www.utextension.utk.edu/publications/spfiles/SP527.pdf

- *Food safety and selection:* Advise clients to follow these tips when selecting products to reduce the risk of foodborne illnesses:
  - ✔ Check produce for bruises, and feel and smell for ripeness.
  - ✔ Look for a sell-by date for breads and baked goods, a use-by date on some packaged foods, an expiration date on yeast and baking powder, and a packaged date on canned and some packaged foods.
  - ✔ Make sure packaged goods are not torn and cans are not dented, cracked, or bulging.
  - ✔ Separate fish and poultry from other purchases by wrapping them separately in plastic bags.
  - ✔ Pick up refrigerated and frozen foods last. Try to make sure all perishable items are refrigerated within one hour of purchase (Table 6-2).

Table 6-2
What to Store Where

Store in Refrigerator			Store on Countertop		Store in a Cool, Dry Place
Apples (storage >7 days)*	Cabbage	Lettuce‡	Apples (storage <7 days)*	Lemons	Acorn squash
Apricots*	Carrots‡	Mushrooms**	Bananas*	Limes	Butternut squash
Cantaloupe*	Cauliflower‡	Okra**	Tomatoes*	Mangoes	Onions (away from potatoes)
Figs*	Celery	Peas‡	Basil	Oranges	Potatoes (away from onions)
Honeydew*	Cherries	Plums	Cucumbers	Papayas	Pumpkins
Artichokes	Corn‡	Radishes‡	Eggplant	Peppers	Spaghetti squash
Asparagus	Grapes	Raspberries†	Garlic	Persimmons	Sweet potatoes
Beets	Green beans	Spinach	Ginger	Pineapple	Winter squash
Blackberries†	Green onions‡	Sprouts	Grapefruit	Plantains	
Blueberries†	Herbs (except basil)	Strawberries†	Jicama	Pomegranates	
Broccoli‡	Lima beans	Summer squash		Watermelon	
Brussels sprouts	Leafy vegetables	Yellow squash			
	Leeks	Zucchini			

Ripen on Counter, Then Refrigerate	
Avocados*	Pears*
Nectarines*	Plums*
Peaches*	Kiwi

*Ethylene producers (keep away from other fruits and vegetables) †Store unwashed and in a single layer ‡Store unwashed and in a plastic bag **Store in a paper bag

Source: Reprinted with permission from Barnes, L. (2013). *How to Keep Fruits and Veggies Fresh: Proper Storage Prevents Spoilage, Saving You Hundreds.* www.sparkpeople.com/resource/nutrition_articles.asp?id=1103. Reprinted courtesy of www.sparkpeople.com

EXPAND YOUR KNOWLEDGE

Do Vegetables and Fruits Have to Be Fresh to Provide the Nutritional Benefit?

Nutrition professionals often recommend a diet high in fresh fruits and vegetables. But what if a client cannot always purchase fresh food—whether due to cost, taste preferences, spoilage risk, or any other of several possible reasons to choose frozen or canned over fresh? It turns out that most of the evidence suggests that frozen fruits and vegetables are just as good (if not better in some cases) than fresh produce.

Unless a client is choosing fresh produce from a farmers' market or his or her own backyard, chances are good that the produce was picked at least several days, or even weeks, earlier—likely not at its peak ripeness (otherwise, it would spoil too quickly en route to the store) and with degradation of some of its nutritional value after picking and during transport. Once fresh fruits and vegetables are harvested, they undergo higher rates of respiration—a physiologic process in which plant starches and sugars are converted into carbon dioxide, water, and other by-products—leading to moisture loss, reduced quality, and susceptibility to microorganism spoilage. Refrigeration during transport helps to slow the deterioration, but still, by the time a person eats a "fresh" vegetable that traveled across the country or a continent to reach the dinner table, a substantial amount of its nutritional value may be lost. Clients can help maximize nutritional value of fresh produce by choosing locally grown produce, refrigerating the fruits and vegetables to help slow down nutrient losses, and steaming rather than boiling to minimize the loss of **water-soluble vitamins.**

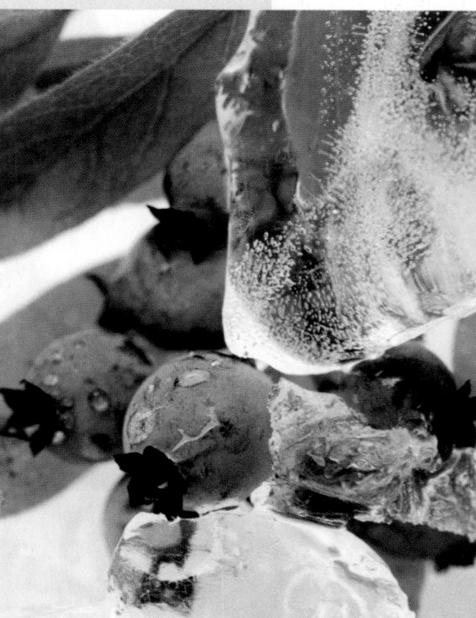

Produce destined for freezing is picked at its maximal ripeness, quickly frozen to a temperature that maximally retains its nutritional value and flavor, and kept frozen until it gets to the freezer in the local store. While some initial nutrient loss occurs with the first steps in the freezing process—washing, peeling, and heat-based blanching (done for vegetables but usually not fruits)—the low temperature of freezing keeps the produce good for up to a year on average. Once a client thaws and eats the frozen food, he or she benefits from the majority of the food's original nutritional value. Be assured, if a client loves blueberries and all their health benefits, for example, the frozen version is just as good as the fresh. And depending on how the food is cooked or prepared, it may taste quite similar to its fresh counterpart.

The process is somewhat different for canned produce, and in some cases, nutritional value may suffer. Similar to the freezing process, in the canning process, the produce is picked at its maximal ripeness, blanched (this time for longer duration and with somewhat increased nutrient loss for heat-sensitive compounds compared with frozen), and then canned. Oftentimes, sugary syrup or juice is added to canned fruit. Salt is added to many vegetables to help retain flavor and avoid spoilage. These additions can take a very healthy fruit or vegetable and make it much less desirable than its fresh or frozen counterpart. But without these additions, the nutritional value of canned fruits and vegetables is generally similar to fresh and frozen. For fruits, look for canned fruit "in its own juice." For vegetables, check the sodium content on the nutritional label and aim for vegetables with "no added salt" and without added butter or cream sauces. Because the canned produce is maintained in an oxygen-free environment, canned foods can last for years (but be weary of dented or bulging cans).

By the time they're consumed, most fresh, frozen, and canned fruits and vegetables seem to be nutritionally similar. Each has the same **fat, carbohydrate,** and protein content as the preharvested fruit. While variable loss in water- and **fat-soluble vitamins** can occur depending on the postharvest processing method, for the most part, clients can feel confident that frozen and canned (without additives) fruits and vegetables are just as good for them and their families as fresh food. Ultimately, clients might find that choosing a mix of fresh, frozen, and canned fruits and vegetables will help them and their families to more easily, inexpensively, and creatively enjoy the nine or more servings per day of fruits and vegetables recommended by the *Dietary Guidelines for Americans* without sacrificing nutritional value.

Source: www.fruitsandveggiesmatter.gov

EXPAND YOUR KNOWLEDGE

Should Clients Be Eating Organic? When Does It Really Matter?

Organic food choices fill supermarket shelves. Many people happily pay almost double for organic foods in some cases, whereas others balk at such a high price for food that usually tastes no different than its conventional counterpart. Clients may ask, "Is organic food healthier and safer than nonorganic food?"

To get the USDA organic seal, foods need to have been grown, handled, and processed by certified organic facilities. These facilities must be wholly organic. Meat, poultry, eggs, and dairy products need to be produced from animals that have never been given antibiotics or hormones and who have been fed organic crops. Organic crops must be grown free of conventional pesticides, free of fertilizers made with synthetic ingredients or sewage sludge, and without bioengineering or use of ionizing radiation. The USDA is careful to note that an organic seal does not mean that a food is healthier or safer than its conventionally grown equivalent.

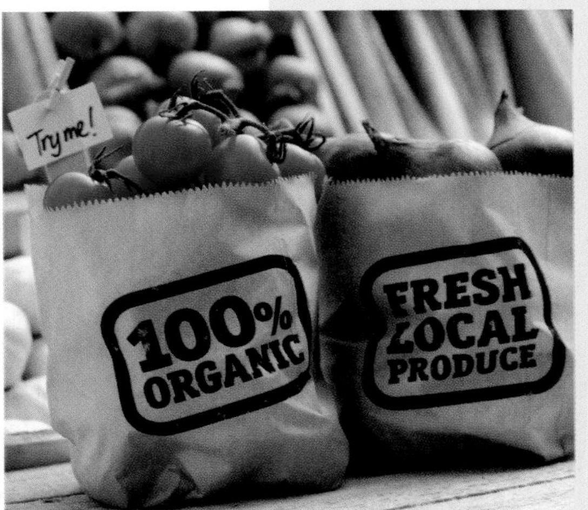

In fact, a 2010 review looking at studies of organic foods and health benefits over the past 50 years determined that there is not enough good data to say one way or the other if organic foods are healthier (Dangour et al., 2010). Of the studies that had been done, the only one that found a health difference showed that the risk of eczema was decreased in infants who ate strictly organic dairy products. A subsequent 2012 review attempted to answer the same question and concluded: "The published literature lacks strong evidence that organic foods are significantly more nutritious than conventional foods. Consumption of organic foods may reduce exposure to pesticide residues and antibiotic-resistant bacteria" (Smith-Spangler et al., 2012).

Pesticide exposure could pose a safety risk. A study of preschool children in Seattle found that kids who ate conventional diets had significantly higher levels of urine pesticides than the kids who ate organic (Curl et al., 2003). However, higher urine pesticides have not been connected to real health outcomes, although intuitively it seems like a good idea to minimize consumption of toxic chemicals.

Ultimately, it may not be the health and safety for the consumer that will tip a client one way or the other with organic foods, but it is worth considering the broader health and environmental outcomes. For example, farm workers overall are afforded minimal rights and often work in horrendous conditions. Those working on conventional farms are often exposed to massive levels of pesticides, which can contribute to serious health outcomes including birth defects and cancers. Furthermore, an extraordinary amount of environmental resources and energy go into shipping a crop from halfway around the world to a local grocery store. However, presently it is not unusual to see organic food that was grown abroad. This will become more common as an increasing number of companies jump on the organic bandwagon.

Clearly, everyone has to make their own decision about whether to buy organic based on the limited information available on whether organic foods are worth it. It may be that the spirit of growing organic foods (which one can often tap into at a local farmer's market or by nurturing a garden)—like good use of natural resources, minimal use of toxic compounds, sustainable farming, and supporting local business—is more important than whether the food is actually grown organic.

The Environmental Working Group (EWG, 2012) conducted a study to see which fruits and vegetables had the highest and lowest levels of pesticides. They declared the following foods to be the "Dirty Dozen" (in other words, try to buy these organic):

- Celery
- Peaches
- Strawberries
- Apples
- Blueberries
- Nectarines
- Sweet bell peppers
- Spinach
- Kale/collard greens
- Cherries
- Potatoes
- Grapes (imported)

The following foods were declared the "Clean 15" (lowest in pesticides, so clients probably do not need to buy organic):

- Onions
- Avocado
- Sweet corn (frozen)
- Pineapples
- Mango
- Sweet peas (frozen)
- Asparagus
- Kiwi fruit
- Cabbage
- Eggplant
- Cantaloupe (domestic)
- Watermelon
- Grapefruit
- Sweet potatoes
- Honeydew melon

Make Informed Purchasing Decisions

Food manufacturers and food marketers are continually devising ways to appeal to consumers. ACE Fitness Nutrition Specialists can help clients to be discerning customers and make informed purchasing decisions. One critical way to do this is to help clients develop skills in reading the nutrition label (refer to Chapter 3).

EATING HEALTHY WHEN EATING OUT

A large proportion of meals eaten in the United States are eaten at restaurants and other establishments outside the home. The difference between making wise and unwise decisions when eating out can make or break a client's weight-management efforts. To avoid excessive caloric intake when eating out, clients should focus on taking steps to control portions and making choices low in added fats and sugars.

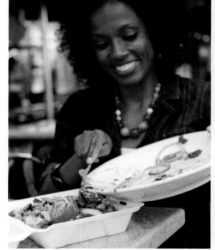

Tips for Reducing Portions

Several strategies can help to control portion sizes. The following list is excerpted from the USDA's "Eat Healthy, Be Active" workshop (USDA, 2010):

- Choose "child's size" portions if possible or choose the smallest size available.
- Eat half of the meal at the restaurant and save the other half for the next day's lunch.
- Order an appetizer-sized portion or a side dish instead of an entrée.
- Share a main dish with a friend.
- Resign from the "clean your plate club." Help clients relearn how to eat based on feelings of hunger and fullness rather than the amount of food left on the plate. Encourage clients to stop eating when they are full and leave the rest. Alternatively, they can ask the server to package up half of the meal when it arrives to ensure portion control.
- Order an item from the menu instead of heading for the "all-you-can-eat" buffet.

Tips for Reducing Calories

One of the major concerns when eating foods that have been prepared by someone else is that it is difficult to know what ingredients have been added to a particular dish and how the calories and saturated fat stack up. Fortunately, many establishments are moving toward including nutrition information on labels to help consumers be better informed when making purchase decisions. Here are a few other tips to try to minimize excess calories when eating out:

- Look for terms such as baked, lightly sautéed, boiled (in wine or lemon juice), poached, broiled, roasted, grilled, and steamed in its own juice (au jus).
- Watch out for terms such as alfredo, casserole, escalloped, au fromage, cheese sauce, fried, au gratin, creamed, gravy, basted in cream or cream sauce, hollandaise, béarnaise, crispy, pastry crust, breaded, deep fried, pot pie, and butter sauce.
- Order calorie-free beverages such as water and unsweetened iced tea. Avoid beverages with added sugar.
- Load sandwiches/subs/pizza with veggies rather than cheese.
- Ask for whole-wheat bread for sandwiches, and ask that it not be prepared with butter or mayonnaise.
- Start with a salad loaded with veggies to meet nutrient needs and curb hunger. This will translate into fewer calories from the main entrée.
- Ask for salad dressing to be served on the side and use sparingly.

Table 6-3 lists several tips for making healthier choices while eating out at various types of establishments, including fast food restaurants, delis, steakhouses, and several types of ethnic restaurants.

Table 6-3
Tips for Choosing Healthier Foods at Restaurants

Look for the terms below on menus for items lower in calories, solid fats (saturated and trans fat), and sodium.	
Fast Food	
• Grilled chicken breast sandwich without mayonnaise • Single hamburger without cheese	• Grilled chicken salad with reduced-fat dressing • Low-fat or fat-free yogurt
Deli/Sandwich Shops	
• Fresh sliced vegetables on whole-wheat bread with low-fat dressing or mustard	• Turkey breast sandwich with mustard, lettuce, and tomato • Bean soup (lentil, minestrone)
Steakhouse	
• Lean broiled beef (no more than 6 ounces)—London broil, filet mignon, round and flank steaks	• Baked potato without butter, margarine, or sour cream • Seafood fishes that are not fried
Chinese	
• Zheng (steamed) • Gun (boiled) • Kao (roasted) • Shao (barbecue) • Lightly stir-fried in mild sauce • Hot and spicy tomato sauce	• Reduced-sodium soy, hoisin, and oyster sauce • Dishes without MSG added • Bean curd (tofu) • Moo shu vegetables, chicken, or shrimp • Hot mustard sauce
Italian	
• Lightly sautéed with onions, shallots, or garlic • Red sauces—spicy marinara sauce (arrabiata), marinara sauce, cacciatore, red clam sauce • Primavera (no cream sauce) • Lemon sauce	• Florentine (spinach) • Grilled (often fish or vegetables) • Piccata (lemon) • Manzanne (eggplant)

Source: U.S. Department of Agriculture (2010). *Eat Healthy, Be Active Community Workshops.* www.choosemyplate.gov/downloads/EatHealthyBeActiveCommunityWorkshops.pdf

SUMMARY

A true test of whether a client will achieve nutrition goals is whether he or she can effectively translate nutrition recommendations into practical strategies to improve the nutritional quality of the eating plan on a daily basis. By coaching clients through the essentials of meal preparation and selection, the ACE Fitness Nutrition Specialist sets the stage for long-term client success and permanent lifestyle change.

REFERENCES

Barnes, L. (2013). *How to Keep Fruits and Veggies fresh: Proper Storage Prevents Spoilage, Saving You Hundreds.* www.sparkpeople.com/resource/nutrition_articles.asp?id=1103

Bennion, M.B. & Scheule, B.S. (Eds.) (1999). *Introductory Foods* (13th ed.) New York: Prentice Hall.

Curl, C.L. et al. (2003). Organophosphorus pesticide exposure of urban and suburban preschool children with organic and conventional diets. *Environmental Health Perspectives,* 111, 377–380.

Dangour, A.D. et al. (2010). Nutrition-related health effects of organic foods: A systematic review. *American Journal of Clinical Nutrition*, 92, 203–210.

Environmental Working Group (2012). *Health/Toxics: Pesticides & Organics.* www.ewg.org/pesticidesorganics

Smith-Spangler, C. et al. (2012). Are organic foods safer or healthier than conventional alternatives? A systematic review. *Annals of Internal Medicine*, 157, 5, 348–366.

University of Tennessee Extension (2002a). *Eat Smart: Get Your Family to the Table. Cooking Basics.* https://utextension.tennessee.edu/publications/Documents/SP732.pdf

University of Tennessee Extension (2002b). *A Guide to Buying Fruits and Vegetables.* www.utextension.utk.edu/publications/spfiles/SP527.pdf

U.S. Department of Agriculture (2015). *2015-2020 Dietary Guidelines for Americans* (8th ed.) www.health.gov/dietaryguidelines

U.S. Department of Agriculture (2010). *Eat Healthy, Be Active Community Workshops.* www.choosemyplate.gov/downloads/EatHealthyBeActiveCommunityWorkshop

SUGGESTED READING

University of Tennessee Extension (2002a). *Eat Smart: Get Your Family to the Table. Cooking Basics.* https://utextension.tennessee.edu/publications/Documents/SP732.pdf

University of Tennessee Extension (2002b). *A Guide to Buying Fruits and Vegetables.* www.utextension.utk.edu/publications/spfiles/SP527.pdf

U.S. Department of Agriculture (2015). *2015-2020 Dietary Guidelines for Americans* (8th ed.) www.health.gov/dietaryguidelines

U.S. Department of Agriculture (2010). *Eat Healthy, Be Active Community Workshops.* www.choosemyplate.gov/downloads/EatHealthyBeActiveCommunityWorkshops.pdf

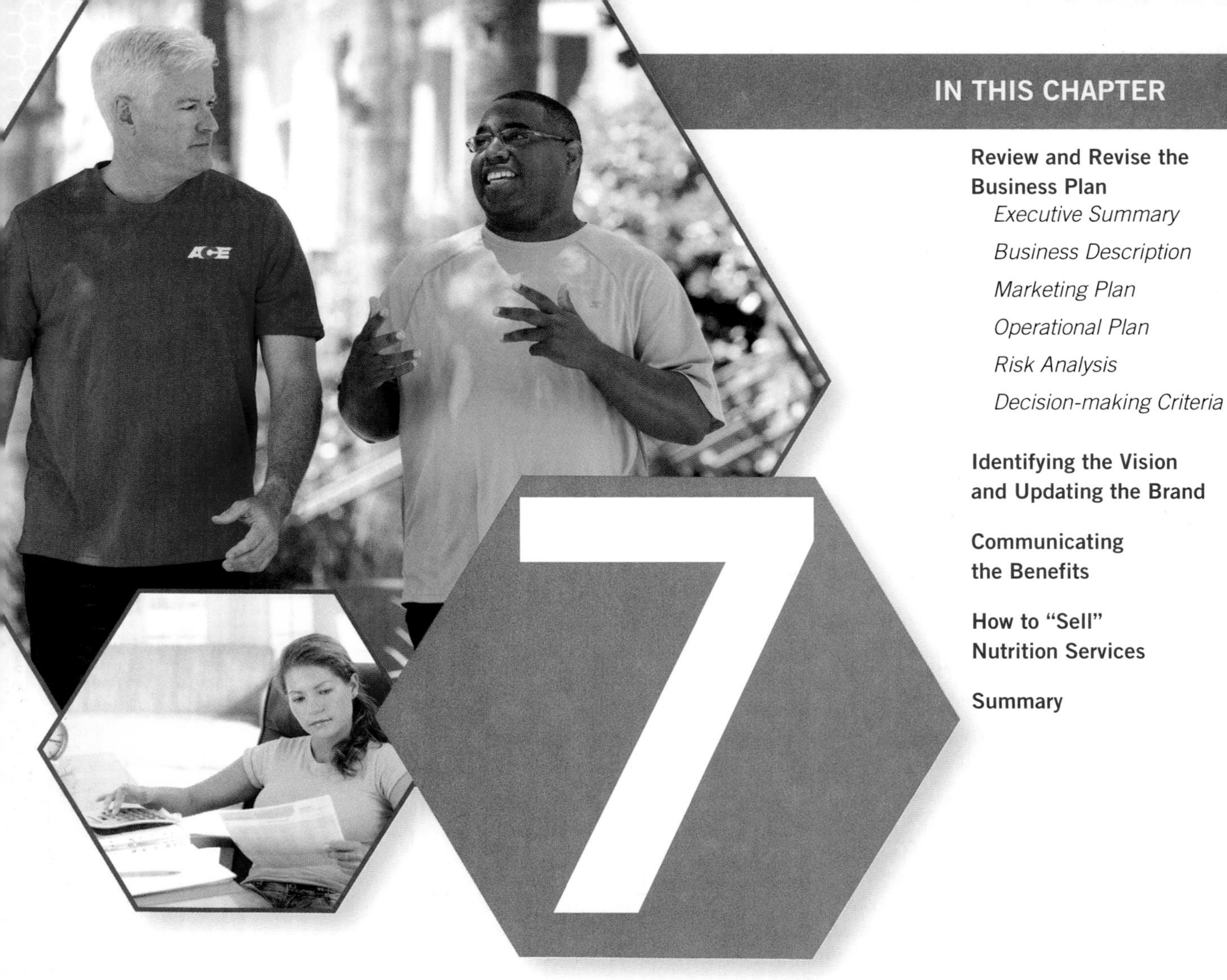

IN THIS CHAPTER

ACE would like to acknowledge the contributions to this chapter made by Pete McCall, M.S., an exercise physiologist with the American Council on Exercise.

LEARNING OBJECTIVES

AFTER READING THIS CHAPTER, YOU WILL BE ABLE TO:

- DESCRIBE THE VARIOUS COMPONENTS OF THE BUSINESS PLAN AND POTENTIAL NUTRITION APPLICATIONS
- DEVELOP A MARKETING PLAN TO PROMOTE THE NEW NUTRITION SERVICES THAT WILL BE OFFERED
- UNDERSTAND HOW TO USE INNOVATIVE TECHNOLOGIES AND SOCIAL MEDIA TO EXPAND REACH AND PROMOTE SERVICES

ESSENTIALS FOR GROWING YOUR BUSINESS

Continuing education in nutrition not only expands a fitness professional's knowledge base and skill set, but it also provides an exceptional opportunity to grow an existing business. Whether someone is a personal trainer who is now more comfortable providing answers to clients' nutrition questions or a health coach who can translate the increased knowledge into a cooking class or nutrition seminar, becoming an ACE Fitness Nutrition Specialist can open up new business opportunities.

REVIEW AND REVISE THE BUSINESS PLAN

The first step to developing a plan for how to incorporate nutrition-related coaching into daily practice is to reassess the original business plan. The business plan serves as an operating guide for achieving specific objectives, such as yearly income and the number of clients needed to achieve that income, as well as a marketing plan for attracting new clients. Each of the six components of the business plan—executive summary, business description, marketing plan, operational plan, risk analysis, and decision-making criteria—is discussed in this chapter, along with considerations for when a fitness professional is expanding his or her services to include nutrition coaching.

Executive Summary

The executive summary is a brief outline of the business and an overview of how the business fills a need within the marketplace. This should be a succinct synopsis of the business, with the rest of the business plan providing the exact specifications in greater detail. A well-written executive summary is one page and includes the following information:

- *Business concept:* A description of the business, the service it provides, the market for that service, and why this particular business holds a competitive advantage
  - ✓ *Nutrition application:* The business plan can be updated to also include nutrition coaching and how it is integrated into the business, the importance of nutrition in achieving health and fitness goals, and the ACE Fitness Nutrition Specialist credential. It is important, however, not to identify oneself as a nutritionist or dietitian.
- *Financial information:* The financial information section of the executive summary includes the key financial considerations for a business, including the start-up costs for the first year of operation (or the first year of provision of new services), the source of capital for initial expenses, and the potential for sales revenue and profits, with an emphasis on the expected **return on investment,** which is the ratio of net income to the average money spent overall on the company or on a specific project. It is usually expressed as a percentage and helps to indicate whether or not a company is using its resources in an efficient manner.
  - ✓ *Nutrition application*: As nutrition is integrated into the business model, it is

important for the fitness professional to plan for the initial expenses related to expanding and promoting new services.

- *Current market position:* The current market position typically includes the products or services being sold, including how they compare to the competition, pricing structure, and promotional activities.
  - ✓ *Nutrition application:* With an expansion of services to include nutrition coaching, the company may be able to develop a competitive edge, upgrade pricing structure, and plan for a promotional campaign to increase awareness of the new services.
- *Major achievements:* This section includes any awards received or clients who have given written permission for their names to be used in marketing materials. This section should identify a specific protocol for exercise program design that is different from competitors, such as sport-specific training, or list any local or national celebrities who will provide an endorsement of the fitness professional's work.
  - ✓ *Nutrition application:* The fitness professional can describe the ACE Fitness Nutrition Specialist credential and services offered in this list of achievements.

Business Description

This section of the business plan provides the details for the business as outlined in the executive summary, including the mission statement, business model, current status of the market, and the management team. When describing the business, the fitness professional should:

- Identify the operating model and how it is different or unique when compared to the competition
- Describe the fitness industry specific to the local market, including the present financial situation and the outlook for future growth
- Provide details such as the number and location of competitors, how many **employees** they have, and the number of clients to whom they provide services
- List the members of the management team, highlighting their knowledge, skills, and experience

The purpose of this section of the plan is to provide information about the structure of the business, the market it will serve, and the people who will run it. Potential lenders or investors will want to review all of this information before making a decision about providing capital.

Marketing Plan

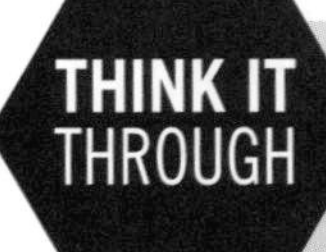

Spend some time thinking about how your business will be different from other existing businesses that offer nutrition-related coaching services. What sets your business apart from the others? What makes your service unique compared to the competition?

This section of the business plan specifies how prospective clients become paying clients. Whether working as an employee or as an **independent contractor,** an ACE Fitness Nutrition Specialist needs to develop a comprehensive marketing plan to communicate with prospective clients. Marketing is the process of promoting a service by communicating the features, advantages, and benefits to potential clients. Marketing tools for a service such as nutrition coaching should tell a story about how that service can enhance a person's life. All marketing pieces should communicate the benefits of working with an ACE Fitness Nutrition Specialist, specifically showing how this expertise will help potential clients meet their health and fitness goals.

An effective marketing campaign will communicate how a specific product or service meets the needs of a potential client. The marketing plan should list the details of the demographics for the area around the business, the demand for nutrition coaching services (possibly by highlighting the rates of **obesity** or lack of access to **registered dietitians**), the specific type of services being offered (such as webinars, in-person cooking demonstrations, or group sessions), and the plan for communicating the benefits of the services to potential customers.

The marketing plan should include a specific audience that the ACE Fitness Nutrition Specialist will target and a process for reaching those individuals. For example, if there is a high rate of obesity in the community, the ACE Fitness Nutrition Specialist may consider reaching out to a major employer in the community and propose a lunchtime weight-management program.

Operational Plan

This portion of a business plan describes the structure for how a business will operate, including an organizational chart that identifies key decision makers and the employees responsible for executing those decisions. This section also describes what has been done already in the development of the business and what is yet to be done. The operational plan is a very important and comprehensive component of the business plan. The details of developing the operational plan are outside the scope of this text.

Risk Analysis

There are a number of risks involved in owning and operating a business. Risks can be categorized into one of the following areas:

- *Barriers to entry:* The costs associated with starting a business, such as rental fees, equipment, employees, and marketing
- *Financial:* The access to the capital required to start or expand a business
- *Competitive:* Other players in the market who are competing for the same pool of customers
- *Staffing:* Issues associated with managing employees and budgeting for a consistent payroll
- *Legal:* Ensuring adherence to best practices and staying within one's professional scope of practice

A simple tool for evaluating risks is a **SWOT analysis,** which stands for strengths, weaknesses, opportunities, and threats. When completing a SWOT analysis, an ACE Fitness Nutrition Specialist should consider the strengths and weaknesses of the business, as well as potential opportunities to advance the business (such as offering nutrition coaching to clients or developing a nutrition workshop or webinar) and threats to the business's success (such as competition or a down financial market). An example of a SWOT analysis for a nutrition specialist is included in Figure 7-1.

Decision-making Criteria

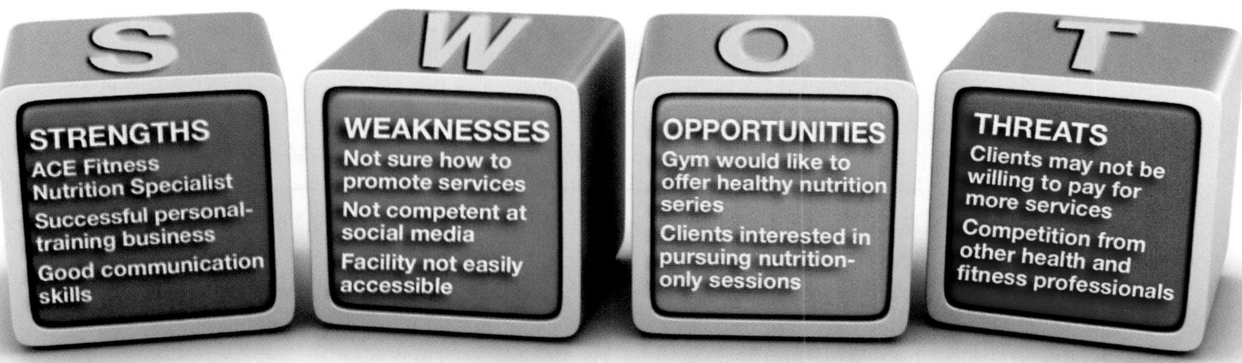

S
W
O
T
STRENGTHS
ACE Fitness Nutrition Specialist
Successful personal-training business
Good communication skills
WEAKNESSES
Not sure how to promote services
Not competent at social media
Facility not easily accessible
OPPORTUNITIES
Gym would like to offer healthy nutrition series
Clients interested in pursuing nutrition-only sessions
THREATS
Clients may not be willing to pay for more services
Competition from other health and fitness professionals

Figure 7-1
SWOT analysis

This component of the business plan includes a detailed cost-benefit analysis that demonstrates that the process of expanding the business to include nutrition coaching services is worth the financial risks. The ACE Fitness Nutrition Specialist should highlight the specifics about the expansion of the business plan that support that it will be a successful venture. A well-written plan will present all of the components of the business in such a way that the final section is simply a conclusion summarizing how the business will be a profitable venture.

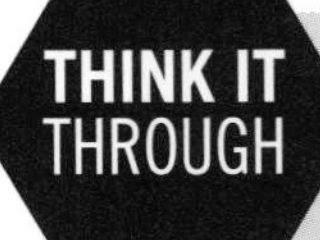

All fitness professionals should have a business plan, even if they are just getting started or are employees in someone else's business. Mapping out your strengths, goals, and opportunities in writing is a great way to get started. If you do not have a business plan, use the guidelines in this chapter to help you create one. If you do, consider how your business plan can be enhanced through the acquisition of the ACE Fitness Nutrition Specialty Certification.

IDENTIFYING THE VISION AND UPDATING THE BRAND

The ACE Fitness Nutrition Specialist should consider using the business-evaluation process to develop a vision statement for the business. This statement should clearly communicate the purpose of the business and what the intended customer can expect to receive. For example, a health coach with the ACE Fitness Nutrition Specialty Certification may have the vision to "Empower individuals to adopt a lifelong commitment to healthy eating and physical activity through effective behavioral change." Once an ACE Fitness Nutrition Specialist has adopted a vision statement, he or she can then take steps to develop an easily identifiable brand.

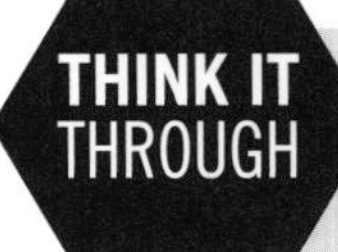

Write a few variations on a vision statement for yourself or your business. Talk with friends, colleagues, and some trusted clientele in order to better focus your vision.

COMMUNICATING THE BENEFITS

The next step is to create a strategy to promote the brand. There are a number of ways to market one's services to prospective clients. It is important to identify the most cost-effective method that will have the greatest reach. For instance, a personal trainer who is just beginning to incorporate nutrition into his business may offer a complimentary nutrition coaching session in which he shows a client how to keep a food log and enter the data into the SuperTracker for analysis and then discusses the results with the client (see Chapter 5). He may offer a nutrition workshop or cooking class to current or prospective personal-training clients. The value-added services or a complimentary workshop allow a client the opportunity to "try out" the services and develop **rapport** with the ACE Fitness Nutrition Specialist. A satisfied prospective client is likely to purchase additional services. Another example is that of a facility interested in offering a nutrition program or workshop as a service to members. An ACE Fitness Nutrition Specialist may consider offering these services as an opportunity to meet people and develop relationships, thus widening the pool of potential clients.

Fitness professionals may consider updating their business cards to mention the ACE Fitness Nutrition Specialist credential so that prospective clients appreciate the additional value from hiring a fitness professional who has invested the time and energy to learn more about nutrition and how to promote healthier nutrition habits.

Incorporating testimonials on a business webpage from satisfied clients who have received help in adopting a healthier eating plan is a powerful tool to attract new clients. The website should also include the ACE Fitness Nutrition Specialist's personal biography to tell a story about who he or she is as a fitness professional and as a person. To serve as an effective tool, the website should be updated periodically. For further reach, an ACE Fitness Nutrition Specialist may consider maintaining a blog or featuring relevant articles and links.

A social media account offers a far-reaching medium to attract and retain clients. At the least, maintaining a Facebook and Twitter account will broaden a professional's network of contacts and can help to build credibility. Many other social media networks such as LinkedIn, Google +, YouTube, and Pinterest (among many others) offer additional opportunities to expand one's reach.

EXPAND YOUR KNOWLEDGE

Virtual Tools for the ACE Fitness Nutrition Specialist

By Ted Vickey, M.A.

Ted Vickey, M.A., is an entrepreneurial strategist whose clients have included the U.S. Department of Commerce, the Securities and Exchange Commission, Fruit of the Loom, and Osram Sylvania. He is currently a Ph.D. candidate at the National University of Ireland Galway in exercise adherence and technology and is a member of the ACE Board of Directors.

Imagine running a business where your website ranks on page one of an internet search, bills are paid, and fees are collected with the touch of a button. In addition, clients' nutrition and physical-activity achievements are wirelessly sent from their mobile phones to your email for tracking. That practice is readily available through the use of technology. There are two types of technology that all fitness professionals should consider as part of their overall practice: business-management tools and connected health tools.

Business-management Tools

Fitness businesses can reap the benefits of various business-management tools, including the creation of a website, engagement with clients, professional relationship management, appointment scheduling, accounting, and online credit card processing.

It can be difficult to decide which platform is most suitable for a particular business. Which platform allows for easy publishing of a site and can also grow with one's practice? Which platform drives engagement and leads to new clients and/or additional appointments? Which platform has reporting capabilities that can show a return on the initial investment? While the task may seem daunting at first, the reality is that with some trial runs, and even beta-testing with friends and family, creating an online business-management platform may offer tremendous return for very little time investment. No longer must a fitness professional hire an expensive design company to create a website, although for best results, consulting a website designer is never a bad idea.

Social media and online marketing are increasingly important for fitness professionals to get a practice noticed and utilized by potential clients on the web. There are a number of good reasons for a business to participate in and maintain an online presence, including the following:

- Connect and engage with current and potential clients
- Get discovered by people searching for fitness- and nutrition-related services
- Create an active and persuasive community around the practice
- Promote content such as webinars, blog articles, or health tips (visit www.ACEfitness.org for free tips you can use in your practice)
- Generate leads for the practice

Fitness professionals around the world are using Facebook as their primary website, not only to attract new business, but also to remain engaged with former and existing clients. On Facebook, "profiles" are meant for people, while "pages" are meant for businesses. To fully engage and leverage the power of Facebook, be sure to create a page for the business. Pages are public and are split into different categories, and are therefore searchable. These "branding" pages also allow anyone to become a fan of (or "like") the page without needing administrator approval. Facebook also provides flexible privacy settings to control who sees what parts of your page (*Source:* Hubspot). For additional information about setting up Facebook as your website, conduct an online search for "Facebook for Business."

Fitness professionals are also using Twitter to stay in touch with clients by sharing short, valuable health-related tips. Twitter is a free service that allows anyone to say anything in 140 characters or less. Twitter allows fitness professionals to promote particular services directed at a target market; connect with other coaches who share their views; get instant access to relevant, timely opinions; receive a steady stream of ideas, content, links, resources, and tips focused on their area of expertise; and monitor what is being said about the practice (*Source:* Duct Tape Marketing). Twitter is more than promotion; it is also about the sharing of valuable information. For every business promotion, consider sharing several health tips. For additional information about using Twitter in your practice, search "Twitter for Business."

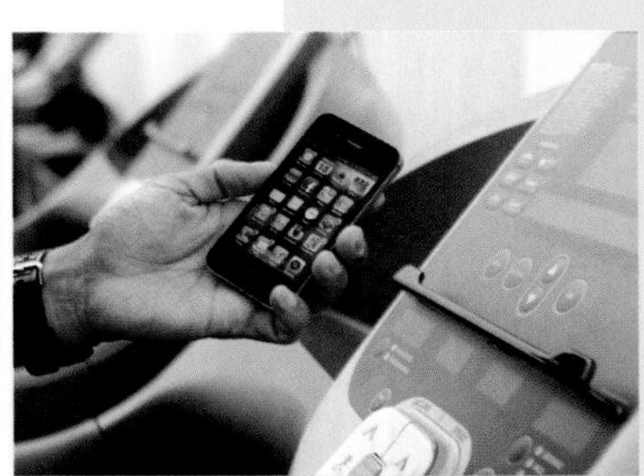

Another easy-to-use website that can add value to a fitness professional's practice is LinkedIn (www.linkedin.com). On LinkedIn, ACE Fitness Nutrition Specialists can connect not only with potential clients, but also with other health and wellness professionals in the area, state, and even around the world. Fitness professionals should be sure to add all relevant information, include a professional picture, request the vanity URL (that can include your name in the URL), and use this resource to connect with other like-minded professionals with a click of the mouse. The LinkedIn help section provides tips to make a profile stand out from the rest. Once a member of LinkedIn, the ACE Fitness Nutritional Specialist should join groups and be active by posting questions, providing answers, and engaging with the rest of the group. There are a number of ACE groups on LinkedIn that ACE Fitness Nutrition Specialists can join, all for free.

Other do-it-yourself websites include Tumblr (www.tumblr.com), Pinterest (www.pinterest.com), Instagram (www.instagr.am), and Tout (www.tout.com). Prior to committing to one site, spend some time planning an online strategy. It helps to have a checklist of features that are both user-friendly and useful. Review other professionals who are currently using these tools effectively.

For additional information about business tools for fitness businesses, consider searching for these terms: social media, online marketing, online appointment scheduler, online accounting, and credit card processing. Also visit the ACE website (www.ACEfitness.org) for additional resources for building, marketing, and expanding your business.

Connected Health Tools

Former Surgeon General C. Evert Koop dreamed of a day where "...cutting-edge technology, especially in communication and information transfer, will enable the greatest advances yet in public health. Eventually, we will have access to health information 24 hours a day, 7 days a week, encouraging personal wellness and prevention, and leading to better informed decisions about health care" (Koop, 1995). That dream is now a reality, as personal trainers and health coaches are using the power of technology (the Internet, social networking services, and mobile phone applications) as persuasive tools to help clients lead healthier lives.

Connected health tools are small, inexpensive client-based mobile applications or websites that eliminate the four walls of a physical building and allow nutrition coaching to take place virtually in real time. These tools can transmit health data from the client to the ACE Fitness Nutrition Specialist, such as heart rate, physical activity, meal logs, body weight, blood pressure, and sleep habits. This allows the fitness professional to not only hold clients accountable between appointments, but also but allows for real-time immediate feedback and encouragement for daily behaviors. By using connected health technology, fitness professionals can provide a more personalized experience and potentially reach more individuals with effective health-related advice and information at a very low cost. Griffiths et al. (2006) suggest five reasons for using connected health tools for delivering web-based health, wellness, and fitness interventions:

- Reduced delivery costs
- Convenience to users

- Timeliness
- Reduction of stigma
- Reduction of time-based isolation barriers

Within the healthcare field, interactive technologies can be effectively deployed to take on multiple roles at the same time. For example, a simple online tool can measure calories while at the same time give a reward upon attainment of a personal goal. This type of self-monitoring is a key ingredient in successful behavioral modification. The power of self-monitoring is not just between client and trainer or coach. Research suggests that if several people are connected through the Internet, social support can be leveraged, which has been shown to impact motivation and behavioral change (Chatterjee & Price, 2009). Fitness professionals should find ways to connect clients with friends, family, or other clients to create an "electronic bond." Accountability emails, online chats, Facebook posts, and Twitter messages can be powerful motivational tools.

Tracking of physical activity is moving away from the paper and pencil of a workout card and more toward digital tracking. Technology allows users to track progress, interact with trainers and coaches who can suggest areas for improvement, and self-administer tests and measures. Blood pressure cuffs that connect to the web, body-weight scales that tweet a person's weight, and even sleep-monitoring systems are allowing people to track their personal health data from the comforts of their own homes (www.withings.com). Tracking tools such as BodyMedia (www.bodymedia.com), FitBit (www.fitbit.com), Jawbone UP (www.jawbone.com/up), and Nike Fuel (www.nike.com/fuelband) empower users to collect and share exercise, nutrition, and sleep data. In-depth nutrition apps such as MyNetDiary (www.mynetdiary.com) and Foodzy (www.foodzy.com) are modern, comprehensive diet services that help users track and monitor food intake while displaying a robust nutritional analysis based on personalized guidelines. These tools can be extremely useful for a client who needs that extra motivation to stay the course.

Mobile fitness applications can offer similar tracking options for a fraction of the cost. Apple and Android software provide data collection and motivational tools. The sharing of data within a private group, on Facebook, or on Twitter can provide additional accountability and support for clients. Health information data portals such as Microsoft's Health Vault (www.microsoft.com/en-us/healthvault) and RunKeeper's HealthGraph (www.runkeeper.com) allow for health data to be collected, monitored, and shared not only with the client, but also with other members of the client's healthcare team, including physicians, nutritionists, and personal trainers.

For more information about connected health tools that fitness professionals can implement in their practice, conduct an online search for mobile fitness applications (or "apps"), personal health-information management, Microsoft Health Vault, and mobile health apps.

HOW TO "SELL" NUTRITION SERVICES

Many health professionals entered the field out of a desire to help people and would prefer to avoid asking for a sale. The term "salesperson" often carries a negative connotation, but the sales process is based on helping others. When a person joins a health club or a potential client inquires about services, the person is looking for the advice and guidance of an expert who can help him or her achieve specific results through exercise and improved nutrition. Selling is the process of sharing information with potential clients about how they can achieve their goals. The sales process requires asking a prospective client to make a commitment to his or her personal goals by investing in the ACE Fitness Nutrition Specialist through the purchase of services.

Marketing fitness or nutrition services involves effectively communicating how the knowledge and skills of the ACE Fitness Nutrition Specialist can meet or exceed the needs of a potential client. The process of selling services to a client involves developing the relationship so that the customer trusts that the fitness professional can help him or her achieve meaningful results. Selling is a win-win process. When an ACE Fitness Nutrition Specialist sells a package to a client, the client "wins" because he or she is purchasing a needed and valuable service, and the fitness professional "wins" because he or she has gained a new client and new source of revenue. While it can take years to develop effective sales techniques, there are two basic components to being a successful sales professional:

- Marketing the service to potential clients
- Asking for the sale

While there are many ways to sell, the most important involves taking the time to gain prospective clients' trust and discover what they need, and then educating them on how they will meet that need when working with the nutrition specialist. The following are seven basic rules for selling (Gitomer, 2003):

- Say it (make the presentation) in terms the client wants, needs, and understands.
- Gather personal information and learn how to use it.
- Build friendships.
- Build a relationship "shield" that no competitor can pierce.
- Establish common ground.
- Have fun and be funny.

Allied health professionals typically enter their professions to help people improve their lives. A successful fitness professional with additional training in nutrition will focus the conversation on how he or she is able to help change a prospective client's life. This is where the desire to help people meets the practical need to earn a living. If an ACE Fitness Nutrition Specialist is sincere in his or her interest in providing a high level of service to change a person's life, the sales process simply becomes a means of discovering what the client needs and then educating the client on the benefits of the services offered. Prospective clients want to understand how their needs, wants, and desires are going to be satisfied.

SUMMARY

Earning the ACE Fitness Nutrition Specialist certification and enhancing one's career can be rewarding personally, professionally, and financially. However, earning the specialty certification is just the beginning. To be successful, it is imperative to think ahead and develop a plan to attract clients and successfully manage a business.

REFERENCES

Chatterjee, S. & Price, A. (2009). Healthy living with persuasive technologies: Framework, issues, and challenges. *Journal of the American Medical Informatics Association,* 16, 2, 171–178.

Gitomer, J. (2003). *The Sales Bible* (revised edition). Hoboken, N.J.: John Wiley & Sons.

Griffiths, F. et al. (2006). Why are health care interventions delivered over the internet? A systematic review of the published literature. *Journal of Medical Internet Research,* 8, 2, e10.

Koop, C.E. (1995). A personal role in health care reform. *American Journal of Public Health,* 85, 6, 759–760. www.pubmedcentral.nih.gov/articlerender.fcgi?artid=1615490&tool=pmcentrez&rendertype=abstract

SUGGESTED READING

Covey, S. (2004). *The Seven Habits of Highly Effective People.* New York: Simon and Schuster.

Peterson, J. & Tharrett, S. (2008). *Fitness Management* (2nd ed.). Monterey Calif.: Healthy Learning.

Plummer, T. (2007). *Anyone Can Sell: Creating Revenue Through Sales in the Fitness Business.* Monterey, Calif.: Coaches Choice.

Plummer, T. (2003). *The Business of Fitness.* Monterey, Calif.: Coaches Choice.

Plummer, T. (1999). *Making Money in the Fitness Business.* Monterey, Calif.: Coaches Choice.

Ries, A. & Ries, L. (2004). *The Origin of Brands.* New York: Harper Business.

Ziglar, Z. (2003). *Secrets of Closing the Sale* (updated edition). Grand Rapids, Mich.: Fleming H. Revell.

ADDITIONAL RESOURCES

American Council on Exercise:

- ACE-certified professionals and their clients can access a variety of client-focused handouts, blogs, and other resources at www.ACEfit.com.
- ACE-certified professionals can access business forms and tools at www.ACEfitness.org. Simply log in and click "Fitness Professional Resources" and then "Business Forms."

Federal Food Safety Information: www.foodsafety.gov

Institute of Medicine: www.iom.edu

The Guide to Community Preventive Services: www.thecommunityguide.org

United States Department of Agriculture:

- *2015-20 Dietary Guidelines for Americans:* www.health.gov/dietaryguidelines
- MyPlate: www.choosemyplate.gov
- SuperTracker: www.supertracker.usda.gov

Academy of Nutrition and Dietetics Position Statements: www.eatright.org/HealthProfessionals

- Food and Nutrition for Older Adults: Promoting Health and Wellness
- Total Diet Approach to Communicating Food and Nutrition Information
- Vegetarian Diets
- Dietary Fatty Acids
- Health Implications of Dietary Fiber
- Weight Management
- Nutrition and Athletic Performance for Adults
- Nutrition Guidance for Healthy Children Aged 2 to 11 Years
- Promoting and Supporting Breastfeeding

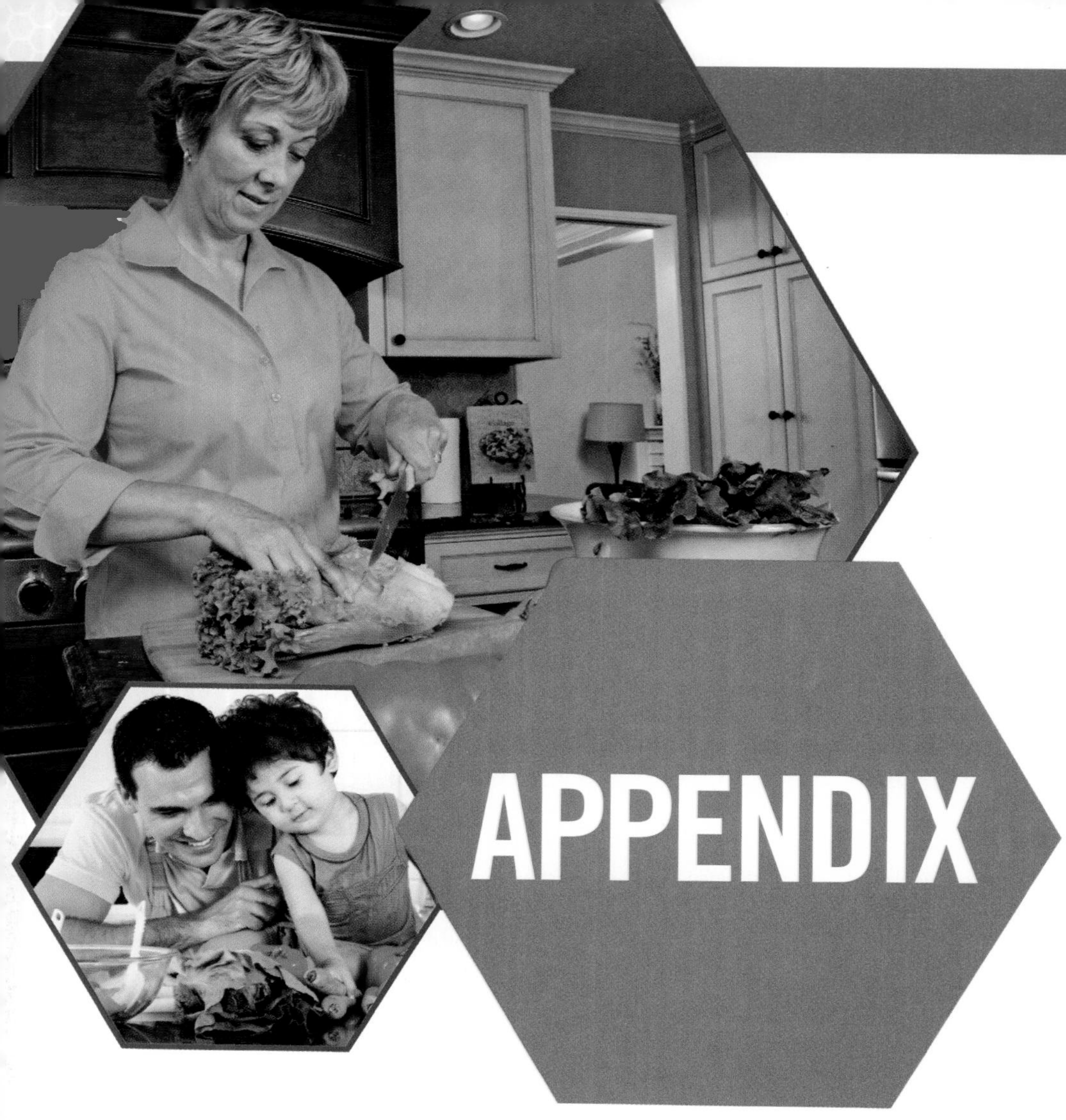

The recipes presented here correspond with the cooking demonstrations offered as part of the ACE Fitness Nutrition Specialty Certification. Visit ACEfitness.org to learn more about this opportunity.

Mary Saph Tanaka, M.D., M.S., developed her love for cooking at a young age, with fond memories of planting and cooking vegetables from the garden with her mother. She regularly utilizes locally grown ingredients and her knowledge of nutrition and herbs to prepare nutritious meals for family and friends. She is completing her pediatrics training at UCLA Mattel Children's Hospital as part of the Community Health and Advocacy Training Program. She developed the recipes for the recently released book *"Eat Your Vegetables" and Other Mistakes Parents Make: Redefining How to Raise Healthy Eaters* written by Natalie Digate Muth, M.D., MPH, R.D. (Healthy Learning, 2012).

HEALTHY RECIPES

MYPLATE

Baked Honey Mustard Chicken With Cauliflower Potatoes and Roasted Asparagus

Baked Honey Mustard Chicken

2 skinless, boneless chicken breasts
2 tablespoons of honey
2 tablespoons of Dijon or whole-grain mustard
2 tablespoons of olive oil
1 teaspoon of ground black pepper

Preheat the oven to 400 degrees. Cut each chicken breast into 3–4 even pieces and place into a medium mixing bowl. In a smaller bowl, mix the honey, mustard, olive oil, and pepper. Pour over the chicken until well coated. Let the chicken marinate for 30–40 minutes in the refrigerator.

Place the chicken evenly on a baking tray. Bake in the oven for 25–30 minutes, until cooked through well.

Cauliflower Potatoes

1 small head of cauliflower
1 medium-sized russet potato
¼ cup of low-fat plain Greek yogurt
1 tablespoon of olive oil

Wash and dry the cauliflower and potato. Cut the cauliflower and potato into small pieces of approximately the same size. Put the cauliflower and potato into a large pot and add water until the vegetables are covered. Bring to boil over medium-high heat, then lower the heat to medium and cook for 15 minutes, until tender. Drain the water and mash the cauliflower and potatoes with a fork (or potato masher). Pour in the yogurt and olive oil and mix well. Sprinkle with salt and pepper.

Simple Roasted Asparagus

1 pound of asparagus, ends trimmed
2 tablespoons of olive oil

Preheat the oven to 400 degrees. Evenly spread the asparagus over a baking sheet and drizzle with olive oil. Bake in the oven for 15 minutes.

Spice up this simple recipe with your favorite herbs. Try lemon pepper or fresh rosemary and chopped garlic.

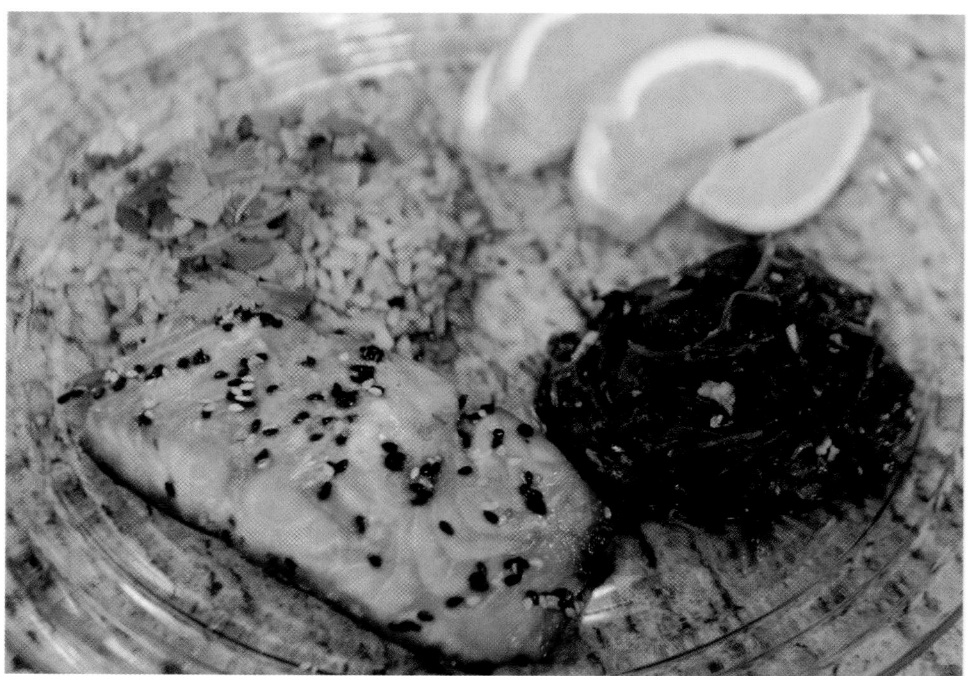

Grilled Teriyaki Salmon With Garlicky Spinach, Cucumber and Carrot Sesame Salad, and Brown Rice

Grilled Teriyaki Salmon

4 3-ounce filets of salmon
1 cup of low-sodium soy sauce
1 inch of fresh ginger, sliced thin
2 cloves of garlic, minced
Juice of ½ orange
1 tablespoon of honey

Mix the soy sauce, ginger, garlic, orange juice, and honey into a small pot over medium heat. Let simmer for 10–15 minutes.

Preheat the oven to 375 degrees. Place the salmon on a baking tray and pour the teriyaki sauce over the salmon. Bake in the oven for approximately 20–25 minutes.

Garlicky Spinach

2 cloves of garlic, minced
2 8-ounce baby spinach bags, washed and dried
2 tablespoons of olive oil

In a large pan, heat the olive oil. Place the garlic into the oil and stir for 1 minute. Next, place the spinach into the pan and stir until spinach leaves are wilted, approximately 3–4 minutes.

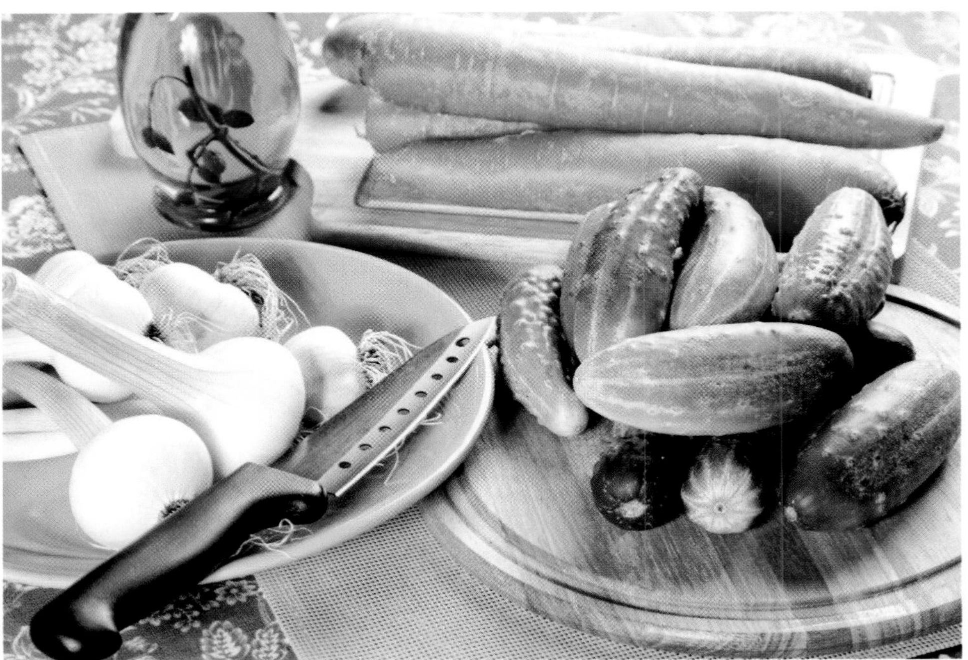

Cucumber and Carrot Sesame Salad

2 medium-sized carrots
1 large cucumber
1–2 stalks of green onions
1 tablespoon of sesame seeds
2 tablespoons of vinegar or juice of one lime

Peel carrots. Slice carrots in half lengthwise, then lay carrots flat and cut into thin slices across. Put into large bowl. Next, cut the cucumber in half lengthwise. Using a spoon, scrape out the seeds and then place the cucumber flat and cut into thin slices across. Place the cucumber into a bowl with the carrots and add green onions and sesame seeds. Mix in vinegar or lime juice and stir. Add salt and pepper.

Simple Brown Rice Recipe

1 cup of brown rice
2.5 cups of water
1 tablespoons of olive oil

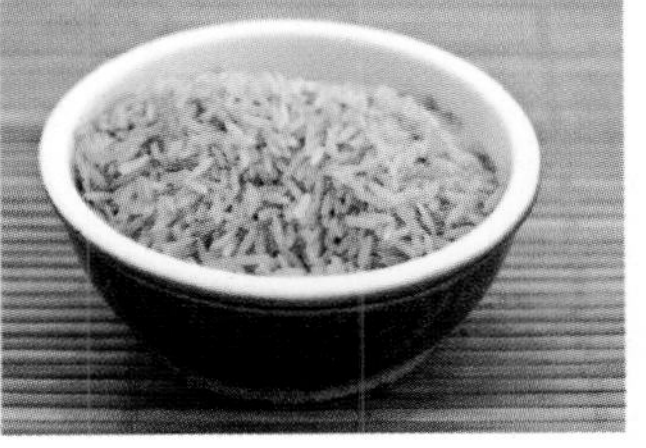

Rinse the brown rice with plenty of water and drain off the water. Place the brown rice into a pot with a fitted lid. Add the water and olive oil to the pot. Bring the pot to a boil and then lower the heat to a gentle simmer at low heat. Place the lid on the pot and let cook for 45–50 minutes.

Cooking brown rice does take more time than white rice, but it is also a much more nutritious whole-grain option packed with vitamins and minerals. Double (or triple) this recipe and freeze the cooked rice for a quick option in the future.

TRY THESE VARIATIONS TO SPICE UP PLAIN RICE:

- **Add a few sprigs of fresh herbs to the rice while simmering, such as thyme or rosemary.**
- **Turn your brown rice into a tasty pilaf by using chicken or vegetable broth to cook the rice instead of water. After the rice is cooked, add ½ cup of cooked onions, ½ cup of slivered almonds, and ¼ cup of raisins and mix well.**

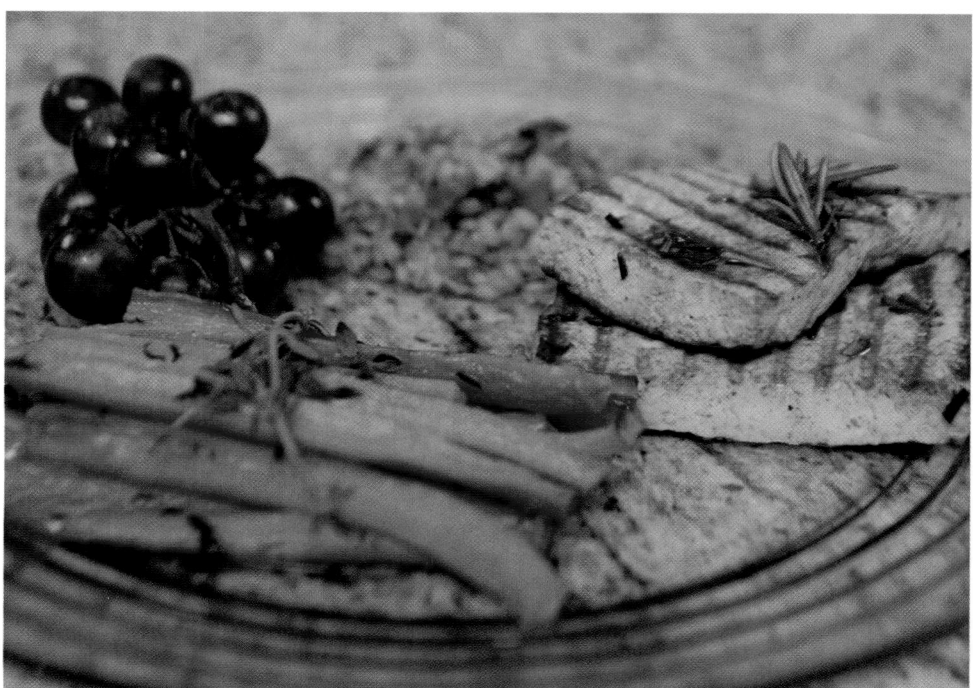

Baked Balsamic Rosemary Tofu With Roasted Carrots, Edamame and Red Pepper Salad, and Barley Black Bean Pilaf

Balsamic Rosemary Tofu

1 package of plain firm tofu
¼ cup of balsamic vinegar
2 sprigs of fresh rosemary
2 tablespoons of olive oil
1 clove of garlic, minced

Remove the leaves of rosemary off of the wooden center and chop. Place the balsamic vinegar, rosemary, garlic, and olive oil in a baking dish. Cut the tofu block into ½-inch-thick slices and place into the vinegar mixture. Marinate for 1 hour in the refrigerator.

Preheat the oven to 400 degrees. Remove the tofu from the refrigerator and place slices onto a baking tray. Bake in the oven for 15 minutes, until golden brown.

Roasted Carrots

8 medium whole carrots
4–5 sprigs of fresh thyme
Olive oil

Preheat the oven to 400 degrees. Wash, dry, and peel the carrots. Cut the carrots widthwise in half. Then cut each piece lengthwise in half and then again into quarters. Place carrot slices onto a baking tray and drizzle olive oil over them. Scatter fresh thyme over the carrots. Bake in the oven for approximately 15–20 minutes (they can be baked alongside the balsamic rosemary tofu).

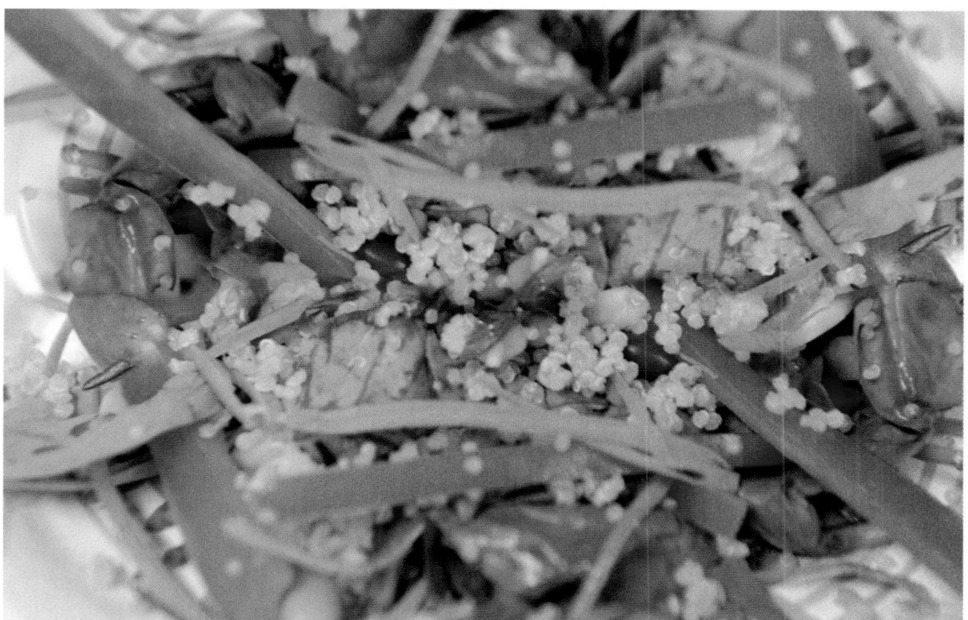

Edamame and Red Pepper Salad

1 cup of shelled edamame
1 cup of frozen corn, defrosted and drained
1 red pepper, diced
¼ cup of diced scallions
2 tablespoons of olive oil
1 tablespoon of lemon juice

Mix all ingredients well in a medium bowl.

Barley Black Bean Pilaf

To prepare the barley:
1 cup of uncooked barley
3.5 cups of water
1 tablespoon of olive oil

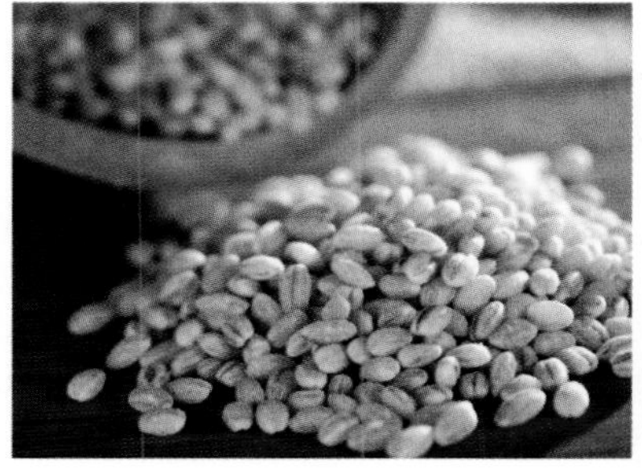

Rinse the barley with plenty of water and drain the excess water. Place the barley into a pot and pour the 3.5 cups of water and olive oil over the barley. Bring to a boil and then reduce the heat to low. Cover the pot with a tight lid and simmer for 50–60 minutes.

Once the barley is cooked:
Add ½ cup of cooked onions, 1 can of black beans, and ½ cup of chopped green onions for a tasty side dish.

Barley is a great whole grain with a deliciously nutty flavor, but it takes some time to cook. Make more than you need for your meal and turn the leftovers into a quick and simple meal for the next day.

What else can I do with barley?
For a quick and simple lunch, add 1 cup of cooked barley to the edamame and red pepper salad!

Barley for breakfast? Instead of oatmeal, try barley as a tasty alternative. Serve the cooked barley with warm milk, cinnamon, and a sprinkle of raisins for a warm and filling breakfast.

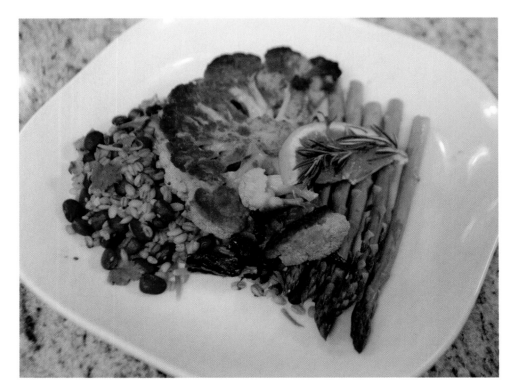

FOOD RESTRICTIONS: VEGAN

Curry Cauliflower "Steak" With Barley Black Bean Pilaf and Roasted Asparagus

Curry Cauliflower "Steak"

1 small head of cauliflower
2 tablespoons of curry powder
3 tablespoons of olive oil

Wash and dry the cauliflower and remove the green leaves. Slice the cauliflower in half. Slice each half into halves again, lengthwise, so you have a total of four "steaks." Place each "steak" onto a baking tray. In a small bowl, mix the curry powder and olive oil together and then drizzle over the cauliflower. Using a brush (or your fingers), spread the olive oil over the cauliflower so that each side is evenly coated. Bake in the oven for 20 minutes or until browned.

Barley Black Bean Pilaf: See page 179.

Roasted Asparagus: See page 175.

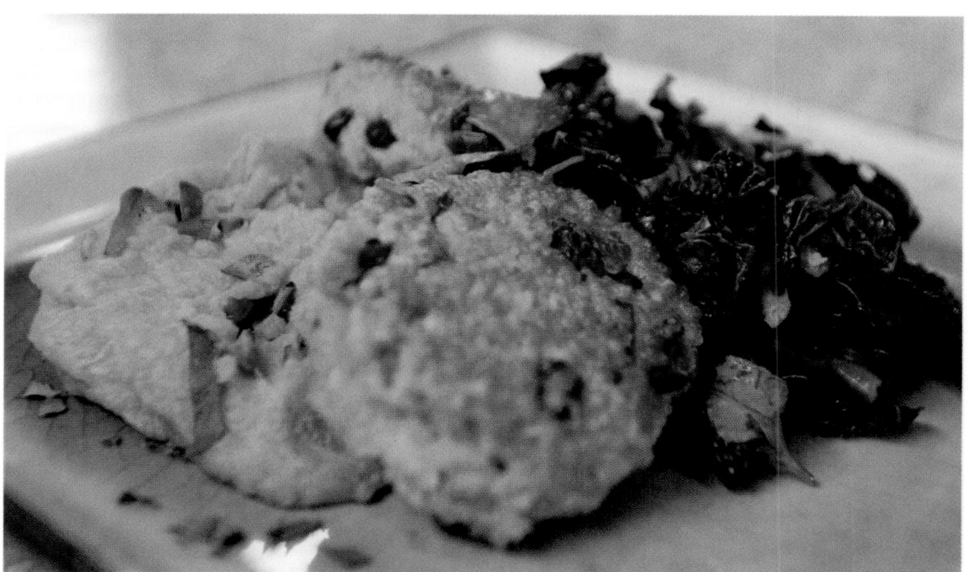

FOOD RESTRICTIONS: GLUTEN-FREE

Quinoa Cakes With Sweet Potato Mash and Garlicky Spinach

Basic Quinoa Recipe

1 cup of dry quinoa
2 cups of water

Rinse quinoa with plenty of water and drain the excess water. Bring water to boil in a pot. Add quinoa and reduce heat to low. Cover and let cook for 20 minutes. Drain excess water if necessary.

Quinoa Cakes

1 cup of cooked quinoa
1 egg
1/3 cup of black beans
3 tablespoons of cornstarch
1 clove of garlic, minced
2 tablespoons of cilantro, chopped

Mix all ingredients well in medium-sized bowl. Scoop approximately 2 tablespoons of the mixture and roll into a ball with your hands. Place a pan over medium heat and drizzle 2 tablespoons of olive oil onto the pan. Place 2–3 cakes on the pan and gently flatten the balls once on the pan. Cook on each side for 6–7 minutes, until browned and crispy on both sides.

Sweet Potato Mash

4 medium-sized sweet potatoes

Wash sweet potatoes well. Peel and cut into 1-inch pieces. Place the potatoes in a pot and add enough water to cover the potatoes. Place on the stove at medium-high heat. Cook until potatoes are tender, approximately 30 minutes. Once tender, drain the water. Mash potatoes with a fork or potato masher, then serve.

Garlicky Spinach: See page 176.

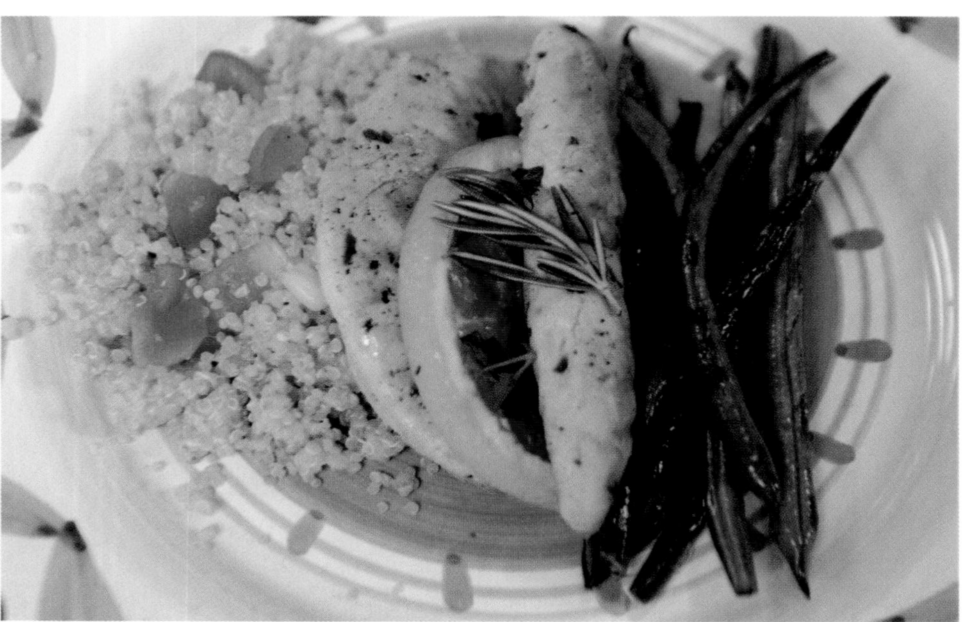

SPECIALIZED EATING PLANS: DIETARY APPROACHES TO STOP HYPERTENSION (DASH)

Orange Rosemary Chicken With Almond Green Beans and Quinoa

Orange Rosemary Chicken

2 skinless, boneless chicken breasts
Juice of ½ orange
2 sprigs of fresh rosemary, leaves removed and chopped
1 tablespoon of red wine vinegar
2 tablespoons of olive oil
1 teaspoon of ground black pepper

Preheat the oven to 400 degrees. Cut each chicken breast into 3–4 even pieces and place into a medium mixing bowl. In a smaller bowl, mix the orange juice, rosemary, vinegar, pepper, and olive oil. Pour over the chicken until it is well coated. Let chicken marinate for 30–40 minutes in the refrigerator.

Space the chicken evenly on a baking tray. Bake in the oven for 25–30 minutes, until cooked through.

Almond Green Beans

1 pound of green beans
¼ cup of slivered almonds (or chopped almonds)
Olive oil

Wash and dry green beans and trim the ends off. Heat a pan over medium heat with 2 tablespoons of olive oil drizzled over the pan. Place green beans into the pan and stir occasionally for 5–6 minutes, until lightly browned.
Remove green beans from heat and sprinkle with almonds. *Optional:* Serve with lemon wedges.

Quinoa: See page 181.

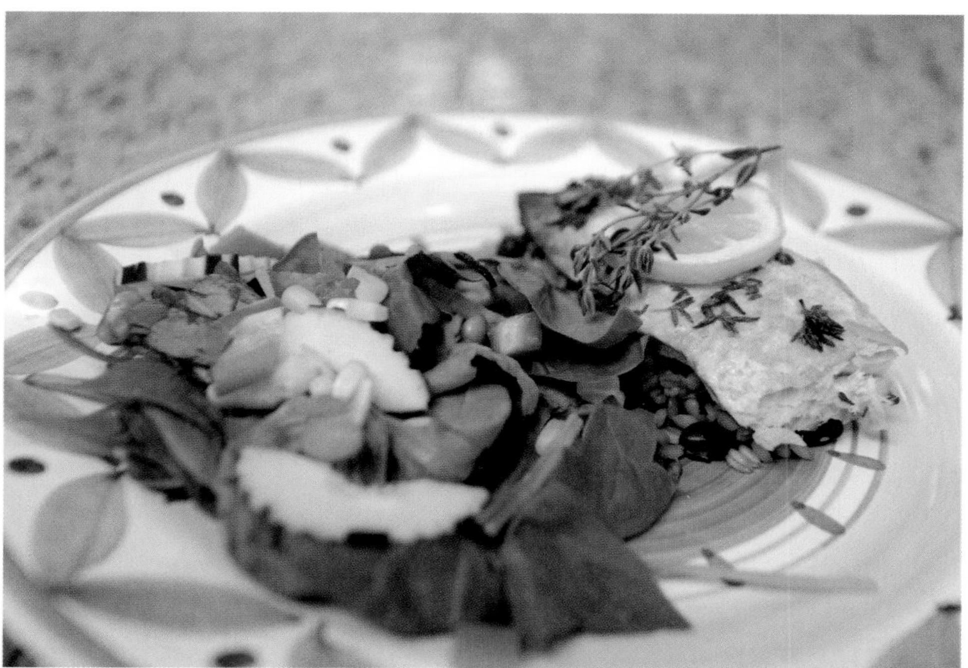

SPECIALIZED EATING PLANS: USDA

Baked Lemon-Thyme Salmon and Barley With Side Salad

Baked Lemon-Thyme Salmon

4 3-ounce filets of salmon (or other fish)
Juice of ½ lemon
3–4 sprigs of fresh thyme (leaves removed)
1 tablespoon of honey
1 tablespoon of Dijon mustard
2 tablespoons of olive oil

Mix the lemon juice, thyme, honey, Dijon mustard, and olive oil in a small bowl.

Preheat the oven to 375 degrees. Place the salmon on a baking tray and pour the lemon-thyme marinade over the salmon. Bake in the oven for approximately 20–25 minutes.

Barley: See page 179.

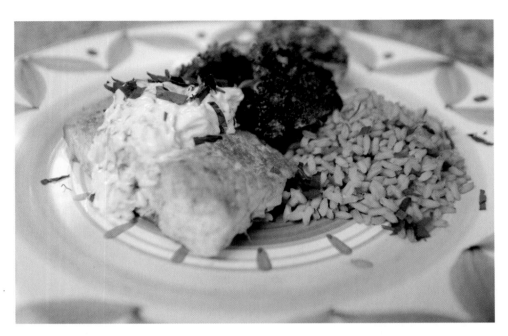

SPECIALIZED EATING PLANS: MEDITERRANEAN DIET

Garlic Cumin Salmon With Tzatziki Yogurt Sauce, Steamed Broccoli, and Brown Rice Pilaf

Garlic Cumin Salmon With Tzatziki Yogurt Sauce

4 3-ounce filets of salmon
2 tablespoons of olive oil
1 tablespoon of ground cumin
2 cloves of garlic, minced
2 teaspoons of pepper

Mix the olive oil, cumin, garlic, and pepper in a small bowl.

Preheat the oven to 375 degrees. Place the salmon on a baking tray and pour the garlic cumin marinade over the salmon. Bake in the oven for approximately 20–25 minutes.

Tzatziki Yogurt Sauce

1 cup of nonfat Greek yogurt
1 small Persian or pickling cucumber (or ½ English cucumber)
1 clove of garlic, minced
¼ cup of chopped green onions
2 tablespoons of chopped fresh mint

Using the larger grating holes, grate the cucumber into a small kitchen towel. Squeeze out the excess water from the cucumber after grating. Place the cucumber into a bowl and add the garlic, onions, and mint. Pour the yogurt into the cucumber mixture and mix until well incorporated.

Brown Rice Pilaf: See page 177.

WITH WHAT OTHER FOODS CAN I EAT THIS YOGURT SAUCE?

Pita sandwiches with yogurt sauce: Use the recipe with baked chicken and chop the chicken up into bite-sized pieces. Cut a pita in half and stuff the middle of the pita with chicken, spinach, chopped tomatoes, and a dollop of the tzatziki sauce.

Mediterranean-inspired burgers: Use this tzatziki sauce on top of veggieful hamburgers (see page 185) as a creamy spread.

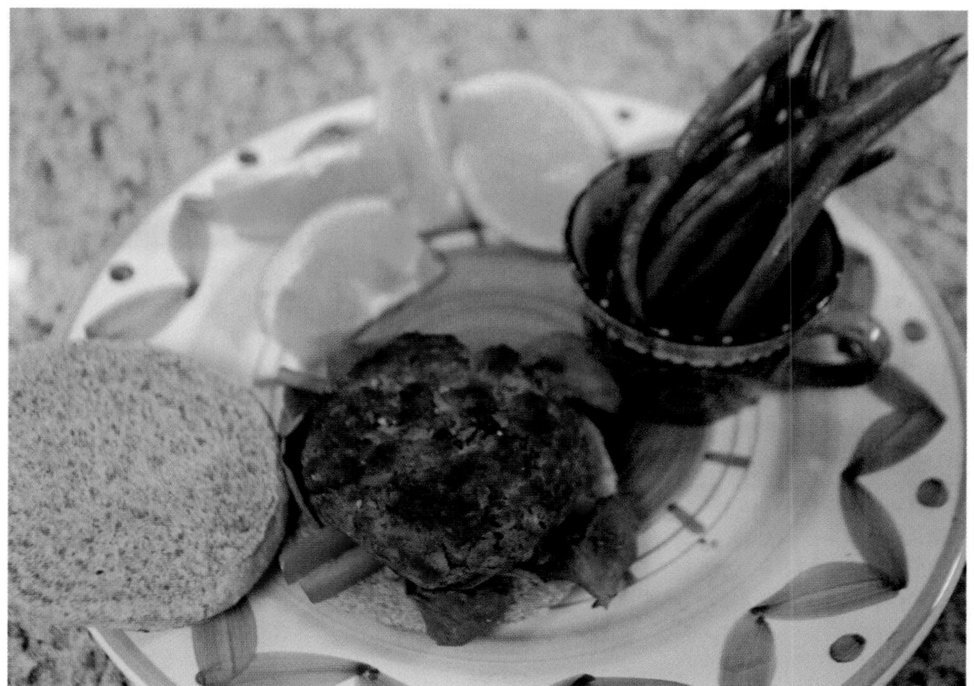

FEEDING KIDS

Veggieful Hamburgers With Crispy Green Bean "Fries"

"Veggieful" Hamburgers

1 pound of lean ground beef or turkey
2 cups of shredded vegetables (carrots, zucchini, peppers)
½ cup uncooked oatmeal
1 teaspoon of salt and pepper
Whole-wheat hamburger buns
Toppings: Lettuce, tomatoes, onions, mushrooms, and cheese

Hamburger patties: Mix vegetables, meat, salt, pepper, and oatmeal in a bowl and stir. Take two large spoonfuls of the mixture and roll into a ball, then flatten to form a patty.

Place a pan on the stove at medium heat. Place 1 tablespoon of olive oil in the pan. Place the hamburger patty on the pan and cook for 5–6 minutes. Turn the patty over and cook for another 5–6 minutes. Serve on hamburger bun with your favorite toppings.

Crispy Green Bean "Fries"

1 pound green beans, washed, dried with ends trimmed
2 tablespoons of olive oil
Salt and pepper

Preheat the oven to 425 degrees. Place green beans on a baking sheet in a single layer. Pour olive oil over the beans. Sprinkle salt and pepper. Bake for 20 minutes, until crispy.

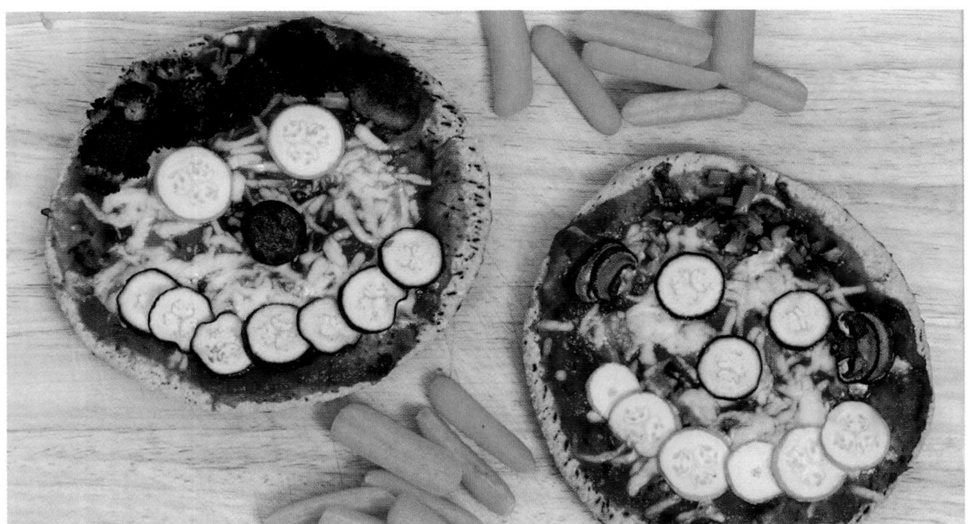

Smiling Faces Pita Pizzas

4 whole-wheat pitas
1 cup of tomato sauce
2 cups of assorted chopped vegetables (mushrooms, spinach, onions, peppers, broccoli)
1 cup of shredded mozzarella cheese

Heat oven to 400 degrees. Place 1–2 tablespoons of tomato sauce on pita bread and spread evenly. Top pita bread with vegetables and/or meat of your choice. Sprinkle 2 tablespoons of cheese on top of vegetables. Place on baking sheet and bake for 10–15 minutes, until cheese is melted.

Baked Honey Mustard Chicken Fingers With Sweet Potato Mash

Baked Honey Mustard Chicken Fingers

2 cups of crispy brown rice cereal
3 skinless and boneless chicken breasts
Salt and pepper
2 teaspoons of dried parsley or oregano
¼ cup Dijon mustard
3 tablespoons of honey
Olive oil

Preheat oven to 400 degrees. Cut chicken breasts lengthwise into ¼-inch-wide strips. Sprinkle the chicken strips with salt, pepper, and the dried parsley or oregano. Mix mustard and honey together in a bowl and then pour into a large resealable plastic bag. Place the chicken strips in the bag and seal. Lightly coat the chicken strips with the mustard/honey mixture on both sides.

Place cereal into a large resealable plastic bag. Gently crush the cereal into smaller bits (but not into a flour-like consistency). Transfer 4–5 chicken strips from the honey mustard mixture into the bag with the cereal. Coat the chicken with cereal and then place on a baking sheet that has been sprayed with nonstick cooking spray. Place the chicken pieces approximately 2 inches apart. Drizzle 2 tablespoons of olive oil over chicken and place in the oven.

Bake for approximately 20–25 minutes (depending on the thickness of your chicken pieces).

Sweet Potato Mash: See page 181.

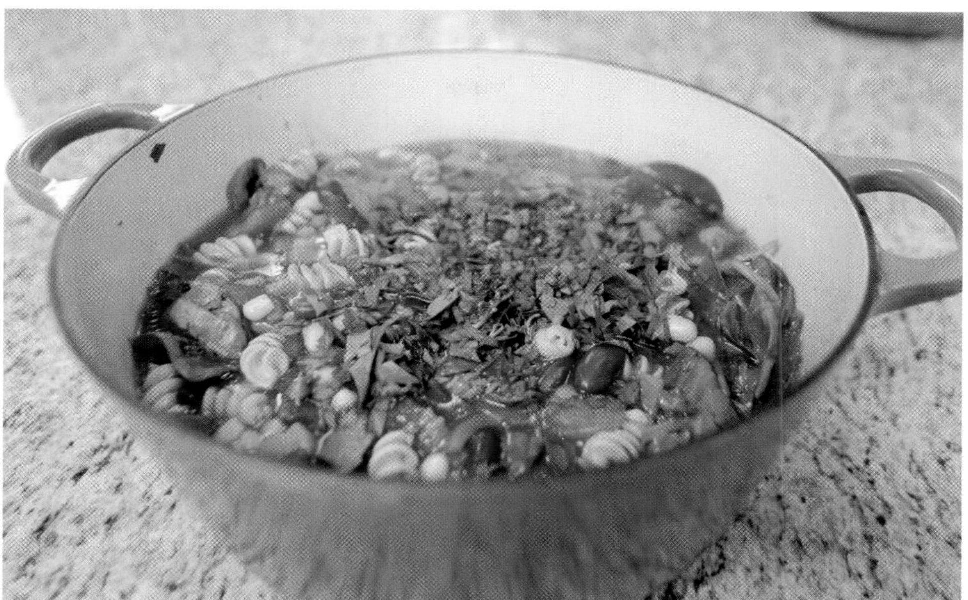

QUICK AND EASY COOKING FOR OLDER ADULTS

Vegetable Minestrone Soup

1 can of red kidney beans, drained
1 can of white cannellini beans, drained
1 package of assorted frozen vegetables, defrosted and drained
1 package of whole-wheat short pasta, cooked
2 cans of low-sodium diced tomatoes
2 cans of low-sodium chicken broth
1 medium onion, chopped

Heat a large pot over medium heat. Place 2 tablespoons of olive oil into the pot. Place onions into the pot and cook until softened. Add all the ingredients into the pot and stir. Let simmer over low heat for 40 minutes.

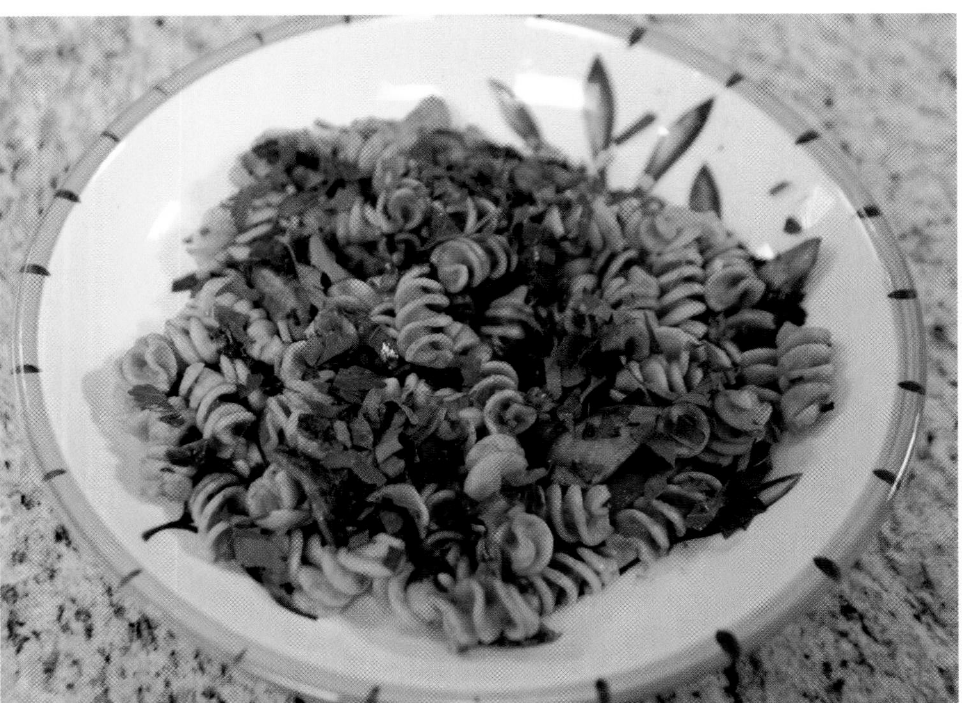

Whole-wheat Spinach Pasta With Chicken Sausage

1 pack of whole-wheat short pasta
2 cups of frozen spinach, defrosted (with excess water squeezed out)
4 links of precooked chicken sausage
1 jar of tomato or marinara sauce
½ cup of grated parmesan or mozzarella

Cook pasta as instructed on the label. Heat a pan over medium heat. Slice the chicken sausage into 1/8-inch rounds and place in the pan. Cook for approximately 5 minutes. Add the spinach to the sausage and stir. Next, add the pasta to the sausage/spinach mixture. Add tomato/marinara sauce and stir well. Pour contents of the bowl into a large baking casserole tray.

Preheat the oven to 375 degrees. Place the dish into oven and cook for 30 minutes. Remove the dish from the oven and sprinkle cheese on top. Return the dish to the oven and cook another 15 minutes, until cheese is melted.

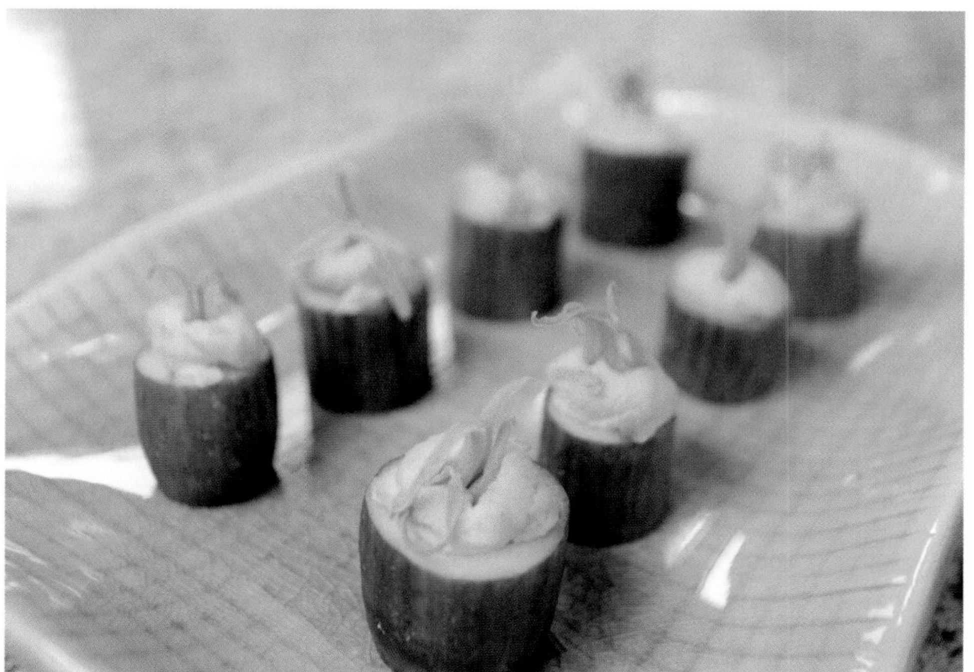

COOKING TO CONTROL WEIGHT

Creamy Hummus Cucumber Bites

1 can of garbanzo beans, drained
2 tablespoons of olive oil
2 tablespoons of water
1 garlic clove
Juice of ½ lemon
1 English cucumber
Shredded carrots

Place beans, olive oil, water, garlic, and lemon juice in a blender until smooth. Cut cucumber into ½ inch slices. Top each cucumber slice with a dollop of hummus and shredded carrots and serve.

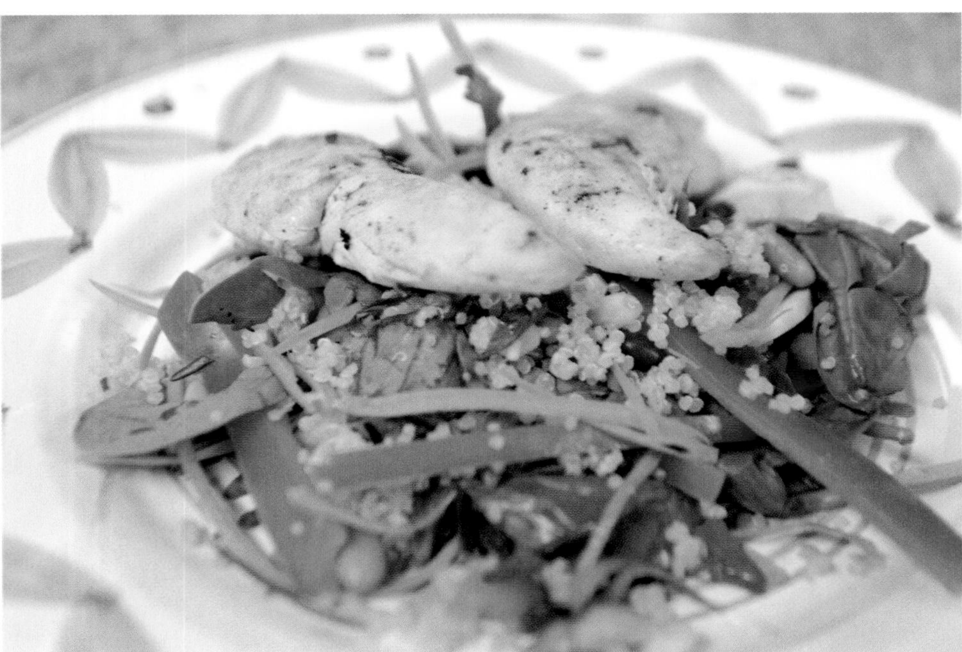

Quinoa Salad With Grilled Chicken

1 cup of cooked quinoa (see page 181)
2 cups of baby spinach
½ cup of shredded carrots
½ cup of red pepper, diced
½ cup of corn
4 pieces of Baked Honey Mustard or Orange Rosemary Chicken (see pages 175, 182)

Divide the ingredients above evenly between two plates. Drizzle with olive oil and either red wine vinegar or balsamic vinegar.

GLOSSARY

Absorption The uptake of nutrients across a tissue or membrane by the gastrointestinal tract.

Acceptable Macronutrient Distribution Range (AMDR) The range of intake for a particular energy source that is associated with reduced risk of chronic disease while providing intakes of essential nutrients.

Action The stage of the transtheoretical model of behavioral change during which the individual is actively engaging in a behavior that was started less than six months ago.

Active listening Mode of listening in which the listener is concerned about the content, intent, and feelings of the message.

Active transport The energy-requiring transfer of a nutrient across a membrane.

Adequate Intake (AI) A recommended nutrient intake level that, based on research, appears to be sufficient for good health.

Adherence The extent to which people follow their plans or treatment recommendations. Exercise adherence is the extent to which people follow an exercise program.

Adulterated A supplement is considered adulterated if it, or one of its ingredients, presents a "significant or unreasonable risk of illness or injury" when used as directed, or under normal circumstances.

Allergen A substance that can cause an allergic reaction by stimulating type-1 hypersensitivity in atopic individuals.

Amino acids Nitrogen-containing compounds that are the building blocks of protein.

Anabolism A state in which the body produces more protein than it breaks down; occurs in times of growth such as childhood, pregnancy, recovery from illness, and in response to resistance training when overloading the muscles promotes protein synthesis.

Anemia A reduction in the number of red blood cells and/or quantity of hemoglobin per volume of blood below normal values.

Angina A common symptom of coronary artery disease characterized by chest pain, tightness, or radiating pain resulting from a lack of blood flow to the heart muscle.

Anion Negative ion.

Anorexia nervosa (AN) An eating disorder characterized by refusal to maintain body weight of at least 85% of expected weight; intense fear of gaining weight or becoming fat; body-image disturbances, including a disproportionate influence of body weight on self-evaluation; and, in women, the absence of at least three consecutive menstrual periods.

Antibody An immunoglobulin molecule produced by lymphocytes in response to an antigen and characterized by reacting specifically with the antigen.

Antioxidant A substance that prevents or repairs oxidative damage; includes vitamins C and E, some carotenoids, selenium, ubiquinones, and bioflavonoids.

Arrhythmia A disturbance in the rate or rhythm of the heartbeat. Some can be symptoms of serious heart disease; may not be of medical significance until symptoms appear.

Atherosclerosis A specific form of arteriosclerosis characterized by the accumulation of fatty material on the inner walls of the arteries, causing them to harden, thicken, and lose elasticity.

Autonomic nervous system The part of the nervous system that regulates involuntary body functions, including the activity of the cardiac muscle, smooth muscles, and glands. It has two divisions: the sympathetic nervous system and the parasympathetic nervous system.

Binge eating disorder (BED) An eating disorder characterized by frequent binge eating (without purging) and feelings of being out of control when eating.

Bioavailability The degree to which a substance can be absorbed and efficiently utilized by the body.

Body composition The makeup of the body in terms of the relative percentage of fat-free mass and body fat.

Body mass index (BMI) A relative measure of body height to body weight used to determine levels of weight, from underweight to extreme obesity.

Bolus A food and saliva digestive mix that is swallowed and then moved through the digestive tract.

Bone mineral density (BMD) A measure of the amount of minerals (mainly calcium) contained in a certain volume of bone.

Brush border The site of nutrient absorption in the small intestines.

Bulimia nervosa (BN) An eating disorder characterized by recurrent episodes of uncontrolled binge eating; recurrent inappropriate compensatory behavior such as self-induced vomiting, laxative misuse, diuretics, or enemas (purging type), or fasting and/or excessive exercise (nonpurging type); episodes of binge eating and compensatory behaviors occur at least twice per week for three months; self-evaluation that is heavily influenced by body shape and weight; and episodes that do not occur exclusively with episodes of anorexia.

Carbohydrate The body's preferred energy source. Dietary sources include sugars (simple) and grains, rice, potatoes, and beans (complex). Carbohydrate is stored as glycogen in the muscles and liver and is transported in the blood as glucose.

Carbohydrate loading Up to a week-long regimen of manipulating intensity of training and carbohydrate intake to achieve maximum glycogen storage for an endurance event.

Cardiovascular disease (CVD) A general term for any disease of the heart, blood vessels, or circulation.

Carotenoid Any of a group of red, yellow, or orange pigments that are found in certain foods (e.g., carrots and sweet potatoes); has antioxidant properties when consumed in the diet.

Casein The main protein found in milk and other dairy products.

Catabolism Metabolic pathways that break down molecules into smaller units and release energy.

Cation Positive ion.

Chelation compound A compound formed from a specific process in which ions and molecules bind metal ions.

Cholesterol A fatlike substance found in the blood and body tissues and in certain foods. Can accumulate in the arteries and lead to a narrowing of the vessels (atherosclerosis).

Chronic Descriptive of a condition that persists over a long period of time; opposite of acute.

Chylomicron A large lipoprotein particle that transfers fat from food from the small intestine to the liver and adipose tissue.

Chyme The semiliquid mass of partly digested food expelled by the stomach into the duodenum.

Cirrhosis A disease of the liver in which normal cells in the liver are replaced by scar tissue. This condition results in the failure of the liver to perform many of its usual functions.

Cofactor A substance that needs to be present along with an enzyme for a chemical reaction to occur.

Complete protein A food that contains all of the essential amino acids. Eggs, soy, and most meats and dairy products are considered complete proteins.

Complex carbohydrate A long chain of sugar that takes more time to digest than a simple carbohydrate.

Congestive heart failure (CHF) Inability of the heart to pump blood at a sufficient rate to meet the metabolic demand or the ability to do so only when the cardiac filling pressures are abnormally high, frequently resulting in lung congestion.

Contemplation The stage of the transtheoretical model of behavioral change during which the individual is weighing the pros and cons of behavioral change.

Coronary heart disease (CHD) The major form of cardiovascular disease; results when the coronary arteries are narrowed or occluded, most commonly by atherosclerotic deposits of fibrous and fatty tissue; also called coronary artery disease (CAD).

Deamination A process by which the liver removes nitrogen from an amino acid; essential before an amino acid can be used by the body.

Decisional balance One of the four components of the transtheoretical model of behavioral change; refers to the numbers of pros and cons an individual perceives regarding adopting and/or maintaining an activity program.

Dehydration The process of losing body water; when severe can cause serious, life-threatening consequences.

Denaturation A process by which a protein loses its unique shape; essential before it can be digested.

Deoxyribonucleic acid (DNA) A large, double-stranded, helical molecule that is the carrier of genetic information.

Diabetes A disease of carbohydrate metabolism in which an absolute or relative deficiency of insulin results in an inability to metabolize carbohydrates normally.

Diastolic blood pressure (DBP) The pressure in the arteries during the relaxation phase (diastole) of the cardiac cycle; indicative of total peripheral resistance.

Dietary Approaches to Stop Hypertension (DASH) eating plan An eating plan designed to reduce blood pressure; also serves as an overall healthy way of eating that can be adopted by nearly anyone; may also lower risk of coronary heart disease.

Dietary fiber Fiber obtained naturally from plant foods.

Dietary Reference Intake (DRI) A generic term used to refer to three types of nutrient reference values: Recommended Dietary Allowance (RDA), Estimated Average Requirement (EAR), and Tolerable Upper Intake Level (UL).

Dietary supplement A product (other than tobacco) that functions to supplement the diet and contains one or more of the following ingredients: a vitamin, mineral, herb or other botanical, amino acid, dietary substance that increases total daily intake, metabolite, constituent, extract, or some combination of these ingredients.

Dietary Supplement and Health Education Act (DSHEA) A bill passed by Congress in 1994 that sets forth regulations and guidelines for dietary supplements.

Digestion The process of breaking down food into small enough units for absorption.

Digestive system The group of organs that break down food and absorb the nutrients used by the body for fuel.

Disaccharide Double sugar units called sucrose, lactose, and maltose.

Diuretic Medication that produces an increase in urine volume and sodium excretion.

Duodenum The top portion of the small intestine.

Electrolyte A mineral that exists as a charged ion in the body and that is extremely important for normal cellular function.

Empathic statement A statement that conveys an attempt at understanding what another person is experiencing from that person's perspective.

Empathy Understanding what another person is experiencing from his or her perspective.

Employee A person who works for another person in exchange for financial compensation. An employee complies with the instructions and directions of his or her employer and reports to them on a regular basis.

Empty calories Calories that provide very little nutritional value; should be limited in the diet.

Enzyme A protein that speeds up a specific chemical reaction.

Esophagus The food pipe; the conduit from the mouth to the stomach.

Essential amino acids Eight to 10 of the 23 different amino acids needed to make proteins. Called essential because the body cannot manufacture them; they must be obtained from the diet.

Essential fatty acids Fatty acids that the body needs but cannot synthesize; includes linolenic (omega-3) and linoleic (omega-6) fatty acids.

Estimated Average Requirement (EAR) An adequate intake in 50% of an age- and gender-specific group.

Estrogen Generic term for estrus-producing steroid compounds produced primarily in the ovaries; the female sex hormones.

Euhydration A state of "normal" body water content.

Facilitated diffusion The passage of molecules or ions across a biological membrane facilitated by specific transmembrane proteins (e.g., the passage of positively charged minerals through the small intestinal border from high concentration to low concentration with a protein carrier).

Fat An essential nutrient that provides energy, energy storage, insulation, and contour to the body. 1 gram of fat equals 9 kcal.

Fat-soluble vitamin A vitamin that, when consumed, is stored in the body (particularly the liver and fat tissues); includes vitamins A, D, E, and K.

Fatty acid A long hydrocarbon chain with an even number of carbons and varying degrees of saturation with hydrogen.

Fiber Carbohydrate chains the body cannot break down for use and which pass through the body undigested.

Folic acid A water-soluble, B vitamin required for breaking down complex carbohydrates into simple sugars to be used for energy; pregnant women have an increased need for folic acid, both for themselves and their child, as it is necessary for the proper growth and development of the fetus.

Food diary A tool used to track food consumption; involves having clients describe a "typical" eating day, including all foods and beverages. Also called a food record.

Food-frequency questionnaire A multipage list of hundreds of different foods or food types; the client is asked to indicate how often each of the foods is consumed on a daily, weekly, or monthly basis.

Food record *See* Food diary.

Fructooligosaccharide A category of oligosaccharides that are mostly indigestible, may help to relieve constipation, improve triglyceride levels, and decrease production of foul-smelling digestive by-products.

Fructose Fruit sugar; the sweetest of the monosaccharides; found in varying levels in different types of fruits.

Functional fiber Fiber obtained in the diet from isolated fibers added to food products.

Functional food Any whole food or fortified, enriched, or enhanced food that has a potentially beneficial effect on human health beyond basic nutrition.

Galactose A monosaccharide; a component of lactose.

Gallbladder A pear-shaped organ located below the liver that stores the bile secreted by the liver.

Gastric emptying The process by which food is emptied from the stomach into the small intestine.

Gastric inhibitory peptide A hormone that slows motility of the intestine to allow foods that require more time for digestion and absorption to be absorbed.

Gastric lipase An enzyme released by the stomach that aids in the digestion of fat.

Gastrin A hormone that maintains the pH of the stomach by signaling the cells that produce hydrochloric acid whenever food enters the stomach.

Glucose A simple sugar; the form in which all carbohydrates are used as the body's principal energy source.

Glycemic index (GI) A ranking of carbohydrates on a scale from 0 to 100 according to the extent to which they raise blood sugar levels.

Glycemic load (GL) A measure of glycemic response to a food that takes into serving size consideration; GL = Glycemic index x Grams of carbohydrate/100.

Glycogen The chief carbohydrate storage material; formed by the liver and stored in the liver and muscle.

Glycogenolysis The breakdown of liver and muscle glycogen to yield blood glucose.

Health claim A statement that describes a relationship between a food or food component and the prevention or treatment of a disease or health-related condition.

Health Insurance Portability and Accountability Act (HIPAA) Enacted by the U.S. Congress in 1996, HIPAA requires the U.S. Department of Health and Human Services (HHS) to establish national standards for electronic healthcare information to facilitate efficient and secure exchange of private health data. The Standards for Privacy of Individually Identifiable Health Information ("Privacy Rule"), issued by the HHS, addresses the use and disclosure of individuals' health information—called "protected health information"—by providing federal protections and giving patients an array of rights with respect to personal health information while permitting the disclosure of information needed for patient care and other important purposes.

Health screening A vital process that identifies individuals at high risk for exercise-induced heart problems that need to be referred to appropriate medical care as needed.

Healthy Mediterranean-Style Eating Pattern One of three USDA Food Patterns featured in the *Dietary Guidelines for Americans;* modified from the Healthy U.S.-Style Eating Pattern to more closely reflect eating patterns that have been associated with positive health outcomes in studies of Mediterranean-style diets.

Healthy U.S.-Style Eating Pattern One of three USDA Food Patterns featured in the *Dietary Guidelines for Americans;* based on the types and proportions of foods Americans typically consume, but in nutrient-dense forms and appropriate amounts.

Healthy Vegetarian Eating Pattern One of three USDA Food Patterns featured in the *Dietary Guidelines for Americans;* modified from the Healthy U.S.-Style Eating Pattern to more closely reflect eating patterns reported by self-identified vegetarians.

Heat exhaustion The most common heat-related illness; usually the result of intense exercise in a hot, humid environment and characterized by profuse sweating, which results in fluid and electrolyte loss, a drop in blood pressure, lightheadedness, nausea, vomiting, decreased coordination, and often syncope (fainting).

Heat stroke A medical emergency that is the most serious form of heat illness due to heat overload and/or impairment of the body's ability to dissipate heat; characterized by high body temperature (>105° F or 40.5° C), dry, red skin, altered level of consciousness, seizures, coma, and possibly death.

Hemoglobin The protein molecule in red blood cells specifically adapted to carry oxygen molecules (by bonding with them).

Heterogenous Nonsimilar or nonuniform in nature, such as a group of lipids with differing basic structures.

High-density lipoprotein (HDL) A lipoprotein that carries excess cholesterol from the arteries to the liver.

High-viscosity fiber A type of fiber that forms gels in water; may help prevent heart disease and stroke by binding bile and cholesterol; diabetes by slowing glucose absorption; and constipation by holding moisture in stools and softening them.

Hormones A chemical substance produced and released by an endocrine gland and transported through the blood to a target organ.

Hypercholesterolemia An excess of cholesterol in the blood.

Hypertension High blood pressure, or the elevation of resting blood pressure above 140/90 mmHg.

Hypertonic Having extreme muscular tension.

Hyponatremia Abnormally low levels of sodium ions circulating in the blood; severe hyponatremia can lead to brain swelling and death.

Ileum One of three sections of the small intestine.

Incomplete protein A protein that does not contain all of the essential amino acids.

Independent contractor A person who conducts business on his or her own on a contract basis and is not an employee of an organization.

Insoluble fiber *See* Low-viscosity fiber.

Insulin A hormone released from the

pancreas that allows cells to take up glucose.

Insulin resistance An inability of muscle tissue to effectively use insulin, where the action of insulin is "resisted" by insulin-sensitive tissues.

Intraluminal stage The phase of mineral digestion that occurs in the uppermost portion of the small intestine, the duodenum.

Iron An essential dietary mineral necessary for the transport of oxygen (via hemoglobin in red blood cells) and for oxidation by cells; deficiency causes of anemia; found in meat, poultry, eggs, vegetables, and cereals (especially those fortified with iron).

Iron-deficiency anemia Anemia that is due to iron deficiency; characterized by the production of smaller than normal red blood cells, which interferes with oxygen transportation and usage throughout the body.

Jejunum One of three segments of the small intestine.

Lactase An enzyme that is needed to break the bond between the glucose and galactose molecules in lactose so that they can be digested; a deficiency of this enzyme leads to lactose intolerance.

Lacto-ovo vegetarian A vegetarian who does not eat meat, fish, or poultry.

Lactose A disaccharide; the principal sugar found in milk.

Lactose intolerance A condition that results from a deficiency in the enzyme lactase, which is required to digest lactose; symptoms include cramps, bloating, diarrhea, and flatulence.

Lacto-vegetarian A vegetarian who does not eat eggs, meat, fish, or poultry.

Large intestine A component of the digestive system where certain minerals and a large amount of water are reabsorbed into the blood.

Lingual lipase An enzyme released in the mouth that marks the beginning of digestion; cleaves short- and medium-chain fatty acids.

Linoleic acid *See* Omega-6 fatty acid.

Linolenic acid *See* Omega-3 fatty acid.

Lipoprotein lipase An enzyme in working cells that cleaves fatty acids so they can be used to produce energy.

Low-density lipoprotein (LDL) A lipoprotein that transports cholesterol and triglycerides from the liver and small intestine to cells and tissues; high levels may cause atherosclerosis.

Low-viscosity fiber The structural part of the plant that does not form a gel in water; it reduces constipation and lowers risk of hemorrhoids and diverticulosis by adding bulk to the feces and reducing transit time in the colon. Also called insoluble fiber.

Lymphatic system A network of lymphoid organs, lymph nodes, lymph ducts, lymphatic tissues, lymph capillaries, and lymph vessels that produces and transports lymph fluid from tissues to the circulatory system.

Macronutrient A nutrient that is needed in large quantities for normal growth and development.

Maintenance The stage of the transtheoretical model of behavioral change during which the individual is incorporating the new behavior into his or her lifestyle.

Medical nutrition therapy The provision of individualized nutrition assessment and dietary recommendations to help manage disease. Medical nutrition therapy is recognized by Medicare as the domain of the registered dietitian.

Mediterranean diet A diet generally

characterized by increased consumption of olive oil, complex carbohydrates, vegetables, and fish, and decreased red meat and pork consumption..

Micelles Aggregates of lipid- and water-soluble compounds in which the hydrophobic portions are oriented toward the center and the hydrophilic portions are oriented outwardly.

Micronutrient A nutrient that is needed in small quantities for normal growth and development.

Mineral An inorganic substance needed in the diet in small amounts to help regulate bodily functions.

Mobilization stage The stage in mineral digestion after the mineral complex has crossed the small intestinal border in which it arrives into the portal blood circulation, which will deliver it to the liver for processing and then distribution to the rest of the body.

Monosaccharide The simplest form of sugar; it cannot be broken down any further.

Monounsaturated fat *See* Monounsaturated fatty acid.

Monounsaturated fatty acid A type of unsaturated fat (liquid at room temperature) that has one open spot on the fatty acid for the addition of a hydrogen atom (e.g., oleic acid in olive oil).

Motivational interviewing (MI) A method of questioning clients in a way that encourages them to honestly examine their beliefs and behaviors, and that motivates clients to make a decision to change a particular behavior.

Myocardial infarction (MI) An episode in which some of the heart's blood supply is severely cut off or restricted, causing the heart muscle to suffer and die from lack of oxygen. Commonly known as a heart attack.

Neurotransmitter A chemical substance such as acetylcholine or dopamine that transmits nerve impulses across synapses.

Niacin A B vitamin found in meat, wheat germ, dairy products, and yeast; used to treat and prevent pellagra.

Nitrogen balance A measure of nitrogen consumed (from dietary intake protein) and nitrogen excreted (from protein breakdown). In a healthy body, the amount of protein taken in is exactly matched by the amount of protein lost in feces, urine, and sweat.

Nonessential amino acid An amino acid that can be made by the body.

Nonsteroidal anti-inflammatory drug (NSAID) A drug with analgesic, antipyretic and anti-inflammatory effects. The term "nonsteroidal" is used to distinguish these drugs from steroids, which have similar actions.

Nutrient A component of food needed by the body. There are six classes of nutrients: water, minerals, vitamins, fats, carbohydrates, and protein.

Nutrient content claim Statement of the implied health benefits of a product that describes the level of a nutrient in a product using terms like "free," "high," or "low," or compared to another product using terms like "more," "reduced," and "lite."

Nutrient density A food that is relatively rich in nutrients for the number of calories it contains.

Obesity An excessive accumulation of body fat. Usually defined as more than 20% above ideal weight, or over 25% body fat for men and over 32% body fat for women; also can be defined as a body mass index of >30 kg/m² or a waist girth of >40 inches (102 cm) in men and >35 inches (89 cm) in women.

Oligosaccharide A chain of about three to 10 or fewer simple sugars.

Omega-3 fatty acid An essential fatty acid that promotes a healthy immune system and helps protect against heart disease and other diseases; found in egg yolk and cold water fish like tuna, salmon, mackerel, cod, crab, shrimp, and oyster. Also known as linolenic acid.

Omega-6 fatty acid An essential fatty acid found in flaxseed, canola, and soybean oils and green leaves. Also known as linoleic acid.

Osteomalacia Softening of the bone.

Osteopenia Bone density that is below average, classified as 1.5 to 2.5 standard deviations below peak bone density.

Osteoporosis A disorder, primarily affecting postmenopausal women, in which bone density decreases and susceptibility to fractures increases.

Outcome-centered goal A goal that can be assessed via a measured outcome [e.g., weight loss of 5 pounds (2.3 kg)].

Overweight A term to describe an excessive amount of weight for a given height, using height-to-weight ratios.

Parasympathetic nervous system A subdivision of the autonomic nervous system that is involved in regulating the routine functions of the body, such as heartbeat, digestion, and sleeping. Opposes the physiological effects of the sympathetic nervous system (e.g., stimulates digestive secretions, slows the heart, constricts the pupils, and dilates blood vessels).

Pepsin An enzyme that breaks the peptide bonds between amino acids to shorten long protein complexes into shorter polypeptide chains.

Peptide bond The chemical bond formed between neighboring amino acids, constituting the primary linkage of all protein structures.

Percent daily value (PDV) A replacement for the percent Recommended Dietary Allowance (RDA) on the newer food labels. Gives information on whether a food item has a significant amount of a particular nutrient based on a 2,000-calorie diet.

Peristalsis The wavelike muscular contractions of the alimentary canal or other tubular structures by which contents are forced onward.

Phospholipid Structurally similar to triglycerides, but the glycerol backbone is modified so that the molecule is water soluble at one end and water insoluble at the other end; helps maintain cell membrane structure and function.

Phytochemical A biologically active, nonnutrient component found in plants; includes antioxidants.

Placenta The vascular organ in mammals that unites the fetus to the maternal uterus and mediates its metabolic exchanges.

Polysaccharide A long chain of sugar molecules.

Polyunsaturated fat *See* Polyunsaturated fatty acid.

Polyunsaturated fatty acid A type of unsaturated fat (liquid at room temperature) that has two or more spots on the fatty acid available for hydrogen (e.g., corn, safflower, and soybean oils).

Portal circulation A circulatory system that takes nutrients directly from the stomach, small intestines, colon, and spleen to the liver.

Portion The amount of a food or beverage consumed by an individual in one sitting.

Precontemplation The stage of the transtheoretical model of behavioral change during which the individual is not yet thinking about changing.

Prediabetes The state in which some but not all of the diagnostic criteria for diabetes are met (e.g., blood glucose levels are higher than normal but are not high enough for a diagnosis of diabetes).

Prehypertension A systolic pressure of 120 to 139 mmHg and/or a diastolic pressure of 80 to 89 mmHg. Having this condition puts an individual at higher risk for developing hypertension.

Prehypertensive *See* Prehypertension.

Preparation The stage of the transtheoretical model of behavioral change during which the individual is getting ready to make a change.

Process-centered goal A goal that is achieved by accomplishing a set of tasks that leads to an outcome-centered goal (e.g., walking for 45 minutes, five days per week).

Processes of change Interventions and strategies that lead to the progression from one stage to the next in the transtheoretical model of behavioral change.

Protein A compound composed of a combination 20 amino acids that is the major structural component of all body tissue.

Provitamin Inactive vitamins; the human body contains enzymes to convert them into active vitamins.

Rapport A relationship marked by mutual understanding and trust.

Recommended Dietary Allowance (RDA) The levels of intake of essential nutrients that, on the basis of scientific knowledge, are judged by the Food and Nutrition Board to be adequate to meet the known needs of practically all healthy persons.

Registered dietitian (RD) A food and nutrition expert that has met the following criteria: completed a minimum of a bachelor's degree at a U.S. accredited university, or other college coursework approved by the Commission on Accreditation for Dietetics Education (CADE); completed a CADE-accredited supervised practice program; passed a national examination; and completed continuing education requirements to maintain registration.

Relapse In behavioral change, the return of an original problem after many lapses (i.e., slips or mistakes) have occurred.

Resting metabolic rate (RMR) The number of calories expended per unit time at rest; measured early in the morning after an overnight fast and at least eight hours of sleep; approximated with various formulas.

Return on investment (ROI) The ratio of the net income (profit minus depreciation) to the average money spent by the company overall or on a specific project. Usually expressed as a percentage, a measure of profitability that indicates whether or not a company is using its resources in an efficient manner.

Riboflavin A yellow, water-soluble, B vitamin that occurs in green vegetables, germinating seeds, and in milk, fish, egg yolk, liver, and kidney; essential for the carbohydrate metabolism of cells.

Ribonucleic acid (RNA) A chemical cousin of deoxyribonucleic acid (DNA), RNA is responsible for translating the genetic code of DNA into proteins; found in the nucleus and cytoplasm of cells.

Saturated fat *See* Saturated fatty acid.

Saturated fatty acid A fatty acid that contains no double bonds between carbon atoms; typically solid at room temperature and very stable.

Scope of practice The range and limit of responsibilities normally associated with a specific job or profession.

Secretin A hormone that signals the pancreas to produce and secrete bicarbonate to neutralize the stomach acid.

Self-efficacy One's perception of his or her ability to change or to perform specific behaviors (e.g., exercise).

Serving The amount of food used as a reference on the nutrition label of that food; the recommended portion of food to be eaten.

Simple carbohydrate A short chain of sugar that is rapidly digested.

Simple diffusion A process by which molecules diffuse across a membrane based on a concentration gradient without the assistance of a protein carrier.

Small intestine The part of the gastro-intestinal system that is the site of the majority of food digestion and absorption.

SMART goal A properly designed goal; SMART stands for specific, measurable, attainable, relevant, and time-bound.

Socio-ecological model An approach to behavioral change that emphasizes the development of coordinated partnerships, programs, and policies to support healthy eating and active living.

Social support The perceived comfort, caring, esteem, or help an individual receives from other people.

Soluble fiber *See* High-viscosity fiber.

Stages-of-change model A lifestyle-modification model that suggests that people go through distinct, predictable stages when making lifestyle changes: precontemplation, contemplation, preparation, action, and maintenance. The process is not always linear.

Starch A plant carbohydrate found in grains and vegetables.

Stimulant A substance that activates the central nervous system and sympathetic nervous system.

Stroke A sudden and often severe attack due to blockage of an artery into the brain.

Structure/function claim A statement that relates a nutrient or dietary ingredient to normal human structure or function such as "calcium builds strong bones," or describes a benefit related to a nutrient deficiency. It must state a disclaimer that the U.S. Food and Drug Administration has not evaluated the claim and that the supplement is not intended to treat, cure, or prevent any disease.

SWOT analysis Situation analysis in which internal strengths and weaknesses of an organization (such as a business) or individual, and external opportunities and threats are closely examined to chart a strategy.

Systolic blood pressure (SBP) The pressure exerted by the blood on the vessel walls during ventricular contraction.

Testosterone In males, the steroid hormone produced in the testes; involved in growth and development of reproductive tissues, sperm, and secondary male sex characteristics.

Thiamin A water-soluble B vitamin found in meat, yeast, and the bran coat of grains; necessary for carbohydrate metabolism and normal neural activity.

Tolerable Upper Intake Level (UL) The maximum intake of a nutrient that is unlikely to pose risk of adverse health effects to almost all individuals in an age- and gender-specific group.

Toxicity The degree to which a substance can be harmful to the body.

Trans fat *See* Trans fatty acid.

Trans fatty acid An unsaturated fatty acid that is converted into a saturated fat to increase the shelf life of some products.

Transamination The reversible exchange of amino groups between different amino acids.

Translocation stage The process of digestion wherein negatively charged minerals pass across the border of the small intestine for absorption through either simple diffusion, facilitated diffusion, or active transport.

Transtheoretical model of behavioral change (TTM) A theory of behavior that examines one's readiness to change and identifies five stages: precontemplation, contemplation, preparation, action, and maintenance. Also called the stages-of-change model.

Triglyceride Three fatty acids joined to a glycerol (carbon and hydrogen structure) backbone; how fat is stored in the body.

Trypsin An enzyme responsible for breaking down proteins into single amino acids or amino acids joined in twos (dipeptides) or threes (tripeptides).

24-hour recall A method of gaining information about a client's eating habits by asking for detailed information about the foods and drinks the client consumed in the past 24 hours.

Type 1 diabetes Form of diabetes caused by the destruction of the insulin-producing beta cells in the pancreas, which leads to little or no insulin secretion; generally develops in childhood and requires regular insulin injections; formerly known as insulin-dependent diabetes mellitus (IDDM) and childhood-onset diabetes.

Type 2 diabetes Most common form of diabetes; typically develops in adulthood and is characterized by a reduced sensitivity of the insulin target cells to available insulin; usually associated with obesity; formerly known as non-insulin-dependent diabetes mellitus (NIDDM) and adult-onset diabetes.

Unsaturated fatty acids Fatty acids that contain one or more double bonds between carbon atoms; typically liquid at room temperature and fairly unstable, making them susceptible to oxidative damage and a shortened shelf life.

Vegan A vegetarian who does not consume any animal products, including dairy products such as milk and cheese.

Vegetarian A person who does not eat meat, fish, poultry, or products containing these foods.

Villi Finger-like projections from the folds of the small intestines.

Vitamin An organic micronutrient that is essential for normal physiologic function.

$\dot{V}O_2$max Considered the best indicator of cardiovascular endurance, it is the maximum amount of oxygen (mL) that a person can use in one minute per kilogram of body weight. Also called maximal oxygen uptake and maximal aerobic power.

Water-soluble vitamin A vitamin that requires adequate daily intake since the body excretes excesses in the urine; dissolvable in water.

Whey The liquid remaining after milk has been curdled and strained; high in protein and carbohydrates.

INDEX

C

D

E

M

N

O

P

Q

R

T

Z

ABOUT THE AUTHOR

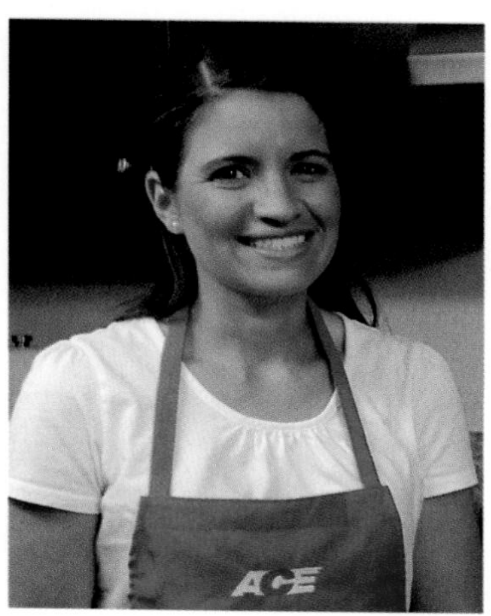

Natalie Digate Muth, M.D., M.P.H., R.D., is a pediatrician, registered dietitian, Board-Certified Specialist in Sports Dietetics (CSSD), and Senior Advisor for Healthcare Solutions at the American Council on Exercise (ACE). She is also an ACE Certified Health Coach, Personal Trainer, and Group Fitness Instructor. She is author of more than 100 articles, books, and book chapters, including the book *"Eat Your Vegetables!" and Other Mistakes Parents Make: Redefining How to Raise Healthy Eaters* (Healthy Learning, 2012) and *Sports Nutrition for Health Professionals* (F.A. Davis, 2014).